Pain Management - Research and Technology

nova
Medicine & Health
New York

Pain Management - Research and Technology

Pain Management: Recent International Research
Joav Merrick, MD, MMedSci, DMSc (Editor), Mohammed Morad, MD (Editor)
2022. ISBN: 978-1-68507-493-7 (Hardcover)
2022. ISBN: 978-1-68507-598-9 (eBook)

Antinociceptive Tolerance to NSAIDs in Brain Limbic Areas: Role of Endogenous Opioid and Cannabinoid Systems
Merab G. Tsagareli, PhD, DSc (Author)
Natia Tsagareli (Author)
Nana Tsiklauri (Author)
2021. ISBN: 978-1-53619-814-0 (Softcover)
2021. ISBN: 978-1-53619-881-2 (eBook)

Interventional Techniques for the Management of Sacroiliac Joint Pain
Nomen Azeem, MD (Editor)
Ajay Antony, MD (Editor)
Miguel Attias, MD (Editor)
Michael Esposito, MD (Editor)
Navdeep Jassal, MD (Editor)
Michael Hanes, MD (Editor)
2020. ISBN: 978-1-53618-767-0 (Softcover)
2020. ISBN: 978-1-53618-864-6 (eBook)

Behavioral Study of Agonist-Evoked Activation of Transient Receptor Potential Channels
Merab G. Tsagareli, PhD (Editor)
2019. ISBN: 978-1-53616-501-2 (Softcover)
2020. ISBN: 978-1-53616-502-9 (eBook)

More information about this series can be found at
https://novapublishers.com/product-category/series/pain-management-research-and-technology/

Indraneil Mukherjee
Editor

Rayna Walburger
and Simer Preet Singh
Co-Editors

Postoperative Pain

From Management to Recovery

nova
Medicine & Health
New York

https://doi.org/10.52305/LKRZ1385

Library of Congress Cataloging-in-Publication Data

ISBN: 978-1-68507-971-0

Published by Nova Science Publishers, Inc. † New York

Contents

Preface

Most patients who undergo surgery will experience acute postoperative pain, making postoperative pain management an important topic. Pain management has shifted towards a multimodal approach and away from the traditional opioid administration due in part to the opioid crisis. As opioids came to be abused, with many starting after initially being prescribed opioids by their physician, the focus on how to manage pain changed. However, a multimodal approach also has benefits outside of decreasing use of opioids such as targeting multiple pathways of pain to lead to more favorable outcomes for patients. A multimodal approach does not consist of the same approach for each patient. It gives the ability to tailor the pain management approach to the patient and the type of surgery. In this textbook, the approach to postoperative pain management for different surgeries will be highlighted. The different modalities used for a multimodal approach will be defined with their underlying pathophysiology explained. This textbook will give a basic understanding of how the combination of multiple medications often results in superior outcomes, with better patient satisfaction and often lower doses being required due the additive effects of different pathways being targeted.

Chapter 1

Enhanced Recovery after Surgery

Jonathan Gardy Alabre*
City University of New York School of Medicine, New York, NY, USA

In 1997, Danish gastrointestinal surgeon Henrik Kehlet first introduced the idea of a fast-track recovery pathway for surgery. He proposed that surgical teams make use of specific methods and procedures that would minimize the physiological stress that surgery places on patients, while also allowing for a safe and efficient return to baseline health. His mechanisms for achieving optimal recovery included pre-operative optimization, intra-operative use of multi-modal anesthesia, and early post-operative mobilization and activity. Dr. Kehlet eventually went on to receive the 2014 Excellence in Research Award by the American Society of Anesthesiologist for his contribution to the anesthetic and surgical world. His ideas became known as a system of protocols termed Enhanced Recovery After Surgery (ERAS), and to this day ERAS continues to be implemented among hospital systems worldwide. With continued research and innovation, ERAS has been standardized into 3 major categories of peri-operative care: the pre-operative, intra-operative, and post-operative stages. Within each branch there are many distinct guidelines that health care teams should consider in order to assure optimal care for their patients.

Prior to having surgery, a patient should be thoroughly evaluated to assess whether they are a proper candidate for the procedure. While different hospital systems have their own protocols for pre-surgical evaluation, ERAS has sought to standardize this stage of care by providing regulations that should support health-care teams in their practice. Though it is not currently mandated

---

* Corresponding Author's Email: jalabre000@citymail.cuny.edu.

In: Postoperative Pain
Editors: Indraneil Mukherjee et al.
ISBN: 978-1-68507-971-0

by any governing body that ERAS should be incorporated into the management plans of patients, there are some minimum standards, that happen to align with ERAS, that all hospitals should follow. Some of these include, but are not limited to, patients receiving adequate education on their scheduled procedure, and implementation of strict intake and outtake procedures to minimize the risk of surgical complication during the procedure. One major standard of ERAS is that all patients should be subject to a thorough pre-operative medical risk and comorbidity screening. Often times the medical risk assessment will be conducted by the patient's primary care physician, and the major focus is to evaluate whether the patient's pulmonary and cardiovascular system are stable enough to withstand the proposed procedure. We focus on the cardiovascular system because cardiac complications like myocardial infarction (MI) are a major risk of even non-cardiac procedures. Thus, initial patient interviewing should include a cardiac specific review of systems, inquiring about symptoms such as palpitations, chest pain, exertional dyspnea, angina, orthopnea etc. The primary care physician should also determine if the patient has a history of cardiac or vascular related disease such as Hypertension, hypertrophic cardiomyopathy, cerebrovascular disease, atherosclerosis, diabetes, or kidney disease. A thorough evaluation of family history and social history should also be obtained, followed by an in-depth physical exam. It is key to obtain the patients' blood pressure and heart rate, while also visually inspecting for signs of edema and vascular compromise. Patients with risk factors such as unstable angina, cardiac arrythmia, heart failure, recent MI, or valvular disease are at most risk for complication. These patients are placed into a high-risk category and should subsequently be referred to a cardiologist for further evaluation and possible optimization of their medical condition.

According to the American College of Cardiology/American Heart Association, it is recommended that an electrocardiogram (ECG) be obtained on all high-risk cardiac patients undergoing non-cardiac surgery prior to the procedure. Though some clinicians may elect to obtain a pre-operative ECG on asymptomatic patients without a pertinent cardiac history, it is not generally recommended because the prognostic capability of this test is not specific in this patient population. Abnormalities found on the ECG in this circumstance may provide minimal certainty as to whether there is increased risk of complication during the procedure, and therefore would not change standard of care. Just as essential to the overall medical risk assessment, is the pulmonary functional status evaluation.

The purpose of the pulmonary evaluation is to minimize the risk of any major known post-operative respiratory complications such as bronchitis, pneumonia, atelectasis, hypoxemia, or respiratory failure. Mitigating the risk of these complications starts with identifying which patient-related and procedure-specific risk factors are present. Once they've all been identified, modifiable risk factors should be addressed so that the patient is in the optimal position for a successful surgical course. Some patient specific risk factors include age, history of smoking, asthma, chronic obstructive pulmonary disease (COPD), obesity, and overall health. Factors related to the nature of the surgery include the duration of the surgery, the site of operation, the mode of anesthesia used, and the type of neuromuscular blockade. These factors can all influence the strength of post-surgical respiratory drive and alveolar patency. Similar to the cardiac pre surgical evaluation, a thorough history of pulmonary disease and active symptoms should be taken. A physical exam to assess for breath sounds, lung expansion, chest shape, and other pulmonary parameters should also be performed. For patients with known history of disease, the primary physician may choose to have the patient perform a Pulmonary Function Test prior to the surgery and based on the results, adjust their current management plan accordingly. After all presurgical requirements have been met, ERAS then offers suggestions on how best to manage patients during the intra-operative stages.

The objective of the intra-operative period is to maintain the patient's vital stability. During surgery patients are subject to tissue trauma, heat-loss, fluid loss, and other stressors that if not properly accounted for, could easily lead to severe complications or even death. Therefore, ERAS has proposed several standards for how to safely and effectively manage a patient throughout a procedure while maintaining optimal hemodynamic stability. The initial step begins with deciding which surgical approach would be best to offer the patient. If possible, laparoscopic surgery is often preferred as it is associated with reduced length of hospital stay, expedited return to physiological organ function, and decreased overall inflammation and trauma. Reported rates of improvement when comparing laparoscopic surgery to open surgery can vary depending on the indication for the procedure however, if a patient is a proper candidate for minimally invasive surgery, they should be offered that option. The choice of administered anesthetic is equally as important during this stage. ERAS typically calls for avoidance of any long-lasting anesthetic agents if possible, as short-acting anesthetics such as propofol are less likely to cause delayed return to normal respiratory function. This quicker return to baseline provides a lower risk of post-operative complications, while simultaneously promoting an early discharge.

Another consideration when choosing the anesthetic of choice is the risk of prolonged gastrointestinal (GI) ileus. Ileus is especially seen with abdominal surgeries, so if possible, it is best to refrain from using opioid analgesics as they are known to decrease GI motility and endorse ileus. A multi-modal pain management plan is often preferred with agents such as NSAIDs, Acetaminophen, or local anesthetic injections. For certain procedures, transverses abdominal plain blocks (TAPB) have also been employed as an alternative form of pain management. In terms of fluid and heat balance, ERAS recommends using a restrictive fluid therapy plan to manage patients. Excessive administration of fluid can lead to coagulopathy, hypothermia, and other complications. Therefore, with a restrictive model we can minimize the risk of volume overload and achieve adequate euvolemia. In addition, for patients undergoing prolonged open abdominal surgery, protocol calls for use of blankets or body warmers in order to minimize heat loss. This is especially important for elderly patients, patients with little body fat, or patients with comorbidities because they are at greatest risk for hypothermia during operations that last more than two hours. Once the patient has completed a successful intra-operative course, the next focus of management is ensuring a safe and efficient discharge.

In the past it was common for patients to remain in the hospital after their surgery for days to weeks until they were deemed to be fully recovered. In the present day, guidelines recommend that patients are prepped for safe discharge as soon as possible. Research has shown that encouraging early oral feedings and ambulation actually improves patient outcomes and enhances recovery. Early ambulation has been found to be associated with decreased risk of developing post-operative deep vein thrombosis, while also decreasing the chances of developing a pneumonia. In addition to mobility incentives, patients should also be given thromboprophylaxis and offered an incentive spirometer to mitigate these risks. In terms of return to feeding, patients are now encouraged to begin eating just a few hours after surgery, even if there is no apparent evidence of resumed bowel function. Traditionally, solid foods would be withheld until signs such as bowel sounds or passing of fluctuance were present. This mindset has shifted as some research has shown that those clinical signs of bowel function are not necessarily associated with tolerance of solid oral intake. While it is expected that patients will report some level of pain, discomfort, nausea, or vomiting while in the initial stages of walking and eating, it is important to only administer non-opioid analgesics if possible.

Offering long-acting opioids while indicated in cases of excessive or refractory pain, can often times exacerbate the discomfort that a patient is experiencing by contributing to the ileus. Though questions arose regarding whether patients were truly safe to be discharged on this expedited track, some studies have actually shown that patients who were discharged prior to resumption of bowel function did not have increased rates of readmission compared to patients who remained in the hospital until there was clear evidence of bowel motility. Once a patient has been deemed stable and is not exhibiting any signs of infection or complication, they should be discharged in less than 5 days maximum. Based on extensive reviews of literature and post-operative statistics, this number has been chosen by ERAS as the marker for accelerated recovery and discharge.

The current evidence regarding the effects of ERAS on hospitalizations is promising, as implementation of these protocols has been shown to decrease overall hospital length of stay, while lowering the overall financial burden of care for patients and hospitals and expediting patient post-operative recovery. As the extensive body of ERAS literature continues to grow, further research is underway to identify areas of improvement in surgical care, and to develop specialized protocols for ERAS depending on the specific procedure type. Based on the nature of the surgery, greater emphasis may be placed on specific portions of the ERAS plan as we can see with DVT precaution in Gynecologic surgery or fluid balance management in Cardiac surgery.

In accordance with the development of general ERAS guidelines overtime, specific protocols for Enhanced Recovery after Gynecological Surgery (ERAGS) have also emerged. The initial intent of ERASGS was to optimize the surgical management plans for women undergoing procedures that required at least one overnight stay however, specific aspects of these programs can be adopted for same-day gynecologic procedures as well. The major pillars of ERAGS are similar to other ERAS protocols in that they can be divided into 3 major categories, the pre-operative, intra-operative, and post-operative stages. With each distinct stage, one must consider the influence that the female anatomy can have on the intended intervention, and how implementation of these protocol can interfere with any ongoing women's-health treatment that the patient may be receiving. One aspects of the pre-operative preparation that is crucial to gynecological surgery is assessment of thrombotic risk and potential cessation of oral contraception prior to surgery Robust evidence regarding the correlation between oral contraceptives (OCPs) and increased risk of post-operative thromboembolism have prompted health care providers to encourage their patients to discontinue use of OCPs prior to surgery. The risk of thrombosis is stratified depending on the type of contraception that the patient is receiving but if possible, patients should be instructed to use an alternative form of contraception during their pre-operative stage. If discontinuation is not possible, continued use of hormonal OCPs in this population is an indication to incorporate thromboprophylaxis into the plan of care. These patients should receive low-molecular-weight-heparin or regular heparin all throughout their peri-operative course, along with additional interventions such as compression stockings post-operatively. Based on the results of a Cochrane analysis on long term hormone therapy, peri-menopausal, post-menopausal, and patients receiving hormone replacement therapy (HRT) all have a well-documented increased risk of developing venous thromboembolism (VTE). While guidelines from various international studies suggest that HRT should be stopped approximately 4 weeks prior to surgery, the benefits and risks of discontinuation must be weighed for each patient on an individual basis. Another high-risk demographic that ERASGS has flagged is women with gynecological malignancies.

According to an institutional database review conducted between 2000-2011, VTE can be seen in up to 8% of surgical patients with endometrial cancer and 38% of surgical patients with ovarian carcinoma. The same study identified serous/clear cell histology, thrombocytosis, elevated CA-125, and Stage III-IV malignancy as independent risk factors for VTE in patients with endometrial carcinoma. An additional report from the Million Women Study revealed that oncological surgery patients were at 90 times increased risk of developing post-operative VTE within the first 6 weeks after surgery. Even at the 12-week mark, women undergoing oncological surgery had a 1/85 risk of developing VTE compared to a 1/365 risk for general gynecologic surgery. While these patients would most definitely be eligible for peri-operative anti-coagulation under ERASGS protocol, they should also be considered for potential long-term anticoagulation therapy as well.

The standardization of ERAGS is evidence-based and thankfully, the overall efficacy of these protocols for gynecologic surgery is well documented. These patients tend to see major improvements in terms of cost reduction, decreased length of stay, decreased opioid use, and improved functional outcomes. A retrospective study conducted from January 2016 to December 2016 sought to review the effects of ERAGS on surgical outcomes. The results showed that patients enrolled in the program required 44% fewer opioids and made 36% less use of patient-controlled analgesia. Despite using less post-operative pharmacologic therapy, these same patients actually reported less pain by post-operative day 3. This was promising data and has contributed to the idea that ERAS protocols are in fact beneficial for gynecologic patients when implemented all throughout the surgical course. Similar studies also found significant reduction in post-operative length of stay for patients in ERAGS programs as compared to traditional post-operative care. Depending on the specific surgery performed, different reductions in LOS have been reported. 2–3-day reductions have been seen for cytoreduction surgery, 1–2-day reductions for open benign gynecologic surgery, and 1 day reduction for surgical staging and vaginal surgery. When compared with patients who receive conventional operative care, ERAGS patients experience faster relief of fatigue in 10 days versus 30 days, and quicker return to mobility with 5 days versus 13 days.

Though the current practice of care has been shifting towards greater adoption of ERAS protocols for gynecologic surgery across the country, more research must be undertaken to identify the potential drawbacks to these interventions as well in order to maximize efficiency of protocol. Another emerging field within the realm of enhanced recovery programs is Cardiac Specific ERAS protocols.

Enhanced Recovery after Cardiac Surgery (ERACS) was developed for the same purpose as other ERAS programs, to optimize care within the perioperative period and prepare the patient for a safe discharge. However, unlike other fields of surgery, cardiothoracic operations often come with increased risk of perfusion and circulation related complications. Thus, the development of ERACS protocol was also rooted in maintaining fluid balance. Currently a standard of care for cardiac surgery patients is to avoid administering excess fluids as to prevent hemodilution and coagulopathy. Additional known risks factors such as pulmonary edema, acute kidney injury, poor wound healing, and increased use of blood products have also been identified as complications of hemodilution.

For certain procedures such as cardiac bypass surgery, mild hemodilution is often unavoidable as there must be an increase in fluid volume for the machinery to function. However, in order to mitigate the risk of deleterious hemodilution, a zero-balance fluid management strategy is often initiated. The goal if this strategy is to minimize surplus water and salt imbalance while maintaining central euvolemia. With a restrictive zero-balance fluid plan, only the estimated fluid that is lost during the procedure is replaced. Patients should receive a balanced electrolyte crystalloid solution at a rate of 1-3 ml/kg/hr. For blood losses, the proposed crystalloid-to-blood volume and colloid-to-blood ratio of administration is about 1.5:1.0 and 1.0:1.0 respectively. In the event that the surgical teams suspects that the patient is hypovolemic, they can administer an IV fluid bolus to assess for the level of fluid responsiveness and correct any abnormalities. Other forms of fluid management strategies such as goal-directed and traditional-liberal fluid management approaches have been contested in the literature as well.

Goal-directed therapy (GDT) was typically reserved for patients scheduled for major invasive procedures which were expected to result in huge blood losses or severe fluid shifts. This strategy allows for a pre-decided fluid balance goal to be achieved. It is typically employed over the old-fashioned conventional fluid management as the traditional protocol is associated with increased patient morbidity. A meta-analysis published in 2018 compared patient outcomes such as development of pneumonia, acute kidney injury, poor wound healing, and mortality between patients who received GDT versus traditional. The study found that GDT was associated with improved clinical outcomes for all specified parameters and more, when compared to standard-management. Ongoing research is currently underway to compare the efficacies of GDT and restrictive therapy (RT). Interestingly, a separate meta-analysis conducted in 2019 examined the mortality and morbidity outcomes between patients treated with restrictive therapy for non-cardiac surgery. While the results showed minor evidence that RT did not affect the risk of complications, there remained a possibility that it could increase the risk of all-cause-mortality for those patients. However, one must be cautious in applying the outcome of this study to cardiac surgeries because there is a significant difference in the physiologic stresses imposed on the body from fluid shifts seen in cardiac versus non-cardiac surgeries. Moreover, review of whether GDT made a significant clinical difference in patients currently enrolled in ERAS programs revealed that there was no additional patient benefit when this strategy was employed.

It is possible that this finding is influenced by the fact that ERAS protocols generally adopt a RT method throughout their peri-operative management to avoid the known complications of hemodilution the standard-therapy or GDT could potentially induce. A reliable indicator that one might use to study intraoperative hemodilution is colloid oncotic pressure (COP) and one major study actually used this index to analyze the effects that different levels of COP would have on cardiac patients intra-/post-operative morbidity. In the study, 61 patients who were undergoing cardiac bypass surgery had their blood samples taken before, during, immediately after surgery, and when transferred to the cardiac intensive care unit. The lowest patient sustained COP value was then juxtaposed with different variables such as post-operative blood loss, blood product transfusion, length of stay, etc. They found that COP was actually inversely proportional to the patient outcomes mentioned above along with other morbidity indexes. This data further supports the established pool of knowledge regarding the risks of hemodilution in cardiac surgery patients and emphasizes that enacting the restrictive fluid management strategies of ERACS has the potential to minimize complications and optimize the patient for a safe and efficient discharge. In addition to fluid management, screening for post-operative delirium is an essential component of ERACS protocol. The majority of patients in the United States who undergo cardiac surgery are of the older-adult and geriatric population, specifically 70 years of age and older. Consequently, this same patient population is the most at risk for developing post-operative delirium. Many institutions assess and diagnose delirium with different parameters; therefore, the estimated incidence of peri-operative delirium is believed to be from 10 to 80 percent. A Canadian study went on to stratify the incidence based on cardiac procedure and found that the incidences are 25%, 31%, and 39% for coronary artery bypass graft, valve replacement, and combined procedures respectively.

While screening tools such as the "confusion assessment method for ICU" and the "Intensive Care Delirium Screening Checklist" exist to assist in identifying post-operative delirium, further study needs to occur in order to better understand what the specific risk factors for cardiac surgery patients at most risk for developing delirium are. Physical "frailty" of a patient has actually been flagged as a measurable risk factor for a patient's risk of developing post-operative delirium and mortality. A pre-operative screening exam to measure a patient gait speed could be used as a marker of frailty and assist with identifying geriatric patients at risk. While it may seem that "frailty" and chronological age could easily cause an issue of confounding bias in this regard, one study found that when accounted for independently frailty could actually have greater influence on risk for delirium than chronological age alone. Some ERACS endorsed interventions used to target this issue range from providing sufficient nutrition and hydration, encouragement of ambulation, providing cognitive stimulation, and addressing any treatable causes of the delirium. Along with several other post-operative goals, recovery from or complete avoidance of acute post-operative delirium is one of the set standards of the rapidly developing enhanced recovery after cardiac surgery protocols.

One must remember that ERAS is dynamic and constantly under review for improvement and innovation; cardiac surgery is simply one field in the realm of developing ERAS protocols, and it can be expected that in the future there will be an abundance of robust evidence-based ERAS protocols for a variety of surgical fields.

References

Bergstrom, Jennifer E., Marla E. Scott, Yewande Alimi, Ting Tai Yen, Deborah Hobson, Karime K. Machado, Edward J. Tanner, et al., 2018. "Narcotics Reduction, Quality and Safety in Gynecologic Oncology Surgery in the First Year of Enhanced Recovery after Surgery Protocol Implementation." *Gynecologic Oncology*. https://doi.org/10.1016/j.ygyno.2018.04.003.

Carter-Brooks, Charelle M., Angela L. Du, Kristine M. Ruppert, Anna L. Romanova, and Halina M. Zyczynski. 2018. "Implementation of a Urogynecology-Specific Enhanced Recovery after Surgery (ERAS) Pathway." *American Journal of Obstetrics and Gynecology*. https://doi.org/10.1016/j.ajog.2018.06.009.

Cavallaro, Paul, and Liliana Bordeianou. 2019. "Implementation of an ERAS Pathway in Colorectal Surgery." *Clinics in Colon and Rectal Surgery*. https://doi.org/10.1055/s-0038-1676474.

Chong, Matthew A., Yongjun Wang, Nicolas M. Berbenetz, and Ian McConachie. 2018. "Does Goal-Directed Haemodynamic and Fluid Therapy Improve Peri-Operative Outcomes?" *European Journal of Anaesthesiology*. https://doi.org/10.1097/EJA.0000000000000778.

Chores, Jeffrey B., and David W. Holt. 2017. "Colloid Oncotic Pressure, Monitoring Its Effects in Cardiac Surgery." *The Journal of Extra-Corporeal Technology*.

Dickson, Elizabeth, Peter A. Argenta, and John A. Reichert. 2012. "Results of Introducing a Rapid Recovery Program for Total Abdominal Hysterectomy." *Gynecologic and Obstetric Investigation*. https://doi.org/10.1159/000328713.

Fleisher, Lee A., Kirsten E. Fleischmann, Andrew D. Auerbach, Susan A. Barnason, Joshua A. Beckman, Biykem Bozkurt, Victor G. Davila-Roman, et al., 2014. "2014 ACC/AHA Guideline on Perioperative Cardiovascular Evaluation and Management of Patients Undergoing Noncardiac Surgery: A Report of the American College of Cardiology/American Heart Association Task Force on Practice Guidelines." *Journal of the American College of Cardiology*. https://doi.org/10.1016/j.jacc.2014.07.944.

Jacob, Matthias, Daniel Chappell, Klaus Hofmann-Kiefer, Peter Conzen, and Markus Rehm. 2008. "A Rational Approach to Perioperative Fluid Management." *Anesthesiology*. https://doi.org/10.1097/ALN.0b013e3181863117.

Joshi, Girish P., and Henrik Kehlet. 2016. "CON: Perioperative Goal-Directed Fluid Therapy Is an Essential Element of an Enhanced Recovery Protocol?" *Anesthesia and Analgesia*. https://doi.org/10.1213/ANE.0000000000001233.

Kalogera, Eleftheria, Jamie N. Bakkum-Gamez, Christopher J. Jankowski, Emanuel Trabuco, Jenna K. Lovely, Sarah Dhanorker, Pamela L. Grubbs, et al., 2013. "Enhanced Recovery in Gynecologic Surgery." *Obstetrics and Gynecology*. https://doi.org/10.1097/aog.0b013e31829aa780.

Kamel, Hosam K., Mohammad A. Iqbal, Ratna Mogallapu, Diana Maas, and Raymond G. Hoffmann. 2003. "Time to Ambulation after Hip Fracture Surgery: Relation to Hospitalization Outcomes." *Journals of Gerontology - Series A Biological Sciences and Medical Sciences*. https://doi.org/10.1093/gerona/58.11.m1042.

Koh, Li Ying, and Nian Chih Hwang. 2019. "Frailty in Cardiac Surgery." *Journal of Cardiothoracic and Vascular Anesthesia*. https://doi.org/10.1053/j.jvca.2018.02.032.

Lenhardt, Rainer, Elvine Marker, Veronika Goll, Heinz Tschernich, Andrea Kurz, Daniel I. Sessler, Edith Narzt, and Franz Lackner. 1997. "Mild Intraoperative Hypothermia Prolongs Postanesthetic Recovery." *Anesthesiology*. https://doi.org/10.1097/00000542-199712000-00009.

Li, Jingyi, Haibei Zhu, and Ren Liao. 2019. "Enhanced Recovery after Surgery (ERAS) Pathway for Primary Hip and Knee Arthroplasty: Study Protocol for a Randomized Controlled Trial." *Trials*. https://doi.org/10.1186/s13063-019-3706-8.

Lourenco, Tania, Alison Murray, Adrian Grant, Aileen McKinley, Zygmunt Krukowski, and Luke Vale. 2008. "Laparoscopic Surgery for Colorectal Cancer: Safe and Effective? - A Systematic Review." *Surgical Endoscopy and Other Interventional Techniques*. https://doi.org/10.1007/s00464-007-9686-x.

Marjoribanks, Jane, Cindy Farquhar, Helen Roberts, and Anne Lethaby. 2012. "Long Term Hormone Therapy for Perimenopausal and Postmenopausal Women." *Cochrane Database of Systematic Reviews*. https://doi.org/10.1002/14651858.cd004143.pub4.

Matsuo, Koji, Annie A. Yessaian, Yvonne G. Lin, Huyen Q. Pham, Laila I. Muderspach, Howard A. Liebman, C. Paul Morrow, and Lynda D. Roman. 2013. "Predictive Model of Venous Thromboembolism in Endometrial Cancer." *Gynecologic Oncology*. https://doi.org/10.1016/j.ygyno.2012.12.014.

Meyer, Larissa A., Javier Lasala, Maria D. Iniesta, Alpa M. Nick, Mark F. Munsell, Qiuling Shi, Xin Shelley Wang, Katherine E. Cain, Karen H. Lu, and Pedro T. Ramirez. 2018. "Effect of an Enhanced Recovery after Surgery Program on Opioid Use and Patient-Reported Outcomes." *Obstetrics and Gynecology*. https://doi.org/10.1097/AOG.0000000000002735.

Nelson, G., A. D. Altman, A. Nick, L. A. Meyer, P. T. Ramirez, C. Achtari, J. Antrobus, et al., 2016. "Guidelines for Pre- and Intra-Operative Care in Gynecologic/Oncology Surgery: Enhanced Recovery after Surgery (ERAS®) Society Recommendations - Part I." *Gynecologic Oncology*. https://doi.org/10.1016/j.ygyno.2015.11.015.

Noss, Christopher, Christopher Prusinkiewicz, Gregg Nelson, Prakash A. Patel, John G. Augoustides, and Alexander J. Gregory. 2018. "Enhanced Recovery for Cardiac Surgery." *Journal of Cardiothoracic and Vascular Anesthesia*. https://doi.org/10.1053/j.jvca.2018.01.045.

Read, Thomas E., Marc Brozovich, Jose E. Andujar, Rocco Ricciardi, and Philip F. Caushaj. 2017. "Bowel Sounds Are Not Associated with Flatus, Bowel Movement, or Tolerance of Oral Intake in Patients after Major Abdominal Surgery." *Diseases of the Colon and Rectum*. https://doi.org/10.1097/DCR.0000000000000829.

Sweetland, Siân, Jane Green, Bette Liu, Amy Berrington De González, Marianne Canonico, Gillian Reeves, and Valerie Beral. 2009. "Duration and Magnitude of the Postoperative Risk of Venous Thromboembolism in Middle Aged Women: Prospective Cohort Study." *BMJ (Online)*. https://doi.org/10.1136/bmj.b4583.

Tashiro, Teruko, Sorin V. Pislaru, Jodi M. Blustin, Vuyisile T. Nkomo, Martin D. Abel, Christopher G. Scott, and Patricia A. Pellikka. 2014. "Perioperative Risk of Major Non-Cardiac Surgery in Patients with Severe Aortic Stenosis: A Reappraisal in Contemporary Practice." *European Heart Journal*. https://doi.org/10.1093/eurheartj/ehu044.

Wrzosek, Anna, Joanna Jakowicka-Wordliczek, Renata Zajaczkowska, Wojciech T. Serednicki, Milosz Jankowski, Malgorzata M. Bala, Mateusz J. Swierz, Maciej Polak, and Jerzy Wordliczek. 2019. "Perioperative Restrictive versus Goal-Directed Fluid Therapy for Adults Undergoing Major Non-Cardiac Surgery." *Cochrane Database of Systematic Reviews*. https://doi.org/10.1002/14651858.CD012767.pub2.

Yates, D. R.A., S. J. Davies, H. E. Milner, and R. J.T. Wilson. 2014. "Crystalloid or Colloid for Goal-Directed Fluid Therapy in Colorectal Surgery." *British Journal of Anaesthesia* 112 (2): 281–89. https://doi.org/10.1093/bja/aet307.

Chapter 2

Multimodal Analgesia

Katrina Kerolus* **and Rayna Walburger, MD**
City University of New York School of Medicine, New York, NY, USA

Introduction

Pain control after surgery plays an important role in the recovery of the patient. Postoperative pain management helps reduce pain, increases early mobilization, decreases hospital stay, and increases patient satisfaction. Opioids have long been the mainstay treatment of acute postoperative pain. However, they are associated with many side effects and have the potential for addiction, abuse, and misuse. The optimal perioperative pain control consists of a multimodal approach. This includes multiple medications aimed at blocking different pathways to achieve the best pain control. Different analgesics can target different phases of the nociceptive pain process, including transduction, transmission, perception, and descending and local modulation. The perioperative period is often accompanied by hyperalgesia and allodynia. This is a result of the neuroplasticity of both peripheral and central neurons.

Many studies have been performed to show the effectiveness of multimodal analgesia on postoperative outcomes in patients undergoing a variety of surgeries. Improved pain control is a commonly reported outcome when multimodal analgesia is compared to opioid use alone. Multimodal analgesia can be individualized to each patient depending on their needs. The type of surgery, projected duration of pain, ability to use regional anesthesia and individual patient factors should all be considered when deciding on the

* Corresponding Author's Email: kkerolu000@citymail.cuny.edu.

In: Postoperative Pain
Editors: Indraneil Mukherjee et al.
ISBN: 978-1-68507-971-0

appropriate pain management regimen. The multimodal approach can involve the use of any of the following medications: opioids, patient-controlled analgesia (PCA) pumps, NSAIDs, ketamine, local anesthesia, steroids, acetaminophen, local anesthetics, neuraxial and peripheral regional anesthesia, and gabapentin. By using a combination of these analgesics, a lower dose of each can be used, reducing the potential side effects of each medication. The multimodal analgesia approach also helps to reduce the need for opioids. The mechanism of action of each of these analgesics should be considered to achieve balanced pain control for the patient.

Nociceptive pain is a type of physical pain that is produced when tissue injuries occur and stimulate nociceptors, which are free nerve endings of primary afferent neurons that sense stimuli, of A-delta and C fibers located throughout the body. Nociceptors are found in somatic structures like skin, muscle, bones, and joints and visceral structures like the liver, spleen, etc. The quality of the pain is also dependent on the type of nerve fiber. A-delta is typically large, myelinated fibers important for acute sharp pain while C fibers are small and unmyelinated responsible for slow, dull, achy pain. This process occurs in four phases which include transduction, transmission, modulation, and perception. Different pain relief medications can be used to block the pain signal within each phase.

The first phase is the transduction phase which occurs when the tissue is injured and usually occurs by one of the three mechanisms: mechanical including pressure or pinch, heat, or chemically. The tissue injury triggers the release of pain-producing chemicals such as prostaglandins, potassium, histamine, serotonin, leukotrienes, and bradykinin. These substances help to trigger an immune response and lead to the exchange of sodium, calcium, and potassium ions at the cell membranes which activate the primary afferent nociceptors to generate the pain impulse. This phase can be interrupted with the use of NSAIDs, membrane-stabilizing agents, and local anesthetics. The primary mechanism of NSAIDs is to block the enzyme cyclooxygenase which converts arachidonic acid to prostaglandins thus, reducing the amount of prostaglandin produced and inflammation. Membrane-stabilizing agents such as gabapentin and pregabalin can be used due to their interaction with voltage-gated calcium channels. These medications lead to the blockage of these channels and consequently pain impulses. Similarly, local anesthetics reversibly inhibit nerve transmission by binding voltage-gated Na channels which will also inhibit the excitation of nerve endings.

The second phase in the process of nociceptive pain is the transmission. This occurs when the pain impulse that was generated is transmitted from the periphery to the central nervous system in the spine and brain. The primary afferent neurons have their cell bodies in the dorsal root ganglia which synapses with secondary neurons found in the dorsal horn of the spinal cord. The action potential crosses over to the other side of the spinal cord within levels of the original stimulus and ascends within the spinal thalamic tract. The secondary neurons synapse with tertiary neurons at the thalamus which then travels to the somatosensory cortex in the brain. These synapses at various levels occur via the release of neurotransmitters such as substance P, glutamate, aspartate, norepinephrine, and serotonin. Opioids work by mimicking endogenous opioid peptides which stimulating opioid receptors which are G-protein coupled receptors found throughout the central and peripheral nervous system. They are mostly Gi receptors therefore they close voltage-gated calcium channels and open calcium-dependent inwardly rectifying potassium channels. This leads to hyperpolarization of the cells and reduced neuronal excitability as well as decreases the concentration of intracellular cAMP which monitors the release of nociceptive neurotransmitters like substance P which would reduce the pain. Alternately, N-methyl-D-aspartate receptors antagonist like ketamine, dextromethorphan, and magnesium can be substituted to decrease pain. These drugs work to interrupt pain transmission at the spinal level by preventing glutamate and aspartate neurotransmitters from binding to NMDA receptors which are responsible for neuropathic pain and hyperalgesia. Local anesthetics can also be used to reduce the transmission of pain.

The third phase in nociceptive pain is modulation. Modulation involves changing or inhibiting the transmission of pain impulses in the spinal cord via the descending modulatory pain pathways. The brain alters the intensity of the signal traveling up the ascending pathway based upon the circumstances that initiated the pain impulse. The gate control theory (GCT), proposed by Patrick Wall and Ronald Melzack in 1965, takes place in the dorsal horn of the spinal cord. Their theory proposes that pain impulses encounter "nerve gates" in the spinal cord that will dictate whether the impulse will be modified, inhibited, or transmitted. If the gates are open, the pain will be transmitted and if they are closed it will be inhibited. Non-painful impulses will close the nerve gates to painful impulses to prevent pain sensation from traveling to the CNS. Conversely, increasing activity of transmission neurons will result in open gates and increased perceived pain. Small and large nerve fibers carry information to the dorsal horn. Large fibers, typically, excite the inhibitory neurons which will diminish the transference of pain and close gates. Small fibers will impede the inhibitory neurons which will allow for pain to travel up the brain through the open gates. Neurotransmitters involved in this process include endogenous opioids, serotonin, norepinephrine, GABA, and acetylcholine. This phase can be influenced by local anesthetics, opioids, NSAIDs, tricyclic antidepressants (TCAs), serotonin-selective reuptake inhibitors (SSRIs), and NDMA antagonists. The use of antidepressants like TCAs and SSRIs work by increasing the effect of excitatory neurotransmitters like norepinephrine and serotonin in the synaptic cleft. Increasing their availability within the dorsal horn will inhibit pain transmission and close the gate.

The fourth phase in nociceptive pain is perception. This phase refers to when the pain impulse reaches the brain, thalamus, cortex and becomes aware of the pain by third-order neurons. There are multiple cortical areas that are activated and respond to the pain impulse. These areas include the reticular system, somatosensory cortex, and limbic system. The reticular system is responsible for autonomic and motor responses to pain. The neurons of the reticular formation can alter heart rate, arterial blood pressure, respiration, and vital functions as well as allow pain stimulus to go unacknowledged when attention is needed elsewhere. The somatosensory cortex works to interpret sensations and identify the intensity, location, type and compares them to past experiences. The limbic system is responsible for the emotional and behavioral response to pain. This phase can be moderated by general anesthetics, opioids, NDMA receptor antagonists, and alpha-2 agonists. The most common alpha-2 agonists are clonidine and dexmedetomidine. They work by direct stimulation of alpha-2 receptors in the central nervous system and spinal cord. This inhibits the cAMP which reduces potassium efflux and calcium influx leaving the neuron in a hyperpolarized state. The hyperpolarization leads to a reduced norepinephrine release which is proposed to be the mechanism of hypnosis and sedation.

Also, direct stimulation of alpha-2 receptors inhibits nociceptive neuronal firing at the dorsal horn by binding to postsynaptic neurons which reduces the release of substance P, leading to less pain. Alpha-2 agonists can also reduce peripheral sympathetic tone and reduce the responsiveness within the brain.

Pain is multifactorial therefore, the approach to pain is also multifactorial. The World Health Organization (WHO) proposed a strategy in 1986 to provide adequate pain relief for cancer patients however it has been modified over the years to incorporate acute and chronic non-cancer conditions including neuropathic pain disorders. The three main principles in the analgesic ladder are "by the clock, by the mouth, by the ladder." This refers to the ability to allow the patient to receive medications on a regular schedule rather than only on demand (PRN). "By the mouth" refers to the fact that medications are preferred when received orally. If there are difficulties with oral administration, less invasive options should be considered such as sublingual or subcutaneous before intravenous administration. "By the ladder" refers to the stepwise order for the administration of drugs to handle pain. The first step in addressing pain involves the use of non-opioids for mild pain. This includes the use of NSAIDs or acetaminophens with or without the use of adjuvants. Adjuvants include antidepressants, anticonvulsants, topical anesthetics, steroids, and other medications previously discussed. If pain persists or is more severe, the second ladder can allow the use of weak opioids such as hydrocodone, codeine, tramadol, with or without the use of non-opioid analgesics and with or without the use of adjuvants. The third step is for severe and persistent pain which allows the use of potent opioids like morphine, methadone, fentanyl, oxycodone, with or without non-opioid analgesics, and with or without adjuvants. Pain is individualized to each patient but this ladder allows healthcare workers to understand pain, be able to address its degree and severity, and prescribe appropriate medications.

References

Anekar, Aabha A., and Marco Cascella. 2021. "WHO Analgesic Ladder." *Journal of the Royal College of Physicians of Edinburgh* 38 (3): 284. https://doi.org/10.1007/978-3-642-28753-4_102537.

Answine, Joseph F. 2019. "A Basic Review of Pain Pathways and Analgesia | Anesthesia Experts." 2019. http://anesthesiaexperts.com/uncategorized/basic-review-pain-pathways-analgesia/.

Institute of Medicine (US) Committee on Pain, Disability, and Chronic Illness Behavior, Marian Osterweis, Arthur Kleinman, and David Mechanic. 1987. "The Anatomy and Physiology of Pain." https://www.ncbi.nlm.nih.gov/books/NBK219252/.

Kirkpatrick, Daniel R., Dan M. Mcentire, Zakary J. Hambsch, Mitchell J. Kerfeld, Tyler A. Smith, Mark D. Reisbig, Charles F. Youngblood, and Devendra K. Agrawal. 2015. "Therapeutic Basis of Clinical Pain Modulation." *Clinical and Translational Science* 8 (6): 848. https://doi.org/10.1111/CTS.12282.

Polomano, Rosemary C., Mechele Fillman, Nicholas A. Giordano, April Hazard Vallerand, Kelly L.Wiltse Nicely, and Carla R. Jungquist. 2017. "Multimodal Analgesia for Acute Postoperative and Trauma-Related Pain." *American Journal of Nursing* 117 (3): S12-26. https://doi.org/10.1097/01.NAJ.0000513527.71934.73.

Schwenk, Eric S. MD, and Edward R. MD MAriano. n.d. "Multimodal Analgesia: The Foundation of a Successful Perioperative Experience." *Anesthesiology News.*

Chapter 3

Intravenous Opioids

Alice Lee*
City University of New York School of Medicine, New York, NY, USA

Introduction

Opioids are the mainstay treatment for postoperative pain management. The most common route of administration is intravenously. The most commonly used Intravenous (IV) opioids are morphine, hydromorphone, and fentanyl (Garimella and Cellini, 2013). All of these are mu-opioid receptor agonists. Many factors contribute to the opioid response, including polymorphisms of the mu-opioid receptor, gender, and age. Elderly patients may require fewer amounts of opioids than younger adults (Golembiewski and Rakic 2010). Opioids are natural, synthetic, or semi-synthetic substances. Morphine is a natural opioid, and to make semi-synthetic opioids, minor modifications can be made to the morphine molecule. Potency, pharmacodynamics, and equilibrium with the plasma will change between the different opioids. If morphine has relative potency of 1, fentanyl is 75-125 times more potent, while meperidine is 0.1 times as potent (Hill 2014).

Although there have been developments in non-opioid analgesics, the use of opioids are still common in the postoperative period. There is wide variability in morphine plasma concentrations amongst individuals. Because there is a delay between administration and analgesic effect, the use of intramuscular or subcutaneous morphine after surgery is usually not appropriate. IV opioid administration ensures 100% bioavailability so the desired drug concentration can be immediately achieved. Intravenous bolus

* Corresponding Author's Email: alee003@citymail.cuny.edu.

In: Postoperative Pain
Editors: Indraneil Mukherjee et al.
ISBN: 978-1-68507-971-0

doses will result in the accumulation of drugs and achieve efficient therapeutic concentration. Although other opioids may be better for achieving rapid pain relief, the use of morphine has been the most studied in the postoperative period (Aubrun, Mazoit, and Riou 2012).

Postoperative pain is inevitable after surgical procedures. Chronic post-surgical pain should be considered, especially after certain types of surgery like thoracotomy and mastectomy. Some predictive factors include preoperative pain, repeat or prolonged surgery, surgical approaches with a higher risk of nerve damage, and psychological and depressive symptoms (Taylor and Stanbury 2009). Managing postoperative pain can be difficult due to low staff numbers, inadequate knowledge, and the subjective nature of pain. Adequate pain management is essential in improving patient satisfaction and reducing the length of stay (Taylor and Stanbury 2009).

Small IV doses of morphine (<5 mg) allow rapid titration in the immediate postoperative period. Administering subsequent doses can be a challenge as the residual effects of the first dose need to be taken into account. A study done by Dahmani et al. identified that ethnicity (Caucasians), emergency surgery, major surgery, surgery exceeding 100 minutes, and a moderate-to-severe pain score on arrival in the PACU were predictive factors of early morphine requirements in the PACU (Dahmani et al. 2001). An example of a titration protocol would be to give boluses in short intervals until pain relief is achieved (Aubrun et al. 2002; Aubrun et al. 2007). If the patient is asleep, they should be considered to have pain relief. If the patient becomes sedated and has a decreased ventilatory rate (<12 breaths per minute or oxygen saturation of <95%), the morphine titration should be stopped (Aubrun, Mazoit, and Riou 2012). Giving small boluses increases the time to pain relief but decreases the risk of adverse events. Patients who are opioid naïve should be given 2-3 mg IV doses rather than 5-10 mg IV doses (Aubrun, Mazoit, and Riou 2012).

Opioid Receptors

Opioid receptors are G protein-coupled receptors that can cause analgesia and sedation when bound. The opioid receptor subtypes include mu, kappa, and delta-opioid receptors. Mu opioid receptors are located in various areas of the brain and are responsible for the feelings of euphoria. However, it is also responsible for physical dependence and respiratory depression. They are located in the regions of the brain, including the nucleus accumbens and basolateral amygdala, which are responsible for the reward stimuli properties and feedback loop that are involved in the development of addictive behavior. Kappa opioid receptors are responsible for dysphoric effects and sedation, and the delta-opioid receptors, which bind enkephalins, are responsible for anxiolytic effects (Wang 2019). Prolonged exposure to opioids can enhance the kappa opioid receptor function, which can cause a depressant effect. The kappa opioid receptors have the opposite impact of the mu-opioid receptor and have anti-reward effects. The increased stress enhances these receptors' function and leads to dysphoric mood during withdrawal and abstinence states, which can lead to relapse (Wang 2019).

Dependence and Tolerance

Individuals who develop dependence and tolerance will have withdrawal symptoms (Wang 2019). Tolerance is the loss of analgesic potency with repeat use. This causes increased dose requirements because of decreasing effectiveness over time (Ricardo Buenaventura, Rajive Adlaka, and Nalini Sehgal 2008). Dependence is the development of physiological symptoms when opioids are not used (Ricardo Buenaventura, Rajive Adlaka, and Nalini Sehgal 2008). Staving off withdrawal symptoms is one of the reasons for continued usage. These symptoms include sweating, abdominal pain, and diarrhea (Wang 2019). Additionally, withdrawal symptoms can include anxiety or irritability, chills, hot flushes, wetness including salivation, lacrimation, rhinorrhea, and piloerection (Hill 2014). A consideration when considering starting patients on long-term opioids is whether efficacy can be maintained over time (Wang 2019).

Preoperative Assessment

Preoperatively, a thorough history, physical, and patient education play a significant role in postoperative pain management. Special consideration should be taken in opioid-tolerant, elderly, or physically limited patients. Opioid-tolerant patients will have a higher postoperative pain requirement (Hill 2014). A baseline pain assessment should also be done even if standardization of pain measurement can be difficult because of the subjective nature of the pain assessment(Lovich-Sapola, Smith, and Brandt 2015).

Morphine

Morphine has a low lipid solubility and will have a slower onset, longer peak effect, and longer duration (Golembiewski and Rakic 2010). The half-life is around 1.5 hours. Because morphine is hydrophilic, its entry into the central nervous system is delayed and does not parallel its disappearance from plasma (Aubrun, Mazoit, and Riou 2012). The half-life of transfer from main to effect compartment for morphine ranges from 1.7 hours in postoperative patients. Therefore, morphine concentration peaks at about 20 minutes after a single IV injection (Aubrun, Mazoit, and Riou 2012). Morphine is metabolized to morphing-6-glucuronide (M-6-G) by the liver, the active metabolite (Golembiewski and Rakic 2010). M-6-G is about 1-8 times more potent than morphine and has a longer elimination half-life. The kidneys eliminate M-6-G. Patients with renal dysfunction will accumulate M-6-G, leading to excessive sedation and respiratory depression (Golembiewski and Rakic 2010).

Fentanyl

Fentanyl is highly fat-soluble and will reach its effect in 5 to 7 minutes. It then will redistribute from the brain to muscle and fat, giving it a short duration of action, between 30-60 minutes after the IV bolus dose is given (Golembiewski and Rakic 2010). The onset is rapid, and there is a short duration of action (Aubrun, Mazoit, and Riou 2012). Fentanyl is metabolized into inactive metabolites by the liver (Golembiewski and Rakic 2010). The half-life of transfer from central to effect compartment for fentanyl is 6 minutes.

Hydromorphone

Hydromorphone has a longer duration than fentanyl but a shorter duration than morphine. When IV opioid doses are titrated in the PACU, enough time must be given for the patient to experience the peak effects (Golembiewski and Rakic 2010). Administering doses before their peak effect can result in a "dose-stacking" (Golembiewski and Rakic 2010). Hydromorphone is metabolized to hydromorphone-3-glucuronide, which is also eliminated renally.

Meperidine, Oxycodone, Tramadol

Meperidine lowers seizure thresholds and has a slower rate of metabolism in elderly patients and patients with hepatic and renal dysfunction. Therefore, the accumulation of meperidine can increase the risk of seizures. The liver metabolizes oxycodone. According to an experimental pain modal, it may be more effective than morphine for visceral pain. Tramadol is used for mild to moderate pain. The risk of respiratory depression is less when compared to other opioids (Lovich-Sapola, Smith, and Brandt 2015).

Adverse Effects

The most common adverse effect is nausea and vomiting. The incidence of nausea and vomiting differs in the PACU and the emergency room. This could be attributed to the use of anesthetic drugs given during surgery before morphine titration. The most serious adverse effect is ventilatory depression. Pulse oximetry ranging from ≤85% to 94% is defined as respiratory depression. However, because patients are commonly on supplemental oxygen postoperatively, pulse oximetry of less than 95% may be considered ventilatory depression. A ventilatory rate of fewer than 12 breaths per minute may be a more reliable measure of respiratory depression (Aubrun, Mazoit, and Riou 2012). Severe respiratory depression should promptly be reversed using naloxone until the respiratory rate I <12 breaths per minute. Sedation is another adverse effect and is a common cause of discontinuation of titration. However, there is a poor relationship between sedation, ventilatory depression, and pain relief. In many patients, titration was discontinued due to sedation before the patient had adequate pain relief (Aubrun, Mazoit, and Riou 2012).

Morphine Titration in the Elderly

Because elderly patients have a 50% reduction in clearance and a decrease in protein binding, the dose of opioids should be reduced (Owen et al. 1983). However, there is no evidence that age should be taken into account when titrating opioids because of the wide variability. Postoperatively, the first IV opioid dose should not differ significantly; however, subsequent doses should be reduced by 40% (Aubrun et al. 2002; Aubrun et al. 2003). Further studies should be done to compare morphine titration in elderly patients and elderly patients >90 years. Small boluses of 1-2mg with more time between them should be studied (Aubrun, Mazoit, and Riou 2012).

Morphine Titration in Children

Morphine in infants <6 months of life is different as phase II metabolism, which morphine undergoes, is immature at birth. Commonly, postoperative pain in children is undertreated because physicians are more reluctant to administer opioid analgesics due to the risk of respiratory depression and difficulty in assessing pain and response to pain medication. There are few studies about morphine titration in children postoperatively. As in adults, pain differs from child to child, and therefore the amount required for analgesia will differ(Aubrun, Mazoit, and Riou 2012). The literature recommends an initial bolus of 100 μg $kg^{-}1$ followed by 20-25 μg $kg^{-}1$ subsequent doses every 5 minutes until there is pain relief (Allegaert et al. 2009; Nandi and Fitzgerald 2005; Duedahl and Hansen 2007; Pop et al. 2007; Gall 2009).

Morphine Titration in Obese Patients

Patients who are obese are more likely to have obstructive sleep apnea. Obstructive sleep apnea increases the risk of opioid-induced respiratory depression. Intravenous injections of morphine can be used; however, it should be taken into account that obesity prolongs the half-life of fentanyl and sufentanil as they are more lipophilic. Morphine should be used with caution in these patients, and they should be monitored closely (Aubrun, Mazoit, and Riou 2012).

Multimodal Approach

IV morphine is an efficient and relatively safe method for pain relief in the PACU. Patients postoperatively are usually in severe pain, and complete pain relief can take between 5-60 minutes (Aubrun, Mazoit, and Riou 2012; Aubrun et al. 2007). Many studies suggest combining opioids with other analgesics to achieve pain relief better while reducing harmful side effects. IV analgesics such as nefopam or a small dose of ketamine could improve the impact of opioids (Kapfer et al. 2005). Opioids in combination with NSAIDs and local anesthetics have also been proven to be effective (Aubrun, Mazoit, and Riou 2012).

Opioid Epidemic

In the mid to late 1990s, the American Pain Society recognized pain as the fifth vital sign, increasing patient autonomy and stressing a patient's rights and involvement in their management of pain. This led to increased prescription of opioids for chronic, noncancer pain (Compton and Volkow 2006). Since the late 1990s, the opioid epidemic has become a public health crisis in the United States. There has been an increase in heroin use, high potency synthetic opioids such as fentanyl, and misuse of prescription opioids (Skolnick 2018). An estimated 245 million prescriptions for opioids were dispensed in 2014 (Volkow and McLellan 2016). It is thought that over 10 million Americans misuse prescription opioids (Saha et al., 2016). Overdose deaths due to heroin have increased by more than 20%, and overdose deaths due to fentanyl have increased by more than 72% between 2014 and 2015 (Rudd et al. 2016). Observational studies have shown that patients who use heroin initially misuse prescription opioids. The incidence of heroin users who misused prescription opioids is 19 times higher than those who did not previously report nonmedical opioid use (Compton, Jones, and Baldwin 2016).

Opioids have been over-prescribed, and the estimated cost is over $700 billion annually. Medical prescription of opioids peaked in 2010 and has declined but overdose due to opioids continues to rise. A CDC report shows that the dose and duration of opioid treatment are important factors that lead to addiction, but other reports suggest that short treatments as short as ten days can lead to opioid dependency. Pain is multidimensional, so a combination of various analgesic medications and nonpharmacological interventions should be used to treat postoperative pain (Wardhan and Chelly 2017).

References

Allegaert, Karel, Sophie Vanhaesebrouck, Rene Verbesselt, and John N van den Anker. 2009. "*In vivo* glucuronidation activity of drugs in neonates: extensive interindividual variability despite their young age." *Therapeutic Drug Monitoring* 31 (4): 411-415.

Aubrun, F, J Amour, D Rosenthal, P Coriat, and B Riou. 2007. "Effects of a loading dose of morphine before iv morphine titration for postoperative pain relief: a randomized, double-blind, placebo-control study." *BJA: British Journal of Anaesthesia* 98 (1): 124-130.

Aubrun, F, JX Mazoit, and B Riou. 2012. "Postoperative intravenous morphine titration." *British Journal of Anaesthesia* 108 (2): 193-201.

Aubrun, Frédéric, Dorothea Bunge, Olivier Langeron, Gérard Saillant, Pierre Coriat, and Bruno Riou. 2003. "Postoperative morphine consumption in the elderly patient." *The Journal of the American Society of Anesthesiologists* 99 (1): 160-165.

Aubrun, Frédéric, Stéphanie Monsel, Olivier Langeron, Pierre Coriat, and Bruno Riou. 2002. "Postoperative titration of intravenous morphine in the elderly patient." *The Journal of the American Society of Anesthesiologists* 96 (1): 17-23.

Compton, Wilson M, Christopher M Jones, and Grant T Baldwin. 2016. "Relationship between nonmedical prescription-opioid use and heroin use." *New England Journal of Medicine* 374 (2): 154-163.

Compton, Wilson M, and Nora D Volkow. 2006. "Major increases in opioid analgesic abuse in the United States: concerns and strategies." *Drug and Alcohol Dependence* 81 (2): 103-107.

Dahmani, S, H Dupont, J Mantz, JM Desmonts, and H Keita. 2001. "Predictive factors of early morphine requirements in the post-anaesthesia care unit (PACU)." *British Journal of Anaesthesia* 87 (3): 385-389.

Duedahl, Tina Hoff, and Ebba Holme Hansen. 2007. "A qualitative systematic review of morphine treatment in children with postoperative pain." *Pediatric Anesthesia* 17 (8): 756-774.

Gall, O. 2009. "Recommended use of morphine in children for postoperative pain relief. Pain and Locoregional Anesthesia Committee and the Standards Committee of the French Society of Anesthesia and Intensive Care." *Annales francaises d'anesthesie et de reanimation* [French Annals of Anesthesia and Resuscitation].

Garimella, Veerabhadram, and Christina Cellini. 2013. "Postoperative pain control." *Clinics in Colon and Rectal Surgery* 26 (3): 191.

Golembiewski, Julie, and Andrei M Rakic. 2010. "Opioids." *Journal of PeriAnesthesia Nursing* 25 (4): 258-260.

Hill, Nicholas B. 2014. "Opioids: Overview, Uses and Management of Acute and Chronic Pain."

Kapfer, Barbara, Pascal Alfonsi, Bruno Guignard, Daniel I Sessler, and Marcel Chauvin. 2005. "Nefopam and ketamine comparably enhance postoperative analgesia." *Anesthesia and Analgesia* 100 (1): 169.

Lovich-Sapola, Jessica, Charles E Smith, and Christopher P Brandt. 2015. "Postoperative pain control." *Surgical Clinics* 95 (2): 301-318.

Nandi, R, and M Fitzgerald. 2005. "Opioid analgesia in the newborn." *European Journal of Pain* 9 (2): 105-108.

Owen, James A, Daniel S Sitar, Lisa Berger, Laurence Brownell, Peter C Duke, and Paul A Mitenko. 1983. "Age-related morphine kinetics." *Clinical Pharmacology & Therapeutics* 34 (3): 364-368.

Pop, Rodica Simona, Renee CB Manworren, Cathie E Guzzetta, and Linda S Hynan. 2007. "Perianesthesia nurses' pain management after tonsillectomy and adenoidectomy: pediatric patient outcomes." *Journal of PeriAnesthesia Nursing* 22 (2): 91-101.

Ricardo Buenaventura, M, M Rajive Adlaka, and M Nalini Sehgal. 2008. "Opioid complications and side effects." *Pain Physician* 11: S105-S120.

Rudd, Rose A, Puja Seth, Felicita David, and Lawrence Scholl. 2016. "Increases in drug and opioid-involved overdose deaths - United States, 2010-2015." *Morbidity and Mortality Weekly Report* 65 (50 & 51): 1445-1452.

Saha, Tulshi D, Bradley T Kerridge, Risë B Goldstein, S Patricia Chou, Haitao Zhang, Jeesun Jung, Roger P Pickering, W June Ruan, Sharon M Smith, and Boji Huang. 2016. "Nonmedical prescription opioid use and DSM-5 nonmedical prescription opioid use disorder in the United States." *The Journal of Clinical Psychiatry* 77 (6): 772-780.

Skolnick, Phil. 2018. "The opioid epidemic: crisis and solutions." *Annual Review of Pharmacology and Toxicology* 58: 143-159.

Taylor, Allison, and Linda Stanbury. 2009. "A review of postoperative pain management and the challenges." *Current Anaesthesia & Critical Care* 20 (4): 188-194.

Volkow, Nora D, and A Thomas McLellan. 2016. "Opioid abuse in chronic pain - misconceptions and mitigation strategies." *New England Journal of Medicine* 374 (13): 1253-1263.

Wang, Shaocheng. 2019. "Historical review: opiate addiction and opioid receptors." *Cell transplantation* 28 (3): 233-238.

Wardhan, Richa, and Jacques Chelly. 2017. "Recent advances in acute pain management: understanding the mechanisms of acute pain, the prescription of opioids, and the role of multimodal pain therapy." *F1000Research* 6.

Chapter 4

Oral Opioids

Chase Skillin*, **DO**
Touro College of Osteopathic Medicine, New York, NY, USA

Abstract

Opioids have been a staple of acute pain management in medicine for decades. They are some of the most efficacious analgesics at our disposal, however, due to their propensity for misuse, their prescription is now under more scrutiny than ever. More centers are beginning to experiment with and adopt the Enhanced Recovery After Surgery (ERAS) model for their perioperative management. And while this protocol involves a number of factors unrelated to pain control, pain control is an integral aspect of ERAS. ERAS is primarily designed to improve outcomes, standardize perioperative care, lead to quicker recovery, and shorter hospital stays. As a byproduct, health care costs when following ERAS should be lower as well. ERAS involves multimodal pain management that minimizes opioid use both intraoperatively and postoperatively. Pain control with NSAIDs, acetaminophen, and regional anesthesia are encouraged, and have led to decreased opioid utilization after surgery, decreased length of hospital stay, and decreased cost (Keller et al., 2017). Nevertheless, oral opioids are still required for pain control after painful procedures, and understanding how and when to use them is essential for all surgeons.

* Corresponding Author's Email: cskillin@student.touro.edu.

In: Postoperative Pain
Editors: Indraneil Mukherjee et al.
ISBN: 978-1-68507-971-0

Mechanism of Action

Opioid analgesics act as agonists at opioid receptors throughout the body. There are three primary types of opioid receptors, Mu, Delta, and Kappa. Delta receptors can also be referred to as OP1, or DOP. Agonism of Delta receptors primarily leads to spinal anesthesia, respiratory depression, and decreased gastric motility. Kappa receptors can be referred to as OP2 or KOP. Agonism of Kappa receptors primarily leads to spinal analgesia, diuresis, respiratory depression, sedation, miosis, and dysphoria. Mu receptors can be referred to as OP3 or MOP. Agonists of the Mu receptor lead to analgesia, sedation, respiratory depression, bradycardia, nausea/vomiting, euphoria, and decreased gastric motility, among other effects (Pathan and Williams, 2012; Trescot et al., 2008). The majority of analgesia comes from the binding of Mu receptors in the central nervous system, and it is important to note that all clinically used opioids are Mu receptor agonists. Opioid receptors are coupled to G proteins that inhibit adenylyl cyclase, and act on ion channels in the cellular membrane. Inhibition of adenylyl cyclase leads to decreased levels of cAMP. Opioid receptors actions on ion channels causes a net increase in potassium conductance, leading to hyperpolarization of neurons. These mechanisms both lead to decreased nociceptive input to the thalamus from the periphery. While the majority of opioid receptors are located in the central nervous system and help provide analgesia, opioid receptors are present in lower concentrations in tissues throughout the body. Systemic administration of opioids stimulates these receptors and can lead to many of the side effects commonly seen with opioid medications.

Choosing a Specific Oral Opioid

In general, there is no evidence favoring one oral opioid over another. Several studies have found that they are equally efficacious, and have similar side effect profiles (Marco et al., 2005; Chang et al., 2014). In a study composed of over 350,000 patients receiving postoperative opioids, hydrocodone was the most common opioid prescription, followed by short acting oxycodone. They all have similar risks for dependence, tolerance, and abuse, with the exception of tramadol, which has a slightly higher risk of dependence and tolerance (Thiels et al., 2019). Despite there being no clear cut answer as to which opioid you should choose over another, certain patient specific factors can favor the use of one opioid over another. For example, hydrocodone is only available in the United States in combination with acetaminophen and ibuprofen whereas oxycodone is available as a sole drug that is not combined with anything else. Therefore, Oxycodone might be preferred in patients taking regular scheduled NSAIDs so there is no duplication of NSAIDs. Short acting opioids are preferred over long acting opioids in opioid naïve patients. A study involving over 800,000 opioid naïve patients from the VA demonstrated that opioid naïve patients started on long acting opioids were more than twice as likely to overdose compared to those started on shorter acting opioids (Miller et al., 2015).

The most commonly prescribed oral opioids postoperatively are hydromorphone, oxycodone, and hydrocodone. Hydromorphone and oxycodone can be prescribed as sole agents since they are not necessarily combined with NSAIDs or acetaminophen. In the United States immediate release hydrocodone is only available in combination with other non-opioid analgesics like acetaminophen. Hydromorphone, brand name Dilaudid, is typically dosed 2-4mg every four hours as needed for opioid naïve patients. It has a half-life of 2-3 hours, and has a duration of action of 3-6 hours. The variation in duration of effect is due to patient specific factors, and is also seen in the other prominent oral opioids. Hydromorphone is metabolized primarily in the liver by phase 2 glucuronidation and is excreted primarily as the glucuronidated conjugate, with small amounts of parent drug and minor amounts of 6-hydroxy reduction metabolites.

Oxycodone is available as a 10mg dose on its low end and administered every 4-6 hours as needed in opioid naïve patients. The half-life is 2-3 hours, and the average duration of action is 3-6 hours. Formulations that combine oxycodone with other non-opioid analgesics such as, Percocet, are also available starting at 5mg in combination with acetaminophen 325mg. Oxycodone is metabolized via the CYP450 system, and careful attention needs to be paid to concomitant medications and other patient factors that can inhibit/induce CYP450.

Hydrocodone/Acetaminophen, is typically dosed 5-10mg every 6 hours as needed. The half-life is 2.5-4 hours, and the average duration of action is 4-8 hours. Like oxycodone, hydrocodone is metabolized by the CYP450 system. Hydrocodone has a weak affinity for the Mu receptor, but it is metabolized into hydromorphone, which has a much stronger affinity. Because of this, some consider it to be a prodrug (Trescot et al., 2008).

Before Prescribing

Several steps should be taken before prescribing oral opioids for patients postoperatively. The patients name and DOB should be entered into your state's opioid prescription database to ensure they have not been receiving opioid prescriptions from other providers. Some states do not require providers to check the database prior to prescription of a controlled substance, however we strongly encourage all providers to ensure the patient has not been receiving opioids from another provider prior to prescription of a new opioid regimen. The patient should be screened for risk factors for opioid abuse. Some risk factors include a personal history of substance abuse, family history of substance abuse, depression, unemployment, poverty, poor follow up etc. Use caution when prescribing opioids to patients with one or more of these risk factors.

Patient Education

Patient education is imperative before prescribing oral opioids. The patient should be educated about the risks and benefits of using opioids for pain control. Benefit is decreased pain and increased comfort after the procedure. Risks include misuse/dependence, overdose potentially leading to death, and side effects including nausea and vomiting, drowsiness, dizziness, and constipation. Because opioids have overdose potential, the patient should also be educated on the availability of Naloxone. The goals of pain control should be defined. It's important that the patient understands that the goal of pain control is not zero pain, but tolerable pain. This will help avoid patient dissatisfaction, and decrease pain medication use. Overdose warning signs should be discussed. These signs include lethargy, confusion, bradypnea/apnea, seizures, and urinary retention. Finally proper storage and disposal should be discussed. While in use, pills should be stored in a safe location that is not accessible to children. Once the pills are no longer needed, pills should be discarded by bringing leftover pills to an FDA takeback location (many pharmacies and police stations) or by flushing them down the sink/toilet.

Patients should be encouraged to not maintain possession of the pills for later use.

Indications: Level of Pain

Opioids are indicated for pain control after surgery. However, the strength and duration of the prescription will vary depending on the type of surgery performed and patient specific factors. In general, procedures involving bones and/or joints are more painful than soft tissue procedures (Kim et al., 2016). Patient specific factors that may influence your decision to prescribe include risk of future abuse, previous opioid use, alcohol use, reliable follow up, age, hepatic/renal/cardiac/pulmonary function, obesity, old age, and the presence of anxiety or depression. It is imperative that non-opioid analgesics including NSAIDs and Acetaminophen are used in conjunction with opioids to treat post-operative pain, and these medications should be maximized before turning to opioids. This allows for adequate pain control with lower dosages, decreased frequency, and decreased duration of opioids. The degree of pain expected after a procedure can be used as a guide for oral opioid prescription postop.

Patients expected to have mild pain should not be given oral opioids for postoperative pain control. It is common for patients to have mild pain after dental procedures, or other minor surgical/percutaneous procedures. Regularly scheduled or as needed NSAIDs and/or acetaminophen are usually sufficient for pain control in patients with mild postoperative pain (Jones, Lamdin, and Dalziel 2020).

Patients expected to have moderate pain after a procedure may be given an opioid prescription, but it should not be for more than 3 days. Procedures expected to produce moderate postoperative pain include laparoscopic procedures, minimally invasive surgery, and soft tissue procedures. With adequate intraoperative pain control (regional/local anesthesia), and multimodal postoperative pain control (NSAIDs/acetaminophen), these patients may not need opioids at all. If opioids are required, the following options are available. Oxycodone 10mg, 3-4 pills/day, for three days. Hydrocodone 5mg, 3-4 pills/day, for three days. Hydromorphone 2mg, 3-4 pills/day, for three days.

Patients undergoing procedures expected to produce more severe pain may receive opioid prescriptions for up to 7 days. Procedures that produce severe pain include major surgery, maxillofacial surgery, and joint replacement. As previously mentioned, multimodal pain control should be utilized, and oral opioids should only be prescribed if needed, and at the lowest dose, frequency, and duration possible. Options for patients expected to experience severe pain include Oxycodone 10mg, 4-6 pills/day, for seven days.

Hydrocodone 5mg, 4-6 pills/day, for seven days. Hydromorphone 2mg, 4-6 pills/day, for seven days. It is important to note that if early follow up can be scheduled (before 3 days post op for moderate pain or before 7 days post op for severe pain), the oral opioid prescription should only cover the days until follow up. If opioid medication is still needed at that time, the prescription can be extended. Patients should also be advised not to take more than one pill every four hours, even for those expected to have severe postoperative pain.

Adverse Effects

Oral opioid side effects are common, even when used short term for acute pain management. The most common side effects include constipation, nausea/vomiting, dizziness, drowsiness, and weakness (Daoust et al., 2020). Constipation is a result of an increase in non-peristaltic smooth muscle tone in the bowel. Nausea and vomiting is a result of direct stimulation of the chemoreceptor trigger zone in the area postrema. It is common practice to also prescribe a stool softener and laxative for patients receiving several days of opioids. More serious side effects are also a possibility. These include hypotension, including orthostatic, bradycardia, and respiratory depression. Opioid induced bradycardia is dose dependent and can result in decreased cardiac output. Opioids work on vasomotor centers in the brain, and on the vagus nerve, leading to a relative increase in parasympathetic activity that causes bradycardia. Hypotension is likely due to depression of the sympathetic nervous system. Some opioids, mostly morphine and meperidine, can lead to increased histamine release from mast cells, leading to further hypotension. Respiratory depression is caused by opioids acting on the respiratory centers in the medulla. This results in decreased respiratory rate, thus decreasing minute ventilation (tidal volumes are less affected by opioids). When initiating opioids to naïve patients, or increasing the dose of opioids, respiratory status should be monitored closely.

Special Populations

Certain special populations may require dosing modifications to achieve pain control and ensure safety. Such populations include patients already taking regularly scheduled NSAIDs or Acetaminophen, the elderly, patients taking concomitant respiratory depressants, and those with comorbidities such as liver and kidney disease. Opioids should be used with caution in patients with renal failure. These patients clear the drug more slowly which leads to an increased risk of prolonged respiratory depression and seizures. Opioids should also be used with extreme caution in obese patients, and patients with OSA, due to the increased risk of respiratory depression.

Excessive Prescribing

Excessive prescription of opioids has been a problem in the United States for several decades, and is a significant contributor to the opioid epidemic we are currently facing.

Prescribing more opioids leads to higher consumption, increased likelihood of dependence/tolerance, and leftover pills if a patient does not complete the prescription. 70% of people partaking in non-medical use of opioids do so without a prescription, and 40-50% of these people get the drug from a friend or family member that has left over pills from a previous prescription (Han et al., 2017).

Decreasing the frequency of opioid prescriptions, and the quantity of pills in prescriptions could help decrease non-medical use.

A study in Michigan including 2392 patients at several medical centers showed that the number of pills prescribed was much higher than the number of pills consumed. Median number of pills prescribed was 30, median number of pills consumed was 9 (Howard et al., 2019). Several other studies have been done with similar findings. Another study comprised of 600 opioid naïve patients undergoing a variety of surgeries compared patients that were treated with an opioid sparing postoperative strategy vs standard postoperative pain control. Patients in the opioid sparing pathway used fewer oral opioids, and reported similar levels of pain management satisfaction (Anderson et al., 2021).

Opioid Epidemic and Risk Factors for Addiction

Prescription opioids have significantly contributed to the current opioid epidemic.

Patients have long been overprescribed opioids, and in some cases these patients develop opioid dependence. Although the percentage of patients that become opioid dependent after surgery is quite small, the impact on public health is significant due to the incredible volume of procedures performed each year. The strongest predictor of opioid misuse is duration of prescription, with longer duration increasing the likelihood of tolerance and dependence (Han et al., 2017). By decreasing the duration of treatment, and providing alternative measures of analgesia, we can ensure that a patient's pain is adequately controlled, and minimize negative outcomes related to opioid misuse.

Summary

Opioids are still indicated for postoperative pain control in certain situations, however they should not be the only agent used to achieve postoperative analgesia. Multimodal pain control decreases the dose of each medication required to achieve successful analgesia, and decreases the likelihood of experiencing side effects from each medication. Before prescribing opioids, it is imperative to educate the patient on the goals of pain management after surgery, and reinforce the risks associated with opioid use. This includes the danger of tolerance, dependence, and addiction. If opioids are required, they should be prescribed in the lowest dose possible and for the shortest period of time. Dose adjustments may be required in certain populations. Advanced age, liver/kidney disease, obesity, OSA, chronic opioid use and concomitant CYP450 medications are some of the factors that should be taken into consideration. Common side effects include nausea and vomiting, drowsiness, and constipation. Respiratory depression is a life threating side effect of opioids, and patients should be monitored closely during drug initiation or when increasing the dose.

References

Anderson Maia, Hallway Alex, Brummett Chad, Waljee Jennifer, Englesbe Michael and Howard Ryan. 2021. "Patient-Reported Outcomes after Opioid-Sparing Surgery Compared with Standard of Care". *JAMA Surgery*. American Medical Association. https://doi.org/10.1001/jamasurg.2020.5646.

Chang Andrew K, Bijur Polly E, Munjal Kevin G and Gallagher E John. 2014. "Randomized Clinical Trial of Hydrocodone/Acetaminophen versus Codeine/Acetaminophen in the Treatment of Acute Extremity Pain after Emergency Department Discharge". *Academic Emergency Medicine* 21 (3): 227-35. https://doi.org/10.1111/acem.12331.

Daoust Raoul, Paquet Jean, Cournoyer Alexis, Piette Éric, Morris Judy, Lessard Justine, Castonguay Véronique, Williamson David and Chauny Jean Marc. 2020. "Side Effects from Opioids Used for Acute Pain after Emergency Department Discharge". *American Journal of Emergency Medicine* 38 (4): 695-701. https://doi.org/10.1016/j.ajem.2019.06.001.

Han Beth, Compton Wilson M, Blanco Carlos, Crane Elizabeth, Lee Jinhee and Jones Christopher M. 2017. "Prescription Opioid Use, Misuse, and Use Disorders in U.S. Adults: 2015 National Survey on Drug Use and Health". *Annals of Internal Medicine* 167 (5): 293-301. https://doi.org/10.7326/M17-0865.

Howard Ryan, Fry Brian, Gunaseelan Vidhya, Lee Jay, Waljee Jennifer, Brummett Chad, Darrell Campbell Jr, et al. 2019. "Association of Opioid Prescribing With Opioid Consumption After Surgery in Michigan Supplemental Content". *JAMA Surg* 154 (1): 184234. https://doi.org/ 10.1001/jamasurg.2018.4234.

Jones Peter, Lamdin Rain and Dalziel Stuart R. 2020. "Oral Non-Steroidal Anti-Inflammatory Drugs versus Other Oral Analgesic Agents for Acute Soft Tissue Injury". *Cochrane Database of Systematic Reviews*. John Wiley & Sons Ltd. https://doi.org/10.1002/14651858.CD007789.pub3.

Keller Deborah S, Pedraza Rodrigo, Tahilramani Reena N, Flores-Gonzalez Juan R, Ibarra Sergio and Haas Eric M. 2017. "Impact of Long-Acting Local Anesthesia on Clinical and Financial Outcomes in Laparoscopic Colorectal Surgery". *American Journal of Surgery* 214 (1): 53-58. https://doi.org/ 10.1016/j.amjsurg.2015.10.035.

Kim Nayoung, Matzon Jonas L, Abboudi Jack, Jones Christopher, Kirkpatrick William, Leinberry Charles F, Liss Frederic E et al. 2016. "A Prospective Evaluation of Opioid Utilization after Upper-Extremity Surgical Procedures: Identifying Consumption Patterns and Determining Prescribing Guidelines". *Journal of Bone and Joint Surgery - American Volume*. Lippincott Williams & Wilkins. https://doi.org/10.2106/JBJS.15.00614.

Marco Catherine A, Plewa Michael C, Buderer Nancy, Black Cheryl and Roberts Alisa. 2005. "Comparison of Oxycodone and Hydrocodone for the Treatment of Acute Pain Associated with Fractures: A Double-Blind, Randomized, Controlled Trial". *Academic Emergency Medicine* 12 (4): 282-88. https://doi.org/10.1197/j.aem.2004.12.005.

Miller Matthew, Barber Catherine W, Leatherman Sarah, Fonda Jennifer, Hermos John A, Cho Kelly and Gagnon David R. 2015. "Prescription Opioid Duration of Action and the Risk of Unintentional Overdose among Patients Receiving Opioid Therapy". *JAMA Internal Medicine* 175 (4): 608-15. https://doi.org/ 10.1001/ jamainternmed.2014.8071.

Pathan Hasan and Williams John. 2012. "Basic Opioid Pharmacology: An Update". *British Journal of Pain* 6 (1): 11-16. https://doi.org/10.1177/ 2049463712438493.

Thiels Cornelius A, Habermann Elizabeth B, Michael Hooten W and Jeffery Molly M. 2019. "Chronic Use of Tramadol after Acute Pain Episode: Cohort Study". *The BMJ* 365. https://doi.org/10.1136/bmj.l1849.

Trescot Andrea M, Sukdeb Datta, Marion Lee and Hansen Hans. 2008. "Opioid Pharmacology". *Pain Physician*. Pain Physician. https://doi.org/10.36076/ ppj.2008/ 11/s133.

Chapter 5

Non-Steroidal Anti-Inflammatory Drugs

Mark El-Miniawi[1,*], Jessica El-Miniawi[2] and Khosrow Kashfi[1], PhD
[1]City University of New York School of Medicine, New York, NY, USA
[2]Memorial Sloan Kettering, New York, NY, USA

Nonsteroidal anti-inflammatory drugs (NSAIDs) are a centuries-old mainstay in the treatment of pain, fever, and inflammation. Records from the 4th century B.C. indicate that plants such as willow bark, which contain the natural forms of these NSAID compounds, were utilized to treat fever and pain. Today, NSAIDs represent a drug class that is highly utilized over a spectrum of conditions, diseases, and pathologies. Due to their analgesic, antipyretic, and anti-inflammatory properties, NSAIDs are an ideal candidate for pain management in the surgical setting. Although they may have diverse chemical structures, they all share the same mechanism of action, which is inhibition of the enzyme cyclooxygenase (COX). They have the added benefit of binding well to proteins like albumin which allows them to concentrate at inflammatory sites. They can be classified into various groups based on structure or by COX selectivity. In this chapter we will present a chronology of their development, effects on the eicosanoid pathway, effects beyond inhibition of COX, common adverse effects, their roles in pain management in the post-operative period, and novel advances in their drug class. We will also highlight the various NSAID hybrids that are in different stages of development.

* Corresponding Author's Email: mark.elminiawi@gmail.com.

In: Postoperative Pain
Editors: Indraneil Mukherjee et al.
ISBN: 978-1-68507-971-0

Chronology of Development and the Overall Mechanism of Action

It was not until the late 1700s that willow bark was published as an antipyretic by Dr. Edward Stone. In the 1800s, it was extracted from the bark, buffered to make salicylic acid, chemically synthesized, and finally introduced to the United States by the Bayer company. In the 1900s, alternative salicylates such as phenylbutazone and indomethacin were produced. In 1982, J. R. Vane achieved the Nobel Prize for discovering its mechanism of action via inhibition of COX (Kolfenbach 2020).

On the cell membrane, arachidonic acid is produced by phospholipase A in response to inflammatory markers as well as other chemical and mechanical stimuli. Arachidonic acid is then subsequently broken down by COX to produce products such as prostaglandins (PGs), leukotrienes, thromboxanes, and toxic oxygen radicals. PGs produce a variety of inflammatory effects such as dolor (pain), rubor (redness), and tumor (swelling). They also modify vascular permeability, induce neutrophil chemotaxis, and have countless effects on multiple organ systems. Their effects on multiple organ systems are achieved through different variations of the COX enzyme. COX-1 is prevalent in platelets, renal collecting ducts, smooth muscle cells, and the gastric mucosa. COX-2 is more prevalent in neurons, smooth muscle cells, and synoviocytes. There is a COX-3 enzyme that is constitutively expressed in heart and brain tissue; however, it cannot be inhibited by NSAIDs. Instead, a high dose of acetaminophen can inhibit its effects (C. Lee, Ishimori, and Wallace 2019).

Effects on the Eicosanoid Pathway

It should be noted that PGs, leukotrienes, and thromboxanes, are classically known as eicosanoids because of the retention of their original 20-carbon unsaturated fatty acid structure and should be thought of as local hormones. PGs, in particular, are immediately released as they are too unstable to be stored. Rather than directly activating sensory receptors for painful stimuli (nociceptors), PGs sensitize them to mechanical and chemical stimuli. PGs E2 in particular is the eicosanoid most affiliated with inflammatory processes and is produced by endothelial cells and small blood vessels. It is a key mediator of peripheral and central pain sensitization (Birmingham and Buvanendran

2014). PGs can be subdivided based on their COX enzyme. COX1 PGs are produced constitutively, considered homeopathic, and express a myriad of functions. Homeopathic PGs are found in gastric mucosa to prevent acid secretion and help produce mucus and bicarbonate (Cohen 1987). They are also found in renal tissue and dilate the efferent arterioles of glomeruli. Other Homeopathic PGs have roles such as epithelial cell migration, goblet cell hyperplasia, dendritic cell migration, and the activation of a diverse immunologic response (K. Lee, Lee, and Kim 2020). COX2 PGs are not produced constitutively and are instead activated in an inflammatory response. COX2 PGs have also been shown, in an oncological context, to have a major role in the development of tumorigenesis. COX2 PGs downregulate apoptosis and promote angiogenesis, tumor invasion, and metastasis (Agarwal, Reddy, and Reddanna 2009). Leukotrienes are produced by eosinophils, basophils, mast cells, macrophages, and myeloid dendritic cells. Leukotrienes trigger smooth muscle cell contraction and increase vascular permeability on endothelial cells. This mechanism is one of the main causes of bronchial constriction in asthma and should be acknowledged in treatment strategies (Woodruff, Bhakta, and Fahy 2016). Thromboxanes are produced by hematopoietic cells such as platelets, macrophages, and leukocytes. It is a potent vasoconstrictor that can increase blood pressure in the body as well as facilitate platelet aggregation. This has the added benefit of reducing blood flow to clots (Breyer, Harris, and Breyer 2013).

Effects beyond Inhibition of COX

The production of each eicosanoid should not be thought of as a linear route to each byproduct. Instead, they should be thought of as a branching system of pipes. If one downstream pipe does not have any flow of water, then the water will back up and flow more into other pipes. If one eicosanoid is inhibited from being produced, the other eicosanoids will be upregulated. For instance, although aspirin (ASA) non-selectively inhibits COX1 and COX2, it is weakly more selective in inhibiting COX1. This has the unintended effect of increasing the catalytic activity of COX2. Which can result in an elevated inflammatory response. This pharmacologic effect is evident in the context of ASA-exacerbated respiratory disease (AERD). It is characterized by a sensitivity to NSAIDs, asthma, and eosinophil attributed nasal polyp formation (K. Lee, Lee, and Kim 2020). When COX1 is inhibited, thromboxane production is blocked and platelet function is compromised. This also decreases mucosal secretion and is evident in exacerbating gastroesophageal reflux disease, bleeding disorders, gastric ulceration, and harm to the kidneys (Stein and Kopf 2020). Several studies have shown that although COX2 plays some role in neoplasia, NSAIDs such as ibuprofen do not mainly acquire their cancer chemoprotective properties by inhibiting this one enzyme. Instead, their chemoprotective properties can be attributed to multiple COX2 independent effects. This can include but is not limited to gene expression, alternate splicing, and actions within the cell cycle as well as apoptosis (Matos and Jordan 2015).

Common Adverse Effects

NSAIDs, as a class, should be differentiated on the basis of their COX selectivity when understanding the adverse effects attributed to them. However, a general point to acknowledge is to use NSAIDs cautiously in the elderly due to the increased risk of toxicity in this population.

NSAIDs that Are Nonselective COX Inhibitors

An overdose of a larger than recommended dose, especially when combined with other analgesics like salicylates and acetaminophen, usually can be tolerated. In the instance a patient becomes symptomatic, it can result in nausea, vomiting, blurry vision, dizziness, and drowsiness. The common gastrointestinal adverse effects include dyspepsia, peptic ulcer disease, and bleeding. Risk factors for its gastrointestinal toxicity include an age great than 60, prior history of gastrointestinal issues, the use of glucocorticoids, *H. Pylori* infection, SSRI use, the use of anticoagulant agents, and the use of antiplatelet agents. They can contribute to renal failure, worsen hypertension, and induce electrolyte abnormalities as a result of their effect on the kidneys. They can also increase the risk of renal cell cancer as well. Therefore, it should be taken into consideration when managing a patient with existing renal diseases or hypertension. They are known to exacerbate existing heart failure and increase the risk for myocardial infarction and stroke. Nonselective NSAIDs can also elevate liver transaminases and have been reported to, rarely, cause hepatocellular injury. Hepatotoxicity usually develops with at least six to twelve weeks of use but can resolve after discontinuing NSAIDs after four to eight weeks. They may cause an anaphylactic reaction including but not limited to angioedema, pruritus, tachycardia, urticaria, and cardiac arrhythmias. As previously discussed, they may cause bronchospasm in the context of AERD, asthma, or general inflammation of the respiratory tract. Several hematologic effects like neutropenia and aplastic anemia rarely occur but should be taken seriously. They generally increase bleeding risk and inhibit platelet function via direct inhibition of platelet adhesion and aggregation. Tinnitus (in high doses), hearing loss, aseptic meningitis, psychosis, and cognitive dysfunction may occur. If tinnitus develops, it is a strong warning sign that there are elevated levels of NSAIDs in the bloodstream. Indomethacin, in particular, is associated with headaches. Skin reactions such as Stevens-Johnson syndrome, toxic epidermal necrolysis, and morbilliform rashes can be seen in this drug class (Solomon 2015).

Selective COX2 NSAIDs

Due to only the selective inhibition of COX2, the adverse effects associated with selective COX inhibitors (gastrointestinal effects, bronchoconstriction, bleeding impairment, and platelet impairment) are tampered in comparison to their nonselective counterparts. Selective COX2 NSAIDs still, however, can cause the same renal effects, cardiovascular effects, and anaphylactoid reactions as their nonselective counterparts (Solomon 2019). Some selective NSAIDs such as celecoxib, valdecoxib, and rofecoxib contain a sulfonamide or sulfone moiety and therefore can cause a sulfa drug allergy.

Role for Pain Management in the Post-Operative Period

NSAIDs may play a large role in the post-operative period depending on the circumstances, indications, and planned surgery. Postoperative pain will influence the quality and length of recovery, ultimately affecting the quality of life for the patient as well. The optimal way to manage a patient in the post-operative period is to apply multimodal analgesia. NSAIDs can easily be utilized as a component in a multimodal plan. The adverse effects of this class of medications should, however, be acknowledged. NSAIDs should therefore be avoided in patients with cardiovascular complications as even short-term administration has been shown to increase the risk of death and recurrent myocardial infarcts (especially in patients with a past history). When used in the right circumstances at the right dose, it can improve pain scores without using narcotics and the undesirable effects related to them. Several studies have shown that patients undergoing spinal surgery can benefit tremendously from using NSAIDs on the first and second postoperative days and reduce the consumptive need for morphine. NSAIDs, particularly lornoxicam, when used in conjunction with morphine or a local anesthetic such as ropivacaine in anterior cruciate ligament repair were shown to reduce pain scores, opioid consumption (and side effects associated with use), and length of hospital stay in comparison to the absence of lornoxicam. In addition, patients were able to start walking earlier when lornoxicam was added to the previously described pain regimen (Gelman et al., 2018). Some concern was raised in animal studies about the risk of bony nonunion as a result of NSAID use. However, in a clinical study of 232 patients undergoing foot and ankle surgery, the NSAIDS ketorolac and ibuprofen showed no strong association with bony nonunion ($p = 0.90$ in ibuprofen and $p = 0.57$ in ketorolac) (Hassan and Karlock 2020). This has also been supported in a Cochrane database study that found no significant outcome was detected in higher-quality studies on NSAID exposure and nonunion in osteotomy, spinal fusion, and fracture cases (Birmingham and Buvanendran 2014). Previous concerns about the use of NSAIDs after gastrointestinal surgery have been otherwise assured based on a metanalysis which did prove that anastomoses leak existed but was not statistically significant. Several studies, including the systematic Cochrane review, have shown that NSAIDs have a synergistic effect when used with acetaminophen in the use of orthopedic and spinal surgery. A regimen of acetaminophen (.5g-1g) plus ibuprofen (200-400 mg) has also been shown to have better postoperative pain relief than in patients who have taken either drug alone. Some have even recommended the combination to be used in all patients after gynecologic or oncologic surgery contingent there are no contraindications (Gelman et al., 2018). In a retrospective cohort of pain management in pediatric acute appendicitis cases, it was found that pain scores and morphine consumption were lower in the early postoperative period for patients receiving intraoperative NSAIDs. Therefore, it is feasible to consider that children with uncomplicated appendicitis may be given intraoperative NSAIDs and can later be managed without the need for patient-controlled analgesia (Ousley et al., 2016).

Novel Advances in NSAIDs

There have been many recent advances in the formulation of newer NSAIDs. One of these newer NSAIDs is nitric oxide (NO) donating NSAIDS (NO-NSAIDS). They consist of a NSAID covalently bound to a NO-releasing moiety. It was created based on the knowledge that prostaglandins have similar properties as NO when acting on the gastric mucosa. Therefore, the NO could repair at the site of NSAID-induced damage. This allows NO-NSAIDS to have fewer adverse gastrointestinal effects in comparison to its traditional NSAID counterpart (Rigas and Kashfi 2004). In an endoscopic study of 40 healthy human volunteers who underwent a seven-day trial of NO-ASA, regular ASA, or placebo, it was evident that the NO-ASA showed only minimal gastrointestinal injury compared to ASA and was virtually identical to the placebo group. Any evident mucosal injuries made by the NO-ASA followed the same topographic damage pattern as regular ASA but lacked any ulceration and nearly complete sparing of the duodenum (Fiorucci et al., 2003). The NO moiety has also been shown to have a series of effects on neoplastic events such as the cell cycle, mismatch repair, and signaling cascades. There have been several studies that have showcased its chemopreventive properties against a variety of cancers including pancreas, colon, prostate, lung, and tongue through the use of NO formulations of ASA, sulindac, ibuprofen, indomethacin, and more through the use of preclinical models such as cell culture systems and animal tumor models. In comparison to ASA, NO-NSAIDs have been proven to be more potent than ASA in preventing colon cancer. In fact, comparisons of NO-NSAIDs to their parent NSAID counterparts in vitro studies showed enhanced potency (even a several hundredfold increase in potency in NO-ASA) (Rigas and Kashfi 2004). A similar medication, NOSH aspirin, utilizes both a nitric oxide moiety and a hydrogen sulfide releasing moiety. It also exhibits more effective anti-inflammatory effects in comparison to parent NSAIDs. It is able to have enhanced antinociceptive effects due to the reduction of pronociceptive cytokine synthesis. It also exhibits a good GI safety profile and possibly enhanced cardiovascular and renal safety profiles (Fonseca et al., 2015). Using a pancreatic cell line and a xenograft mouse model, NOSH aspirin has been shown to inhibit tumor growth of both pancreatic cell xerographs as well as pancreatic cell lines with strong potency (Chattopadhyay et al., 2020).

NSAIDs have proven themselves a great class of medications to be used for centuries. Despite their safety profile, their ability to alleviate pain without the use of narcotics makes them a staple in the management in the post-operative period for numerous procedures. Recent advances may one day eliminate the concern affiliated with them and may make them a more readily feasible drug choice in all patient populations regardless of their comorbidities.

References

Agarwal, S., Gorla Venkateswara Reddy, and Pallu Reddanna. 2009. "Eicosanoids in Inflammation and Cancer: The Role of COX-2." *Expert Review of Clinical Immunology*. Expert Rev Clin Immunol. https://doi.org/10.1586/1744666X.5.2.145.

Birmingham, B., and Asokumar Buvanendran. 2014. "Nonsteroidal Anti-Inflammatory Drugs, Acetaminophen, and COX-2 Inhibitors." In *Practical Management of Pain*, Fifth Edit, 553-68. Elsevier Inc.

Breyer, M., Raymond Harris, and Richard Breyer. 2013. "Eicosanoids and Renal Function." In *Seldin and Giebisch's The Kidney*, Fifth Edit, 487-509. Elsevier Inc.

Chattopadhyay, M., Ravinder Kodela, Gabriela Santiago, Thuy Tien C. Le, Niharika Nath, and Khosrow Kashfi. 2020. "NOSH-Aspirin (NBS-1120) Inhibits Pancreatic Cancer Cell Growth in a Xenograft Mouse Model: Modulation of FoxM1, P53, NF-KB, INOS, Caspase-3 and ROS." *Biochemical Pharmacology* 176 (June). https://doi.org/10.1016/j.bcp.2020.113857.

Cohen, M. M. 1987. "Role of Endogenous Prostaglandins in Gastric Secretion and Mucosal Defense." *Clinical and Investigative Medicine*.

Fiorucci, S., Luca Santucci, Paolo Gresele, Roberto Maffei Faccino, Piero Del Soldato, and Antonio Morelli. 2003. "Gastrointestinal Safety of NO-Aspirin (NCX-4016) in Healthy Human Volunteers: A Proof of Concept Endoscopic Study." *Gastroenterology* 124 (3): 600-607. https://doi.org/10.1053/gast.2003.50096.

Fonseca, M. D., Fernando Q. Cunha, Khosrow Kashfi, and Thiago M. Cunha. 2015. "NOSH-Aspirin (NBS-1120), a Dual Nitric Oxide and Hydrogen Sulfide-Releasing Hybrid, Reduces Inflammatory Pain." *Pharmacology Research and Perspectives* 3 (3). https://doi.org/10.1002/prp2.133.

Gelman, D., Arūnas Gelmanas, Dalia Urbanaitė, Ramūnas Tamošiūnas, Saulius Sadauskas, Diana Bilskienė, Albinas Naudžiūnas, Edmundas Širvinskas, Rimantas Benetis, and Andrius Macas. 2018. "Role of Multimodal Analgesia in the Evolving Enhanced Recovery after Surgery Pathways." *Medicina (Lithuania)*. MDPI AG. https://doi.org/10.3390/medicina54020020.

Hassan, M. K., and Lawrence G. Karlock. 2020. "The Effect of Post-Operative NSAID Administration on Bone Healing after Elective Foot and Ankle Surgery." *Foot and Ankle Surgery* 26 (4): 457-63. https://doi.org/10.1016/j.fas.2019.05.016.

Kolfenbach, J. 2020. "Nonsteroidal Antiinflammatory Drugs." In *Rheumatology Secrets*, 4th ed., 646-54.

Lee, C., Mariko Ishimori, and Daniel Wallace. 2019. "Principles of Therapy, Local Measures, and NSAIDs." In *Dubois' Lupus Erythematosus and Related Syndromes*, Ninth Edit, 640-49. Elsevier Inc.

Lee, K., Sang Hag Lee, and Tae Hoon Kim. 2020. "The Biology of Prostaglandins and Their Role as a Target for Allergic Airway Disease Therapy." *International Journal of Molecular Sciences* 21 (5). https://doi.org/10.3390/ijms21051851.

Matos, P., and Peter Jordan. 2015. "Beyond Cox-Inhibition: 'Side-Effects' of Ibuprofen on Neoplastic Development and Progression." *Current Pharmaceutical Design* 21 (21): 2978-82. https://doi.org/10.2174/1381612821666150514104608.

Ousley, R., Laura L. Burgoyne, Nicola R. Crowley, Warwick J. Teague, and David Costi. 2016. "An Audit of Patient-Controlled Analgesia after Appendicectomy in Children." *Paediatric Anaesthesia* 26 (10): 1002-9. https://doi.org/10.1111/pan.12964.

Rigas, B., and Khosrow Kashfi. 2004. "Nitric-Oxide-Donating NSAIDs as Agents for Cancer Prevention." *Trends in Molecular Medicine*. Elsevier Current Trends. https://doi.org/10.1016/j.molmed.2004.05.004.

Solomon, D. H. 2015. "Nonselective NSAIDs: Overview of Adverse Effects." *UptoDate*. 2015.

———. 2019. "Overview of COX-2 Selective NSAIDs." *UpToDate*. 2019.

Stein, C., and Andreas Kopf. 2020. "Management of the Patient with Chronic Pain." In *Miller's Anesthesia*, Ninth Edition, 1604-21. Elsevier Inc.

Woodruff, P., Nirav Bhakta, and John Fahy. 2016. "Asthma: Pathogenesis and Phenotypes." In *Murray and Nadel's Textbook of Respiratory Medicine*, Sixth, 713-30. Saunders, an imprint of Elsevier Inc.

Chapter 6

Ketamine: Nonopioid Perioperative Analgesia

Rayna Walburger*, MD
Icahn School of Medicine at Mount Sinai, New York, NY, USA

NMDA Receptors

N-methyl-D-aspartate (NMDA) receptors play a role in nociception and the central sensitization during pain states. Central sensitization is a state of spinal neuronal hyperexcitability. There is an increased and prolonged response to noxious stimuli that can spread beyond the injury site causing secondary hyperalgesia. Repeated stimulation of nociceptors results in an increase in pain intensity, a phenomenon called "wind up."

The primary neurotransmitter that acts on this receptor is glutamate. The NMDA receptors are closed in the resting state due to the binding of magnesium. A nociceptive input results in the release of glutamate into the synaptic cleft. Upon binding of glutamate and glycine, the NMDA receptor opens. However, depolarization does not occur as long as the magnesium remains bound to the receptor. Once there is sufficient depolarization magnesium is released from the channel and the receptor is activated allowing for the influx of calcium into neurons. Numerous intracellular pathways are then activated, leading to maintenance of central sensitization.

* Corresponding Author's Email: rayna3208@gmail.com.

In: Postoperative Pain
Editors: Indraneil Mukherjee et al.
ISBN: 978-1-68507-971-0

History of Ketamine

Ketamine is a derivative of phencyclidine (PCP), which was used experimentally in laboratories on animals for surgery in the 1950s. Studies on animals showed that ketamine had analgesic effects with animals keeping their eyes open and having poor muscle relaxation. Administration of PCP did not result in depression of the cardiorespiratory systems and laryngeal and pharyngeal reflexes were maintained; however, there were reported intense psychotomimetic effects. Further research was performed to find a derivative of PCP with minimal side effects. With the discovery of ketamine in 1962, it had the beneficial effects of analgesia and anesthesia, with a decrease in the hypnotic properties that were associated with PCP and other derivatives.

Ketamine was initially a veterinary drug and trials were conducted to study its effects on humans. With participants describing their experience as floating and dreaming, ketamine was coined as a dissociative anesthetic. In 1970, Ketamine was approved by the United States Food and Drug Administration. Ketamine was distributed to soldiers during the Vietnam War due to its sympathomimetic effects and safety profile. Due to concerns over its psychedelic effects and the introduction of new anesthetics, the use of ketamine decreased over the years. The combination of ketamine abuse arising during the Vietnam War and the publication of books reflecting on the authors' psychedelic experiences, resulted in ketamine being classified as a class III substance in the US Controlled Substances Act in 1999. With the continued research into ketamine, its safety and efficacy have been shown over the last several years and its analgesic, anesthetic, and antihyperalgesic effects have been reported in numerous studies.

Ketamine Pathophysiology

Ketamine is a derivative of phencyclidine. Ketamine is primarily a noncompetitive, reversible N-methyl-D-aspartate (NMDA) receptor antagonist; however, it has a wide range of actions, exerting effects on mu, delta, and kappa opioid receptors, monoaminergic sensitive and voltage sensitive calcium channels, sodium channels, and nicotinic and muscarinic receptors. The additive effects of these actions of ketamine result in anesthesia, analgesia, hypnosis, psychotomimetic effects, and antidepressant effects.

Ketamine is a dissociative anesthetic. Dissociative anesthetics produce a state of distorted sensory perceptions likely secondary to interrupting the transmission of sensory signals to the cerebral cortex and disrupting communication within the central nervous system. In this dissociative state, patients do not necessarily lose consciousness, but have feelings of detachment from reality. Their eyes may be wide open and their corneal and light reflexes conserved. This makes it a great drug to use for procedures where skeletal muscle relaxation is not required.

The mechanism of action of ketamine makes it the preferred drug of use in various settings. Ketamine exerts sympathomimetic effects on the respiratory and the cardiovascular systems. This sympathetic activity leads to increases in both the heart rate and blood pressure in the cardiovascular system and bronchodilation in the respiratory system. Its hemodynamic profile allows for its use in emergency situations with unstable patients. Patients presenting with hemodynamic instability from hypovolemia, vasodilation, or severe myocardial dysfunction can be safely induced with ketamine. The bronchodilator effects of ketamine allow for induction of patients with life-threatening asthma and intense acute bronchial constriction. Ketamine usage has also been associated with a lower risk of respiratory depression, maintenance of spontaneous ventilation, and relatively more conserved airway reflexes. This is important for patients at risk for opioid induced respiratory depression, such as those with Obstructive Sleep Apnea.

By targeting NMDA receptors as an antagonist, ketamine helps block the intracellular pathways that are activated leading to central sensitization and "wind up," explaining their role in analgesia. This makes ketamine a rational drug choice for perioperative pain management for patients. However, there are mixed results when it comes to ketamine for preemptive analgesia, or improved pain relief with pre-surgical administration versus post-surgical administration. A study on preemptive analgesia with ketamine for laparoscopic cholecystectomy showed a definitive role of ketamine in reducing postoperative pain, while a study conducted on patients undergoing colon surgery showed no preemptive analgesic effect of ketamine.

Uses

Ketamine can be used for many reasons but is only FDA approved for induction and maintenance of anesthesia. Ketamine is used off-label for procedural sedation, rapid sequence intubation outside of the operating room, management of acute pain, agitation, mechanically ventilated patients in the ICU, depressive episodes with MDD, and refractory status epilepticus.

Ketamine may be used at sub-anesthetic doses off label for management of acute pain. At subanesthetic doses, there are minimal physiologic effects. The use of ketamine was associated with reduction in the use of opioid medications, improvement in pain scores despite decrease in opioid use, improved mobilization, and increase in time to first analgesic use.

Hyperalgesia

Opioids used for pain relief can cause hyperalgesia in a dose dependent manner by activating NMDA receptors. Despite the initial pain relief associated with opioids, delayed hyperalgesia is a side effect that can lead to continued seeking of opioids. The administration of opioids results in neuroplastic changes in both the peripheral and central nervous systems that lead to central sensitization. Ketamine, by blocking NMDA receptors, plays a role in reducing hyperalgesia caused by opioid administration. Several studies have shown benefit in administering ketamine along with opioids. Both immediate and delayed hyperalgesia has been prevented with repeated ketamine administration.

Adverse Effects

Ketamine is not without its side effects. These include sympathomimetic effects such as tachycardia and increased intracranial pressure. Due to its sympathetic effects, there is an increase in myocardial oxygen demand, which can result in acute coronary syndrome in patients with cardiovascular risk factors.

The side effects of dissociative anesthesia and psychotomimetic effects such as vivid dreams, hallucinations, and disorientation have been described. The psychotomimetic effects may occur during emergence and include vivid dreams, "out-of-body" experiences and illusions and can be associated with a wide range of emotions such as excitement, confusion, euphoria, or fear. Administration of ketamine with benzodiazepines, such as midazolam, has shown to minimize the psychotomimetic effects. However, if an emergence reaction does occur and requires pharmacologic intervention, benzodiazepines may also be used as treatment.

Other effects include laryngospasm, hypoxia, and sialorrhea. Laryngospasm is an uncommon side effect. It mostly occurs in infants and self resolves within one minute. However, supportive care should be provided with administration of supplemental oxygen and positive-pressure ventilation by bag valve mask if needed. Preparation for endotracheal intubation should take place in case the laryngospasm does not resolve with basic airway support. Sialorrhea is a known side effect of ketamine. It may be severe enough to result in laryngospasm or intubation. Suction and positioning should be performed in order to decrease the chances of aspiration. If the sialorrhea cannot be controlled with suction and positioning and respiratory compromise develops, administration with an anticholinergic, such as glycopyrrolate, can help reduce the production of saliva.

Ulcerative cystitis has also been described with the use of ketamine. Cases have been reported mostly with chronic abuse; however, there are reported cases associated with medical analgesic use. Other urological symptoms include urinary tract damage and renal impairment, which do not always improve after cessation of ketamine.

Increased opening pressures in children having lumbar puncture after administration of ketamine has been reported. However, administration of benzodiazepines, like Midazolam, can help reduce the incidence.

Ketamine Dosing

Ketamine can be administered both intravenously and intramuscularly. An induction dose for general anesthesia of 0.5 to 2mg/kg IV can be used for most patients. The onset of action is within seconds of administration and the duration of effects is between 10 to 20 minutes. Dose adjustments can be made for certain patient populations. Patients presenting with profound hypotension or shock should receive an induction dose of 0.5 to 1mg/kg. If the patient does not have IV access, an intramuscular induction dose of 4 to 6mg/kg may be used. The onset of action for intramuscular administration is approximately four minutes.

Analgesia for acute pain can be achieved with subanesthetic doses. An initial 0.25 to 0.5mg/kg bolus, with a maximum bolus of 35mg, followed by 0.05 to 0.25mg/kg/hour continuous infusion should provide adequate analgesia. This dose should be titrated to achieve analgesia. Patients who are opioid tolerant or have opioid induced hyperalgesia may require higher dosing.

Special Populations

There is no adjustment in dosing for renal impairment. The hepatic dosing is not defined; however, caution should be used in patients with hepatic impairment. Liver enzyme elevation days within infusions of ketamine have been reported. Hepatotoxicity has also been reported with subanesthetic doses and low dose continuous infusions. NMDA receptor binding decreases in the elderly population, so they should receive lower doses than the adult population; while children metabolize ketamine faster than adults and require higher doses. Due to the lack of evidence, ketamine should be avoided in pregnant and breastfeeding patients as there is not enough data to determine safety in these patients.

Contraindications

The contraindications to Ketamine usage include hypersensitivity reaction to ketamine or situations where an increase in blood pressure would be hazardous such as aortic dissection, uncontrolled hypertension, myocardial infarction, or aneurysm. Other groups in which ketamine is contraindicated include infants less than three months of age and patients with a known or suspected history of Schizophrenia, even if controlled on medications. For operations that require muscle relaxation, ketamine should be avoided as it increases muscle tone.

References

Chu, Larry F., Martin S. Angst, and David Clark. 2008. "Opioid-Induced Hyperalgesia in Humans: Molecular Mechanisms and Clinical Considerations." *Clinical Journal of Pain* 24 (6): 479–96. https://doi.org/10.1097/AJP.0b013e31816b2f43.

Gorlin, Andrew W., David M. Rosenfeld, and Harish Ramakrishna. 2016. "Intravenous Sub-Anesthetic Ketamine for Perioperative Analgesia." *Journal of Anaesthesiology Clinical Pharmacology* 32 (2): 160–67. https://doi.org/10.4103/0970-9185.182085.

Laskowski, Kevin, Alena Stirling, William P. McKay, and Hyun J. Lim. 2011. "A Systematic Review of Intravenous Ketamine for Postoperative Analgesia." *Canadian Journal of Anesthesia*. https://doi.org/10.1007/s12630-011-9560-0.

Laulin, Jean Paul, Pierre Maurette, Jean Benoît Corcuff, Cyril Rivat, Marcel Chauvin, and Guy Simonnet. 2002. "The Role of Ketamine in Preventing Fentanyl-Induced Hyperalgesia and Subsequent Acute Morphine Tolerance." *Anesthesia and Analgesia* 94 (5): 1263–69. https://doi.org/10.1097/00000539-200205000-00040.

Nistal-Nuño, Beatriz, Enrique Freire-Vila, Francisco Castro-Seoane, and Manuel Camba-Rodriguez. 2014. "Preoperative Low-Dose Ketamine Has No Preemptive Analgesic Effect in Opioid-Naïve Patients Undergoing Colon Surgery When Nitrous Oxide Is Used - a Randomized Study." *F1000Research* 3 (226). https://doi.org/10.12688/f1000research.5258.1.

Pendi, Arif, Ryan Field, Saifal Deen Farhan, Martin Eichler, and S. Samuel Bederman. 2018. "Perioperative Ketamine for Analgesia in Spine Surgery." *Spine* 43 (5): E299–307. https://doi.org/10.1097/BRS.0000000000002318.

Perumal, DeepaKameswari, Nitya Selvaraj, Mangaiarkkarasi Adhimoolam, SuneethPullikotil Lazarus, and MeherAli Raja Mohammed. 2015. "Midazolam Premedication for Ketamine-Induced Emergence Phenomenon: A Prospective Observational Study." *Journal of Research in Pharmacy Practice* 4 (2): 89. https://doi.org/10.4103/2279-042x.155758.

Singh, Harsimran, Sandeep Kundra, Rupinder M. Singh, Anju Grewal, Tej K. Kaul, and Dinesh Sood. 2013. "Preemptive Analgesia with Ketamine for Laparoscopic Cholecystectomy." *Journal of Anaesthesiology Clinical Pharmacology* 29 (4): 478–84. https://doi.org/10.4103/0970-9185.119141.

Sunder, Rani A., Gokul Toshniwal, and G. P. Dureja. 2008. "Ketamine as an Adjuvant in Sympathetic Blocks for Management of Central Sensitization Following Peripheral Nerve Injury." *Journal of Brachial Plexus and Peripheral Nerve Injury* 3 (22). https://doi.org/10.1186/1749-7221-3-22.

Zhu, Xiaoying, Lynn R. Kohan, and Robert B. Goldstein. 2020. "Substantial Elevation of Liver Enzymes During Ketamine Infusion: A Case Report." *A&A Practice* 14 (8): e01239. https://doi.org/10.1213/XAA.0000000000001239.

Chapter 7

Local Anesthetics

Joseph Kennedy*, MD

City University of New York School of Medicine, New York, USA

Abstract

Since the chemical isolation of cocaine from the coca plant and the development of synthetic local anesthetics, these medications have had varied uses in the clinical setting. In this chapter, we will review the pharmacological basis of local anesthetics, the clinical uses of local anesthetics, and the important side effects of this class of medications. Additionally, we will discuss avenues for further research as well as some of the gaps in the literature in their usage for regional anesthesia and pain medicine.

Pharmacology

Local anesthetics can be defined as a class of medications that cause localized loss of pain sensation via inhibiting conduction of action potentials in peripheral nerves. They are typically structured with a lipophilic benzene ring and a hydrophilic tertiary amine group joined either by an ester or amide based linking group. The tertiary amine, a weak base, (or sometimes a secondary amine as seen in prilocaine or a piperidine group in bupivacaine) is able to receive a hydrogen ion to create a conjugate acid. Local anesthetics are then further classified by which linker group is contained within the molecule: an ester (e.g., cocaine, procaine, chloroprocaine, tetracaine) or amide (e.g., lidocaine, prilocaine, bupivacaine) group. While exceptions exist, this linker

* Corresponding Author's Email: joekennedy96@gmail.com.

In: Postoperative Pain
Editors: Indraneil Mukherjee et al.
ISBN: 978-1-68507-971-0

group does influence the pharmacodynamic profile of the medications. For example, the amide local anesthetics undergo enzymatic degradation in the liver with subsequent excretion via the kidneys (with the exceptions of prilocaine, which is metabolized in the kidney, and articaine, which is inactivated by plasma carboxylesterase), while ester local anesthetics are hydrolyzed by plasma cholinesterases (with the exception of cocaine, which, as an ester, is metabolized primarily in the liver by carboxylesterase). Additionally, the immunogenic profiles of the two groups are different, with ester compounds being thought to be more immunogenic than amide compounds. This is because the metabolite of ester local anesthetics, p-aminobenzoic acid (PABA), is immunogenic, which is what contributes to ester local anesthetics being significantly more prone to allergic reactions as compared to amide compounds.

Furthermore, the amide-type anesthetics possess a chiral center in the amide piperidine ring, which makes these compounds racemic where they contain an equal amount of two possible stereoisomers (either in a levo [left] or dextro [right] configuration). This is important as these two enantiomers can possess different pharmacological properties. As an example, bupivacaine is a racemic mixture, and levobupivacaine is the enantiomer in the levo (left) geometric configuration, both of which are used clinically. While both demonstrate comparable potency and efficacy, the significant difference between the two lie in their side effect profiles.

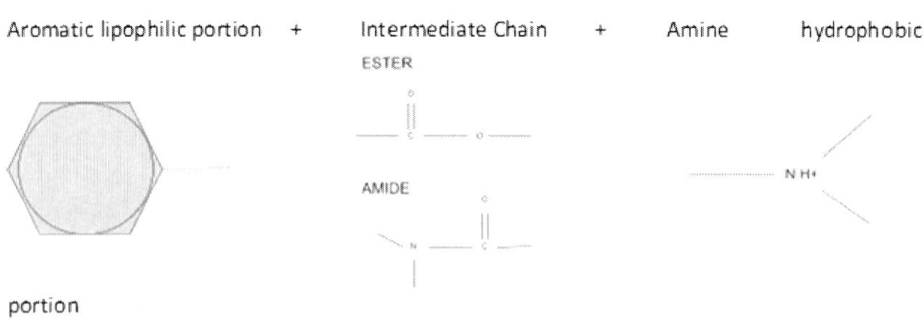

Figure 1. Chemical Structure of Local Anesthetics.

Levobupivacaine, as compared to racemic or the dextro configuration of bupivacaine, has significantly less cardiac and central nervous system (CNS) toxicity [1]. This is attributed to the fact that racemic and the dextro configuration of bupivacaine have a much higher affinity to the sodium channels located in both the heart and the CNS [2]. Another pure enantiomer that was developed from bupivacaine due to the concern for toxicity is ropivacaine. Ropivacaine is also a pure left configuration enantiomer of bupivacaine, and, much like levobupivacaine, the significant difference between ropivacaine and its parent compound lie in the toxicity profiles of each medication [3]. Studies have also demonstrated considerable pharmacological differences between the enantiomers of mepivacaine [4]. On the other hand, the enantiomers of prilocaine, while exhibiting some pharmacological differences, do not seem to possess any clinically significant differences [5]. Additionally, it is important to note that lidocaine, an amide-type local anesthetic, does not contain a chiral center.

While differences exist in the pharmacological profiles of amide- and ester-containing local anesthetics, the basic mechanisms of action remain the same. Through the lipophilic portion of the chemical compound, local anesthetics penetrate through the lipid-rich myelin sheath and cell membrane to inhibit voltage-gated sodium channels, which are multi-subunit transmembrane proteins composed of a single alpha subunit and varying beta subunits. As the binding site for local anesthetics is within the channel pore, the local anesthetic can enter the binding site in either one of two ways: either through a hydrophilic pathway where the compound diffuses through the lipid bilayer in its uncharged form to enter the pore from the intracellular side, where it becomes charged (due to the lower pH intracellularly than the pKa of the compound, leading to the protonated form of the compound), or through a hydrophobic pathway where the compound diffuses laterally through the lipid bilayer. The speed of diffusion of the local anesthetic across the lipid membrane is in large part determined by the pKa of the local anesthetic. The unionized base form of the compound is more lipophilic. Local anesthetics, as weak bases, exist in either the protonated acid form or the neutral base form, depending on the ambient pH and the relative pKa of the compound, as determined by the Henderson-Hasselbach equation:

Local anesthetic (weak base)-H+ $\leftrightharpoons$ Local anesthetic (weak base) + H+
pH - pKa = log (unionized form/ionized form)

As the pKa of a compound approaches physiologic pH, a greater percent of the compound exists in the unionized form, allowing a greater percentage of the compound to diffuse across the membrane. Then, when entering the cytosol, the lower pH shifts the equilibrium toward the protonated form of the compound, which is the form that ultimately inhibits the sodium channel as the channel protein is negatively charged. Thus, the closer the pKa of a local anesthetic is to physiologic pH, the faster the compound is able to diffuse through the lipid membrane, allowing for a faster onset of action.

When the channel is in either an activated (open) state or an inactivated (pore is open but is closed from the intracellular side by an inactivation gate) state, the local anesthetic is able to bind with a higher affinity as its binding site is more available in these two conformations. When the local anesthetic binds within the channel pore, it stabilizes the inactive state of the channel, preventing further activation of the channel. The blocking of the sodium channels at the peripheral nerve prevents the inward rushing of sodium that raises the electrochemical potential from its resting potential, which would trigger the opening of the other ion channels (including voltage gated potassium and calcium channels) that are opened secondary to depolarization. It is important to note that as one moves further away from the origin point of an action potential, the depolarization of the membrane decays in a proportional manner until an impulse can no longer be transmitted due to the depolarization falling below the threshold needed to generate an action potential. This concept is defined as decremental conduction. Thus, when a local anesthetic is injected to block a nerve, sufficient volume must be given to inhibit the critical length of the axon to prevent the regeneration of an action potential by facilitating decremental conduction. In general, in a myelinated nerve fiber that relies on saltatory conduction for faster impulse conduction, at least three nodes of Ranvier, or the nodes between the myelin sheaths that facilitate this expedited conduction, need to be inhibited for there to be a reliable inhibition of nerve conduction.

In addition to the pKa of the compound, the onset of action of a local anesthetic can also be influenced by the route of administration, the dose, and the concentration of local anesthetic used. For example, in a peripheral nerve block, the closer the anesthetic is injected to the nerve, the greater the volume of anesthetic injected, and the smaller the lipid barrier between the nerve and anesthetic injected, the faster the onset of action will be for that local anesthetic. Additionally, higher concentrations can provide more rapid onset, as is the case of chloroprocaine, which is administered at a 3% concentration, allowing for a rapid onset of action despite a relatively high pKa as compared to other local anesthetics.

Duration of action, on the other hand, is largely determined by the protein binding as well as the rate of removal of the local anesthetic from the injection site by vascular uptake. The degree to which a local anesthetic is protein bound to usually either albumin or alpha-1-acid glycoprotein reflects the ability of said drug to bind to the target channel protein as it indicates a higher degree of affinity for general protein binding. For example, bupivacaine and its derivatives, levobupivacaine and ropivacaine, are all very highly protein bound, with percent protein binding being 96, 98, and 94%, respectively. This is, in turn, reflected in these three compound's increased duration of action as compared with chloroprocaine, which has virtually no protein binding. Additionally, highly vascular areas, such as the intercostal space, will result in a decreased duration due to an increased uptake of the medication. This can also occur in highly inflamed tissue, where vascularity will be increased. Local anesthetics can lead to vasoconstriction at lower doses but at higher doses may cause vasodilation, with the exception of cocaine which causes pure smooth muscle contraction and subsequent vasoconstriction.

Thus, to further lengthen the duration of action, a vasoconstrictive agent, such as epinephrine, can be used in combination with the local anesthetic to decrease the vascular removal of the agent in the tissue.

Table 1. Properties of local anesthetics

Agent	**Type**	**pKa**	**Ionization at pH 7.4 (%)**	**Lipid solubility (Partition coefficient)**	**Protein bound (%)**
Procaine	Ester	8.9	97	1.7	6
Chloroprocaine	Ester	9.1	95	9.0	n/a
Tetracaine	Ester	8.5	93	221	76
Lidocaine	Amide	7.9	76	43	65
Prilocaine	Amide	7.9	76	25	55
Mepivacaine	Amide	7.6	61	21	78
Bupivacaine	Amide	8.1	83	346	96
Levobupivacaine	Amide	8.1	83	346	98
Ropivacaine	Amide	8.1	83	115	94

Adopted from: 1) Suzuki S, Gerner P, Lirk P. Local Anesthetics. In: Hemmings HC, Egan TD. Pharmacology and Physiology for Anesthesia. 2nd Edition. Saunders Elsevier; 2018:390-411. 2) Lin Y, Liu SS. Local Anesthetics. In: Barash PG et al. Clinical Anesthesia. 8th Edition. Wolters Kluwer; 2017; 1432-1479. 3) Strichartz GR, Sanchez V, Arthur GR, Chafetz R, Martin D. Fundamental properties of local anesthetics. II. Measured octanol:buffer partition coefficients and pKa values of clinically used drugs. Anesth Analg. 1990 Aug;71(2):158-70. doi: 10.1213/00000539-199008000-00008. PMID: 2375517.

While the pharmacodynamic properties of local anesthetic are important to keep in mind to determine the different pharmacological profiles of each medication, it is also important to consider the differing anatomy of the different nerve types (A, B, and C) being inhibited by the local anesthetic. For example, when applying a local anesthetic, sensory functions are inhibited prior to motor functions, which can be attributed to the different fiber types' anatomy and function, including differing axon size, myelin sheath thickness, and even ion channel composition.

Clinical Applications

Local anesthetics are predominantly used for a wide variety of regional nerve blocks, including peripheral, truncal, spinal and epidural nerve blocks, which are discussed in further detail in the following chapters of this book. Additionally, they can be used for subcutaneous infiltration or applied topically to provide local anesthesia either for procedures or for acute pain relief. Table 2 lists some of the common uses of the local anesthetics with their corresponding concentrations, dosing, and the range of the duration of action in those said applications.

Mixtures

Interestingly, local anesthetics in these clinical applications have been combined with other medications for a variety of purposes. As mentioned prior, vasoconstrictive agents, such as epinephrine and phenylephrine, can be mixed with local anesthetics to reduce their clearance via vascular uptake and thus prolong their duration of action. In addition to increasing the duration of action, they also allow for decreased risk of systemic toxicity as the local anesthetic uptake into the systemic circulation is decreased. They increase the intensity of the block through direct alpha agonist action on anti-nociceptive pathways within the spinal cord and they allow for detection of intravascular injection which allows for prevention of inadvertent intravascular injection of local anesthetic. It is important to note that the use of vasoconstrictive agents in combination with local anesthetics should be avoided in areas with low collateral blood flow, such as the digits, nose, or penis, as the vasoconstrictive effect can cut off direct blood supply to the tissue. Additionally, epinephrine should not be used over the maximum allotted dosing as this may increase the risk of ventricular arrhythmia formation. Of note, phenylephrine can also be used much like epinephrine, with no particular benefit for either vasoconstrictive agent.

Table 2. Clinical applications and doses

Agent	Techniques	Concentrations (%)	Max Dosing (mg/kg; mg)	Duration (hr)
Chloroprocaine	Epidural, infiltration, peripheral nerve block	1, 2, 3	12 mg 800 mg (1 g w/ epinephrine)	0.5 - 1
Tetracaine	Spinal, topical	0.2, 0.3, 0.5, 1, 2	3 mg/kg	1.5 - 6
Cocaine	Topical	4, 10	3 mg/kg	0.5 - 1
Procaine	Spinal, infiltration, peripheral nerve block	1, 2, 10	12 mg/kg	0.5 - 1
Lidocaine	Epidural, spinal, infiltration, peripheral nerve block, IV, regional, topical	0.5, 1, 1.5, 2, 4, 5	4.5 mg/kg 7 mg/kg (with epinephrine) 200 mg 500 mg (w/ epinephrine)	0.5 - 3
Prilocaine	Peripheral nerve block (dental)	4	6 mg/kg 8 mg/kg (w/ epinephrine 400 mg 600 mg (w/ epinephrine)	0.5 - 3
Mepivacaine	Epidural, infiltration, peripheral nerve block	1, 1.5, 2, 3	4.5 mg/kg 7 mg/kg (with epinephrine) 400 mg 550 mg (w/ epinephrine)	1 - 4
Bupivacaine	Epidural, spinal, infiltration, peripheral nerve block	0.25, 0.5, 0.75	3 mg/kg (with/without epinephrine) 150 mg	2- 12
Levobupivacaine	Epidural, infiltration, peripheral nerve block	0.125, 0.5, 0.75	3 mg/kg 150 mg	2 - 17
Ropivacaine	Epidural, spinal, infiltration, peripheral nerve block	0.2, 0.5, 0.75, 1	3 mg/kg	2 - 8

Adopted from: 1) Suzuki S, Gerner P, Lirk P. Local Anesthetics. In: Hemmings HC, Egan TD. Pharmacology and Physiology for Anesthesia. 2nd Edition. Saunders Elsevier; 2018:390-411. 2) Lin Y, Liu SS. Local Anesthetics. In: Barash PG et al. Clinical Anesthesia. 8th Edition. Wolters Kluwer; 2017; 1432-1479.

An additional additive compound that can be mixed with local anesthetics is bicarbonate. Bicarbonate will raise the pH of the solution, which, as demonstrated by the Henderson-Hasselbach equation above, will shift the equilibrium such that there is more unionized local anesthetic within the solution, making it more lipophilic. This will allow more of the anesthetic agent to diffuse across the lipid bilayer, increasing its onset of action. However, it is important to note that excess alkalinization of the mixed solution can lead to precipitation of the local anesthetic as most agents are in slightly acidic preparations.

Other alpha receptor agonists, including clonidine and dexmedetomidine, have also been combined with local anesthetics with varied results. Clonidine, when combined with local anesthetics in epidural injections, is thought to have multiple mechanisms of action, including alpha 2 receptor agonism in the dorsal horn to reduce pain transmission, local vasoconstriction to reduce vascular uptake of the local anesthetic leading to prolonged duration of action, and can enhance neuraxial opioids when those are used concurrently as well [6]. Clonidine has also been used in combination with local anesthetics for peripheral nerve blocks, but these have shown variable results as to their effectiveness, as at higher doses clonidine can lead to sedation and hypotension. Much like with epinephrine, the additive effect of clonidine is most pronounced with shorter acting local anesthetics such as lidocaine and mepivacaine, and two-to-four-hour prolongation of analgesia in the setting of a peripheral nerve block has been reported in the literature. Dexmedetomidine, a more selective alpha 2 receptor agonist with some independent analgesic effects, has also been shown to prolong the effects of local anesthetics in peripheral nerve blocks [7].

Opioids are another class of medications that have been frequently combined with local anesthetics, especially for neuraxial anesthesia, as they have been shown to increase the duration and quality of analgesia, with the potential of using a lower dose of local anesthetic agents. In peripheral nerve blocks, only buprenorphine, a partial opioid agonist, has been used with some effectiveness, as the side effects of nausea and vomiting have limited their use. Table 3 shows some of the common opioids, and their doses, that are used in combination with local anesthetics in neuraxial anesthesia, as well as some of the other medications used in combination with local anesthetics.

Another medication used in combination with local anesthetics includes dexamethasone, an antiinflammatory glucocorticoid. While their precise mechanisms remain unclear, they have been shown to increase both motor and sensory block, as well as overall analgesia, with a decreased incidence of postoperative nausea and vomiting. However, one of the detrimental side effects of combined use has been undesirable prolonged motor blockade. Additionally, with some local anesthetics (such as ropivacaine and bupivacaine), dexamethasone, as well as other steroids such as betamethasone, can precipitate and form crystals, which can lead to embolic infarcts within the central nervous system. This is believed to be due to the increase in pH caused by corticosteroids when mixed with certain local anesthetics, which each have a certain pKa at which they are likely to crystalize; thus, as the pH of the solution increases when mixed with corticosteroids, the risk of precipitation increases [8].

Other combinations with local anesthetics include ketamine, tramadol, neostigmine, and benzodiazepines such as midazolam, but there is limited evidence as to their clinical effectiveness and safety profiles, and so more evidence is needed before they can be recommended for clinical use.

Table 3. Common additives to local anesthetics

Additive Medication	**Indications**	**Dosing**
Epinephrine Phenylephrine	Peripheral nerve blocks	Epinephrine 3 - 5 microg/mL
	Infiltration Epidural Marker for intravascular injection	
Opioids	Neuraxial anesthesia	*Intrathecal:* Morphine 100 - 200 microg Fentanyl 10 - 25 microg Sufentanil 5 microg *Epidural:* Fentanyl 2 - 10 microg/mL Sufentanil 0.25 - 1 microg/mL Hydromorphone 20 microg/mL
Corticosteroids	Peripheral nerve blocks	Dexamethasone 2 - 4 mg
Clonidine	Neuraxial anesthesia Peripheral nerve block	Max dose 1 microg/kg IBW
Dexmedetomidine	Neuraxial anesthesia Peripheral nerve block	Spinal anesthesia 10 microg Epidural anesthesia 0.5 microg/kg 0.5 -1 microg/kg

Adopted from Suzuki S, Gerner P, Lirk P. Local Anesthetics. In: Hemmings HC, Egan TD. Pharmacology and Physiology for Anesthesia. 2nd Edition. Saunders Elsevier; 2018:390-41.

Side Effects

While relatively safe when administered correctly, local anesthetics do have side effects, ranging from mild to life threatening, especially with inadvertent intravascular or intraneural injection or with giving more than the maximum allotted dose. The most classic, and one of the most severe, side effects of local anesthetics is local anesthetic systemic toxicity (LAST). LAST has an estimated rate of 1-2 events per 1000 nerve blocks [9]. Patients who appear to be at an elevated risk of this syndrome are those with underlying hepatic and renal dysfunction, in which the drugs are not metabolized and excreted properly, resulting in increasing levels of local anesthetics into toxic levels. Additionally, patients who have underlying cardiac dysfunction are more prone to developing more severe complications from LAST as the cardiac toxicity may be more detrimental on already diminished cardiac reserve. Patients who are pregnant may also be at elevated risk due to both an underlying hyperdynamic circulation which stimulates more vascular uptake of local anesthetics, as well as reduced alpha-1-glycoprotein with resultant increased free non-protein bound local anesthetic in the bloodstream. Other medical conditions that alter local anesthetic pharmacology, such as acidotic states and low protein states, can also increase the risk of developing LAST. Usually, LAST is associated with high volume nerve blocks and prolonged local anesthetic infusions, either via a catheter or intravenously (in the case of lidocaine). Additionally, it appears that there may be an increased risk of LAST with bupivacaine as compared with ropivacaine (which has less selectivity for cardiac or CNS sodium channels) or lidocaine (which is shorter acting).

The presentation of LAST in the literature is quite heterogeneous, and with a low incidence the clinician must maintain a high level of suspicion for this syndrome in the appropriate clinical setting. Typically, the onset of symptoms can occur rapidly within minutes, especially in the case of inadvertent vascular infusion, but LAST can present in a delayed fashion, especially with cumulative doses and with gradual systemic absorption. Clinically, CNS toxicity can present first, with symptoms ranging from anxiety, dizziness, circumoral numbness, lightheadedness, and tinnitus to shivering, tremors, and eventually generalized tonic-clonic seizures, which was found to be the most common presentation [10]. At higher blood levels, LAST can eventually result in coma and respiratory suppression. The onset of CNS symptoms is usually followed by cardiac findings (although this may be reversed in a significant proportion of patients). Initially these symptoms may include sympathetic activation, but may later manifest with bradycardia, AV block, QRS widening, negative inotropy resulting in hypotension, and possibly cardiac arrest (pulseless ventricular tachycardia, ventricular fibrillation, pulseless electrical activity, or asystole). The proposed mechanisms by which local anesthetics are toxic to the heart include blockade of cardiac sodium channels leading to negative inotropy and arrhythmias, inhibiting fatty acid metabolism with subsequent energy loss, reducing calcium influx and release from the sarcoplasmic reticulum of cardiac myocytes, mitochondrial respiratory chain disruption, and prolonging conduction through the Purkinje fibers and cardiomyocytes. Local anesthetics can also exert their cardiac effects indirectly via the CNS and autonomic nervous systems by causing central disinhibition, which can ultimately result in cardiocirculatory collapse in LAST. As mentioned prior, bupivacaine, as well as the other more lipophilic agents including tetracaine and etidocaine, have a greater propensity to lead to cardiac toxicity as opposed to the less lipophilic agents as these more lipophilic agents tend to be more proarrhythmogenic in addition to their negative chronotropic effects.

Treatment of LAST requires immediate discontinuation of the offending local anesthetic and emergency management of the airway, ventilation, and circulation [11, 12]. Treatment of seizures, along with proper airway management and cardiovascular support, is of utmost importance and can be accomplished with benzodiazepines, such as lorazepam or midazolam, with other possibilities including ketamine, propofol, or thiopental if more rapid onset for seizure breakthrough are needed or the seizures are refractory to benzodiazepines. However, no quality evidence exists for the use of these secondary agents for the treatment of seizures secondary to LAST, and medications such as propofol should be used with caution in this setting as they may further promote cardiovascular collapse. Additionally, phenytoin should be avoided as it exerts sodium channel inhibitory actions and thus may promote toxicity from local anesthetics.

In regards to the hemodynamic management for LAST, significant arrhythmias and cardiovascular collapse should be treated according to ACLS guidelines with some notable exceptions. In the event of ventricular arrhythmias, amiodarone is considered the safest option, but it is important to note that during lipid emulsion, amiodarone may be sequestered with unpredictable effects on dosing. Additionally, lidocaine and procainamide should be avoided as these may exacerbate LAST, and calcium channel blockers and beta blockers should also be avoided as these may further exacerbate any present hypotension. If epinephrine is to be administered (eg.

pulseless electrical activity), it is recommended that it be used at smaller than the recommended dose in the ACLS pathway as epinephrine, at its standard dose, is arrhythmogenic, can increase afterload, and can directly interfere with lipid-based resuscitation [13]. If cardiovascular collapse secondary to LAST is refractory to these therapies, cardiopulmonary bypass or extracorporeal membrane oxygenation may be indicated.

The mainstay of treatment for LAST is lipid emulsion therapy [11, 12, 13]. While it remains unclear as to the precise mechanism of action of lipid emulsion therapy for local anesthetic toxicity, it is theorized to possibly involve sequestration (termed as "lipid sink") of the local anesthetic, which explains the therapeutic benefit of lipid emulsions for other lipophilic drug toxicities such as beta blockers, calcium channel blockers, and tricyclic antidepressants, as well as enhancing fatty acid metabolism of cardiac myocytes. While indications and optimum dosing have not been elucidated as the treatment is primarily based off of case reports in the literature, expert guidelines for the indications for lipid emulsion therapy for the treatment of LAST include substantial neurologic toxicity, substantial cardiovascular toxicity, and rapid clinical deterioration with high suspicion for local anesthetic toxicity. It is important to note that cumulative doses above the upper limit of therapeutic dosing for lipid emulsions should be avoided as potential side effects may include allergic reactions, pancreatitis, thrombocytopenia, and clogging of ECMO and dialysis circuits.

As mentioned prior, local anesthetics can be directly neurotoxic, leading to several possible side effects, including transient neurologic symptoms (TNS) and cauda equina syndrome [14]. TNS is characterized by a transient pain in the low back, buttocks, or thighs after intrathecal local anesthetic administration. It usually presents within a few hours of administration, lasting as long as ten days but it is not a permanent finding. TNS, while associated with all local anesthetics, is most often associated with lidocaine and mepivacaine, with a purported incidence of one in seven cases of intrathecal lidocaine or mepivacaine use [14]. Additionally, reports of cauda equina syndrome after local anesthetic injection through microcatheters have been reported, which appears to be due to poor distribution of the local anesthetic through these catheters, resulting in pooling of the local anesthetic and higher than normal concentrations localized to specific spots, leading to direct neuronal toxicity; ultimately these microcatheters were withdrawn. The use of ultrasound guided injections has greatly decreased the necessary volume of local anesthetic used, decreasing the incidence of direct neuronal toxicity.

Another important side effect of local anesthetics include allergic reactions, which, while rare, is thought to occur more frequently with the ester group of local anesthetics. This is because the metabolite of esters includes p-aminobenzoic acid (PABA), which, as mentioned previously, is immunogenic, and thus can potentially lead to allergic reactions [2]. Some amino amides are produced with a preservative which has a metabolite similar to PABA known as methylparaben that can be immunogenic, but this is much less commonly seen. Another side effect seen with some local anesthetics is methemoglobinemia, in which the iron element of a heme group is oxidized, decreasing its affinity to oxygen while increasing the affinity of normal hemoglobin to oxygen, resulting in a left shift on the oxygen hemoglobin dissociation curve, which in turn leads to less oxygen delivery to peripheral tissue due to decreased release of oxygen from normal hemoglobin. This is commonly seen with prilocaine, which is metabolized to *o*-toluidine in the liver which then subsequently oxidizes hemoglobin to methemoglobin, and benzocaine. The mainstay of therapy for methemoglobinemia is methylene blue, which converts methemoglobin back into hemoglobin.

Advancements/Gaps in Research

One new local anesthetic formulation, liposomal bupivacaine, has made recent advances within the literature. Liposomes are bilayer lipid vesicles that can contain a specific compound to increase the duration of release of a target medication, and Exparel (bupivacaine liposome injectable suspension) has recently gained FDA approval for single dose postsurgical wound infiltration in patients six years or older for postsurgical pain management as well as for interscalene brachial plexus nerve blocks. However, results have been mixed as to the effectiveness of liposomal bupivacaine, and a recent editorial has criticized the cost-effectiveness of Exparel, which resulted in the manufacturing company of Exparel, Pacira Biosciences, to file a lawsuit against *Anesthesiology* and the American Society of Anesthesiologists for libel against the medication. Thus, as it is currently a very divisive issue as to the effectiveness of bupivacaine for certain regional nerve blocks and for postoperative pain, more high quality research will be needed going forward to determine its true effectiveness in these clinical settings.

Other avenues of research regarding local anesthetics has included specific targeting of specific sodium channels as some sodium channels are very specific to certain nociceptive nerve fibers; however, to date, there are no specific sodium-channel antagonists that are within clinical use, and more research is required in this field before such a pharmaceutical is available within the market. Additional research and advancement of ultrasound technology has allowed for visualization of real-time injection of local anesthetic within tissue planes to target specific nerves, and as imaging modalities improve, so will the delivery of regional and neuraxial anesthesia all while avoiding iatrogenic harm to patients.

References

[1] Burlacu, Crina L., and Donal J. Buggy. 2008. "Update on Local Anesthetics: Focus on Levobupivacaine." *Therapeutics and Clinical Risk Management*. https://doi.org/10.2147/tcrm.s1433.

[2] Riazi, Sheila, and Carlos A. Ibarra Moreno. 2019. *Pharmacology and Physiology for Anesthesia. Anesthesia & Analgesia*. 2nd ed. Vol. 129. Saunders Elsevier. https://doi.org/10.1213/ane.0000000000004232.

[3] Casati, Andrea, and Marta Putzu. 2005. "Bupivacaine, Levobupivacaine and Ropivacaine: Are They Clinically Different?" *Best Practice and Research: Clinical Anaesthesiology*. https://doi.org/10.1016/j.bpa.2004.12.003.

[4] Burm, Anton G. L., Imca M. C. Cohen, Jack W. Van Kleef, Arie A. Vletter, Wim Olieman, and Kees Groen. 1997. "Pharmacokinetics of the Enantiomers of Mepivacaine after Intravenous Administration of the Racemate in Volunteers." *Anesthesia and Analgesia* 84 (1): 85–89. https://doi.org/10.1097/00000539-199701000-00016.

[5] Meer, Auke Dirk Van Der, Anton G. L. Burm, Rudolf Stienstra, Jack W. Van Kleef, Arie A. Vletter, and Wim Olieman. 1999. "Pharmacokinetics of Prilocaine after Intravenous Administration in Volunteers: Enantioselectivity." *Anesthesiology* 90 (4): 988–92. https://doi.org/10.1097/00000542-199904000-00010.

[6] Yasaei, R, and A Saadabadi. n.d. "Clonidine." *StatPearls [Internet]. StatPearls Publishing*. https://www.ncbi.nlm.nih.gov/books/NBK459124/.

[7] Pöpping, Daniel M., Nadia Elia, Emmanuel Marret, Manuel Wenk, and Martin R. Tramèr. 2009. "Clonidine as an Adjuvant to Local Anesthetics for Peripheral Nerve and Plexus Blocks: A Meta-Analysis of Randomized Trials." *Anesthesiology* 111 (2): 406–15. https://doi.org/10.1097/ALN.0b013e3181aae897.

[8] King, Wade, Zachary McCormick, and Clark Smith. 2020. "Risks of Precipitate Formation When Combining Corticosteroids with Local Anesthetic for Use during Interventional Pain Procedures." *Pain Medicine (United States)* 21 (2): 423–24. https://doi.org/10.1093/pm/pnz315.

[9] Macfarlane, A. J. R., M. Gitman, K. J. Bornstein, K. El-Boghdadly, and G. Weinberg. 2021. "Updates in Our Understanding of Local Anaesthetic Systemic Toxicity: A Narrative Review." *Anaesthesia* 76 (S1): 27–39. https://doi.org/10.1111/anae.15282.

[10] Anderson, Douglas M., and Jerry A. Beyer. 2006. "Local Anesthetic Toxicity." In *Decision Making in Pain Management*, 242–45. https://doi.org/10.1016/B978-0-323-01974-3.50092-9.

[11] Gitman, Marina, Michael R. Fettiplace, Guy L. Weinberg, Joseph M. Neal, and Michael J. Barrington. 2019. "Local Anesthetic Systemic Toxicity: A Narrative Literature Review and Clinical Update on Prevention, Diagnosis, and Management." *Plastic and Reconstructive Surgery*. https://doi.org/10.1097/PRS.0000000000005989.

[12] El-Boghdadly, Kariem, Amit Pawa, and Ki Jinn Chin. 2018. "Local Anesthetic Systemic Toxicity: Current Perspectives." *Local and Regional Anesthesia* 11: 35–44. https://doi.org/10.2147/LRA.S154512.

[13] Neal, Joseph M., Michael J. Barrington, Michael R. Fettiplace, Marina Gitman, Stavros G. Memtsoudis, Eva E. Mörwald, Daniel S. Rubin, and Guy Weinberg. 2018. "The Third American Society of Regional Anesthesia and Pain Medicine Practice Advisory on Local Anesthetic Systemic Toxicity: Executive Summary 2017." *Regional Anesthesia and Pain Medicine* 43 (2): 113–23. https://doi.org/10.1097/AAP.0000000000000720.

[14] Zaric, Dusanka, Christian Christiansen, Nathan L. Pace, and Yodying Punjasawadwong. 2005. "Transient Neurologic Symptoms after Spinal Anesthesia with Lidocaine versus Other Local Anesthetics: A Systematic Review of Randomized, Controlled Trials." *Anesthesia and Analgesia* 100 (6): 1811–16. https://doi.org/10.1213/01.ANE.0000136844.87857.78.

Chapter 8

Alvimopan: Peripheral Mu-Opioid Receptor Antagonist

Jonathan Gardy Alabre*
City University of New York School of Medicine, New York, NY, USA

Introduction

Alvimopan, brand named Entereg®, is a non-central mu-opioid receptor antagonist that binds competitively at the gastrointestinal (GI) receptors. It binds with a very high affinity for mu-receptors but has significantly limited interaction with kappa and delta receptors as evidenced by their respective inhibition constants [Mu Ki =.4nM, Delta Ki= 4.4nM, Kappa Ki =40nM]. All 3 of these opioid receptors are present within the central nervous system but are also found within the myenteric and submucosal bowel plexus. Apart from those 3 receptor types, Alvimopan is also known to have minimal affinity for non-opioid serotonergic, dopaminergic, adrenergic receptors. Compared to its subclinical affinity for central receptors, Alvimopan binds 200 times stronger to its peripheral receptors. Thus, the selectivity of Alvimopan's interactions to the GI mu system specifically results in the inhibition of any circulating opiates from exerting their peripheral effects. These effects occur due to combination of opioid agonism and inhibition of acetylcholine in the myenteric plexus resulting in diminished smooth muscle tone and decreased peristaltic activity. The resultant bowel distention causes stimulation of mechanoreceptors and other physiological mechanisms that produce and release emetogenic factors into circulation. Ultimately the absent enteric

* Corresponding Author's Email: jalabre000@citymail.cuny.edu.

In: Postoperative Pain
Editors: Indraneil Mukherjee et al.
ISBN: 978-1-68507-971-0

motility and uncoordinated bowel dysfunction cause symptoms of nausea, vomiting, and ileus in patients receiving prescription narcotics. Post-operative ileus (POI) specifically is a highly unfavorable, yet all too common complication seen in patients who've undergone abdominal surgery and are subsequently treated with opioids for pain management. While POI is generally considered to be a multi-faceted issue which can result from a variety of factors such as electrolyte imbalance, inflammation, and mechanical manipulation of the bowel itself, the activity of opiates at the mu receptors seems to be the major root cause of the problem. As a result, during the late 2000s Alvimopan became a highly contested agent in the peri-operative management of patients due to its potential to counter post-operative ileus.

In addition to limiting the side-effect profile of opiates, the utility of Alvimopan was also bolstered by its lack of influence on their centrally derived analgesic effects. Narcotics are able to enter the central nervous system where they primarily interact at the brain stem, rostral anterior cingulate cortex, and dorsal horn of the spinal cord to mediate pain-relief because they have the ability to cross the blood brain barrier (BBB). The BBB is an intricate interface of endothelial cells, gap junctions, and other components that prevent the passage of various agents and noxious compounds into the CNS. Certain characteristics such as molecular size, polarity, and lipid solubility all contribute to whether a compound can pass via simple diffusion, transport mediated diffusion, or not pass at all. Alvimopan's large molecular size and high polarity result in its inability to cross the BBB, thereby allowing for the intended analgesic effect of the administered opiates to occur.

Investigations into the pharmaco- kinetics/dynamics of Alvimopan have revealed that in vitro, it's noted to have a slow rate of dissociation from its target receptors which may contribute to enhanced potency when competing with exogenous opioids. It has limited bioavailability at a range of 1% - 19%, a time to maximum concentration of 2 hours after a single oral dose, and a mean volume of distribution (Vd) of 11 – 98 liters. After absorption, Alvimopan is converted by gut-flora to its active metabolite "ADL 08-0011". However, unlike many other drugs, the active metabolite is actually not required for efficacy in patients experiencing post-operative ileus. Moreover, Alvimopan is primarily excreted via the biliary route at 65% while the remaining 35% is via renal excretion.

Currently, there are several unanswered questions regarding the safety profile and efficacy of Alvimopan in various patient populations and demographics. Many of the studies regarding the drug have been performed in animal models with questionable applicability to human beings. Among those unanswered questions was whether Alvimopan may have unforeseen effects on fertility. Studies were performed in which pregnant rats were given oral and intravenous doses that greatly exceeded the recommended human doses at 68 to 136 times and 3.4 to 6.8 times respectively. The results showed that there was no identifiable effect on reproduction, nor was there any harm done to the rat fetus. However, an insufficient amount of random controlled trials has been conducted in pregnant human receiving Alvimopan, so its use is cautioned in this population unless explicitly necessary. Furthermore, Alvimopan and ADL 08-011 is present in the breast milk of lactating rats, but it is unknown whether the drug can be found in the milk of nursing human mothers. Nor is it known if the presence of the drug in breast milk would be detrimental for a human baby. Nevertheless, Alvimopan's use is also cautioned in woman who currently breast feed unless clearly necessary. Long term carcinogenicity studies were conducted in mice and rats to assess whether Alvimopan had potential to cause cancer. It was found that when female mice received oral doses of Alvimopan at over 600 times the recommended human dose for 104 weeks, there was a significant incidence of fibromas, fibrosarcomas, osteomas, and osteosarcomas in that test population. Interestingly, the female rats who received the exact PO doses for the same amount of time did not exhibit any significant incidence of sarcoma formation. Further investigation into whether these carcinogenicity results can be noteworthy in human models is still necessary.

When compared with adult aged populations, human geriatric patients have not been found to experience any adverse effects of the drug at increased or altered rate. Though efficacy and safety are reported to be clinically similar between both demographics, it should not be ruled out the sensitivity to the drug is possibly greater in geriatric patients. Due to its major methods of excretion, understanding the safety profile of Alvimopan in patients with various comorbidities was also of great importance. In patients with mild hepatic dysfunction, it is generally to use Alvimopan with no dosage adjustments despite the potential for increased circulating plasma levels. However, these patients should be continuously monitored while on Alvimopan and in the event that they experience any major adverse effects, the drug should be discontinued immediately. There are no current guidelines for use in patients with severe hepatic impairment because the drug is simply not recommended in this population. In terms of renal impairment, Alvimopan has not been studied in patients with end-stage renal disease and thus is not recommended. Patients with mild to moderate and even severe renal disease can receive Alvimopan without requiring dosage adjustments, but they too should be closely monitored for any adverse effects. Patients who experience adverse effects due to Alvimopan toxicity should be managed supportively as there is no specific antidote for the drug. Additional evaluations of potential for abuse and dependence of Alvimopan revealed that there is no risk. Though a thorough understanding of the drug has been established thorough extensive trial and research, concrete results of longitudinal research regarding the long-term side effects of Alvimopan has yet to be established. While further studies are underway to evaluate Alvimopan, the FDA, since approving the drug in 2008, has continued to place extensive restriction on the availability, administration, and application of the drug.

Approval

Alvimopan was originally approved by the FDA in 2008 in order to reduce the incidence and intensity of post-operative ileus in patients undergoing small bowel resections with primary anastomosis. As time has passed, expansions to its indications have been made to include any procedures that "include bowel resection and primary anastomosis". Thus, radical cystectomies, total abdominal hysterectomies, and other abdominal procedures are now eligible as well. Initially, the agent seemed very promising in its ability to decrease the risk of POI however, concerns over its use began to arise after a 12-month study in which a higher number of myocardial infarctions (MI) was reported in patients who received 0.5mg twice daily as compared to the placebo group. All of the patients in the study were receiving opioids for non-cancer chronic pain management. Subsequent investigations into the matter failed to reveal a causal relationship between the increased incidence of MI and the use of Alvimopan, but in the interest of patient safety the FDA created strict criterion for eligibility in terms of who could administer the drug and how it was to be dosed. Thus, Alvimopan only became accessible to institutions who enrolled in the newly established ENTEREG Access Support and Education (E.A.S.E.) program.

The requirements for entry into the E.A.S.E program mandate that program materials must be received by the hospital and properly distributed among any health care professionals who are responsible for prescription, administration, or dispensing of the drug. This would include physicians, nurses, pharmacists and anyone else involved in the care plan. In addition, the hospitals must demonstrate that they have protocols in place to limit the use of Alvimopan to more than 15 doses per patient within the hospital. Finally, the hospital must agree to not offer Entereg to any patient as an outpatient medication, while also refusing to offer the drug to any hospital not currently enrolled in the E.A.S.E program. If an institution could strictly follow these requirements, they could legally receive Entereg for use at their facility. Once in possession of the drug, there were further dosing rules that had to be adhered too as well. Entereg is to be taken PO and is produced in 12mg capsule form. Patients are to receive a 12mg dose 30 minutes to 5 hours prior to surgery, and then can receive 12mg doses twice daily for 7 days post-surgery. Alvimopan is not as effective if administered after the onset of post-operative ileus which is why recommendations call for its administration all throughout the peri-operative process. Furthermore, any patient who's received therapeutic doses of opioids for more than 7 consecutive days prior to surgery are not eligible to receive Alvimopan because anyone whose been recently exposed to narcotics is expected to be more sensitive to the drug. Rendering those patients more likely to experience unwanted side effects such as nausea vomiting abdominal pain and diarrhea. The other most commonly reported side effects include but are not limited to anemia, hypokalemia, dyspepsia, urinary retention, and back pain. However, these side effects tend to occur less than only 5% and the drug is generally well tolerated. When used according to the guidelines presented by the FDA and in accordance with the E.A.S.E program, Alvimopan is a highly efficacious tool in preventing post-operative ileus in patients who've undergone abdominal surgery.

Post-operative ileus defined as the extended cessation of coordinated bowel motility that occurs in patients who've undergone surgery involving bowel resection and manipulation. Though ileus can occur to some extent after any surgery, the severity of POI is greatly influenced by the location, duration, and characterization of the procedure. Though the average incidence of POI is approximately 10% worldwide, this number has been reported to range from even 2% to 60% depending on the procedure and criteria for diagnosis. Criteria can differ depending on the duration of latency in return to bowel function or whether clinicians also consider time to tolerance of oral intake. Irrespective of how its described, there is no singular cause for POI, but rather it is the combination of several factors that each individually increase a patient's risk of adequate peristalsis. An imbalance of electrolytes whether from decreased oral intake or malnutrition prior to surgery can result in paralytic ileus. Intraoperative release of inflammatory mediators within the bowel can also cause cessation of bowel movement. Studies have even suggested that mechanical manipulation of the bowel during the procedure itself can result in ileus as well. However, the use of narcotics for pain management post-operatively has been identified as the dominant cause of POI in patients. The health consequences of POI are generally mild with the patient experiencing small bowel obstruction like symptoms such as abdominal pain, distention, nausea and vomiting. However, when caring for these post-operative patients it is best to mitigate the occurrence of these symptoms because in rare situations, they can have catastrophic consequences for the patient. Nausea and vomiting in high-risk patients can lead to aspiration and pneumonia, increasing patient morbidity post-operatively. Severe abdominal distention and inability to tolerate oral intake can result in decreased respiratory reserve and malnutrition, which can promote poor wound healing, infection, and dehiscence. In order to prevent these outcomes, prophylactic interventions with prokinetic agents such as metoclopramide, erythromycin, vasopressin, and cholecystokinin-like drugs can be performed. A study in which several randomized controlled trials were performed in order to evaluate the efficacy of these drugs showed that Alvimopan was the only agent with considerable evidence of improvement of bowel motility and function.

However, there is currently no evidence to support that Alvimopan has any effect on mortality in patients who receive it. Additional prophylactic protocol includes optimization of patient electrolytes, encouragement of postoperative ambulation, and early enteral feedings. With ongoing data emerging regarding the benefit of incorporating Alvimopan into surgical patients plan of care, we have seen an upwards trend in the number of patients receiving Alvimopan since its approval in 2008. Between 2014 and 2016 there was a 24% increase in the use of Alvimopan in patients who underwent radical cystectomy. While this shift has been positive for patient health outcomes in general, hospital systems have also mitigated large costs of stay by joining the E.A.S.E program because of the positive association between decreased cost of hospitalization and prevention of post-operative ileus.

When analyzing the overall financial burden of hospitalization for surgical patients, there are generally two major categories of cost: the operative procedure itself and the post-operative management. While the cost of performing the surgery is usually a fixed sum, hospitals have directed their attention towards developing strategies to maintain the post-operative standard of care while simultaneously diminishing modifiable costs. The cost of hospitalization is intrinsically linked to the length of stay (LOS) for the patient and many studies have consistently found that in patients who've undergone abdominal surgery, the biggest driver for length of stay has been the development of post-operative ileus. Secondary to managing POI a patients LOS may be increased by 2 to 8 days, increasing the cost per patient by $5,000 on average, culminating in an annual national cost of 1.47 billion dollars. Other reviews of phase 3 trials have shown that Alvimopan only decreases the cost of stay by a monetary amount that simply cancels out the cost of paying for the medication. This outcome greatly depends on the individual costs of care set by each institution, and in these situations the hospital may seek alternative agents to manage their patients POI. Overall, the majority of analyses regarding the cost effectiveness of Alvimopan has proven profitable for the hospital and the patient.

Other studies evaluating radical cystectomy patients have shown that use of Alvimopan is associated with decrease in LOS by 1.9 days which correlated with a 20% diminished cost of stay from approximately $40,000 USD to $32,000 USD. In comparison with a placebo in multiple phase 3 trials, Alvimopan has been shown to accelerate GI recovery by 11 hours in patients who received a partial bowel resection. The benefit of using Alvimopan in laparoscopic procedures is variable where some studies stating that it decreases LOS by 1.5 days while other studies suggesting there is no change in outcome. Furthermore, Alvimopan has the potential to decrease time to first flatulence to by 21 hours, decrease time to first bowel movement by 41 hours, and decrease time until a patient is ready for discharge by 23 hours. Alvimopan can indirectly decrease the onset of pain in patients by preventing the discomfort associated with paralytic ileus, however when assessed for its direct ability to influence pain scores, there was no significant difference in patients who received the drug versus the placebo. As it stands Alvimopan remains to be an optimal agent in combating post-operative ileus and should be incorporated into any recovery protocols for treating patients who've received opiates for management of their pain. However, since the advent of the national opioid crisis, providers have sought out alternative methods for establishing peri-operative analgesia which often times use non-opiate drugs such as non-steroidal anti-inflammatory drugs (NSAIDs), glucocorticoids, and spinal epidurals. The role of Alvimopan in these new pain management protocols must then be assessed to see if it can remain of practical benefit to the patient and the hospital.

The United States Opioid Epidemic has been a nationwide crisis for several decades now. Though it initially began due to increasing availability of prescription opiates, the epidemic has continued to be fueled by the widespread usage of illicit narcotics among Americans. Within just a 9-year span between 2005 and 2014, the national rate of hospitalizations secondary to opioid use had increased by 64%. Based on the results from the National

Survey on Drug Use and Health conducted in 2016, 11.8 million Americans aged 12 and older had reported misuse of opioids. 92% of those who admitted to abusing opioids had only used pharmaceutical agents, while the remaining 8% had either used a combination of heroin and pharmaceuticals, or just heroin. Between 2015 and 2016 alone there was a 27% increase in opioid-related deaths at 42,000 Americans.

The Center for Disease Control and Prevention had estimated that 80% of those deaths in 2016 had involved the use of some illicit synthetic opioid. While these figures themselves are already alarming, they do not even begin to capture the full extent of the damage that the opioid epidemic has inflicted upon our society. Combatting this national crisis has required a multi-modal approach to decreasing the availability of these prescription drugs to the public, while also increasing access to resources for individual suffering from drug addiction and abuse.

Within the medical community specifically, many societies have focused their attention towards incorporating non-opiate pharmaceutical agents into the management of their patient's pain.

It is now recommended that providers first attempt to use agents such as acetaminophen, NSAIDs, glucocorticoids, local anesthesia, and spinal epidurals prior to offering patients opioid pharmaceuticals. The development of Enhanced Recovery After Surgery (ERAS) protocols have created a foundation for peri-operative management of patients who've undergone procedures in order to maximize their pain control while avoiding unnecessary administration of opioid drugs. Under ideal circumstances, a post-operative patient would then manage their pain appropriately without narcotics, diminishing the risk for development of POI. Thus, the role of Alvimopan in these emerging ERAS procedures is questionable as the drug is often used in association with opioids. Some institutions have even begun to test Ultrarestrictive Opioid Prescription Protocol (UROPP) for pain management. The goal of these programs is to drastically minimize the quantity of opiates prescribed to patients after gynecologic and abdominal surgery.

However, these alternative methods of pain control are often not 100% effective and many patients still receive a minimal number of opioids for their post-operative pain. Some studies have even shown that in addition to preventing POI, Alvimopan can even promote peristalsis even in the absence of opioid use. Though the mechanism of this phenomenon is not fully understood, it may have to do with Alvimopan's coemption with endogenous endorphins released within the GI system. As the medical community continues to improve upon their current methods of non-opiate pain control, time can only tell whether or not Alvimopan will continue to be of utility in the future. In this current day, a considerable amount of research is being performed to evaluate for the utility of Alvimopan in non-gastrointestinal surgeries.

While initial studies often looked at Alvimopan's efficacy in relation to bowel resection surgery, many clinicians are now researching the effects of these drugs in urologic, gynecologic, and even spinal surgery. In patients who underwent radical cystectomy for malignancy or benign disease, Alvimopan was shown to decrease the time to tolerance of oral intake and reported bowel movement. In addition, it was shown to reduce the time to hospital discharge and decrease the rate of nasogastric tube placement. However, there was no evidence to support that Alvimopan reduced the readmission ate or altered the mean narcotic use in these patient populations. Furthermore, these results came from evaluation with an open surgical approach; Alvimopan use with robotic-assisted radical cystectomy, which is becoming an increasingly popular procedure, has not yet sufficiently been researched.

Research into the use of different mu-opioid receptor antagonist in cancer patients receiving palliative care is now also underway. These patients often experience bowel dysfunction secondary to their opiate use for chronic pain management. It is possible that Alvimopan could have a significant role as an adjunct agent in the future treatment plans of these patients. In addition, research has also been conducted to assess the role of Alvimopan for patients who've undergone spinal surgery. Pain management in this patient population requires high doses of opioids which is why the incidence of post-operative ileus and opioid-induced constipation is very high in this patient subgroup. Opioid induced constipation (OIC) has the same foundational pathogenesis as post-operative ileus however, the time frame and setting in which the two occur is different. POI is diagnosed within the immediate post-operative period whereas OIC can occur at any point during opiate treatment. Compared with placebo groups, patients who received Alvimopan were reported to have earlier time to first solid intake. As it stands now, Alvimopan remains to be a very effective agent in combating the opioid induced cessation of bowel activity often seen after abdominal surgery. As ongoing research continues to evaluate for the potential of Alvimopan's role in non-abdominal surgery, we in the medical community can expect to see many original and creative applications for this drug in the future.

References

Coussens NP, Sittampalam GS, Jonson SG, Hall MD, Gorby HE, Tamiz AP, McManus OB, Felder CC, and Rasmussen K. n.d. "The Opioid Crisis and the Future of Addiction and Pain Therapeutics". *Journal of Pharmacology and Experimental Therapeutics* 371 (2): 396-408. https://doi.org/10.1124/jpet.119.259408.

Delaney C. n.d. "Management of Postoperative Ileus: Focus on Alvimopan". *Therapeutics and Clinical Risk Management* 4: 965-973. https://doi.org/10.2147/tcrm.s3147.

Duncan C, Teh J and Lawrentschuk N. n.d. "Alvimopan for Post-Radical Cystectomy Ileus: What Should We Know?" *Translational Andrology and Urology* 8 (S1): 96-98. https://doi.org/10.21037/tau.2019.02.01.

Dunn LK, Thiele RH, Lin MC, Nemergut EC, Durieux ME, Tsang S, Shaffrey ME, Smith JS, Shaffrey CI and Naik BI. n.d. "The Impact of Alvimopan on Return of Bowel Function after Major Spine Surgery – A Prospective, Randomized, Double-Blind Study". *Neurosurgery* 85 (2): 233-239. https://doi.org/10.1093/neuros/nyz005.

Hensley P, Higgins M, Rasper A, Ziada A, Strup S, Coleman C, Ruf K and Gupta S. n.d. "Efficacy and Safety of Alvimopan Use in Benign Urinary Tract Reconstruction". *International Urology and Nephrology* 53 (1): 77-82. https://doi.org/10.1007/s11255-020-02621-9.

Itawi EA, Savoie LM, Hanna AJ and Apostolides GY. n.d. "Alvimopan Addition to a Standard Perioperative Recovery Pathway". *JSLS : Journal of the Society of Laparoendoscopic Surgeons* 15 (4): 492-498. https://doi.org/10.4293/108680811x13176785204076.

Keller DS, Flores-Gonzalez J-R, Ibarra S, Mahmood A and Haas EM. n.d. "Is There Value in Alvimopan in Minimally Invasive Colorectal Surgery?" *The American Journal of Surgery* 212 (5): 851-856. https://doi.org/10.1016/j.amjsurg.2016.02.016.

Lyden J and Binswanger IA. n.d. "The United States Opioid Epidemic". *Seminars in Perinatology* 43 (3): 123-131. https://doi.org/10.1053/j.semperi.2019.01.001.

Mark J, Argentieri DM, Gutierrez CA, Morrell K, Eng K, Hutson AD, Mayor P et al. n.d. "Ultrarestrictive Opioid Prescription Protocol for Pain Management after Gynecologic and Abdominal Surgery". *JAMA Network Open* 1 (8): 185452. https://doi.org/10.1001/jamanetworkopen.2018.5452.

Sultan S, Coles B and Dahm P n.d. "Alvimopan for Recovery of Bowel Function after Radical Cystectomy". *Cochrane Database of Systematic Reviews* 1. https://doi.org/10.1002/14651858.cd012111.pub2.

Chapter 9

Epidural and Spinal Anesthesia

Chikadibia Agoha*
City University of New York School of Medicine, New York, NY, USA

Introduction

Epidural anesthesia and spinal anesthesia are two common types of neuraxial anesthesia. They both provide regional blockade for procedures involving the pelvis, hips and/or lower limbs, making it possible to perform many major procedures without the use of general anesthesia. Neuraxial anesthesia bypasses the risks associated with general anesthesia including airway management, allowing for a more rapid recovery from surgery in regard to motor and bowel functions. It also provides better postoperative pain control in comparison to intravenous narcotics. When combined, a technique called a CSE (combined spinal-epidural), benefits of both techniques can be combined and shortcomings of each avoided.

In this chapter, we will discuss epidural and spinal anesthesia, its differences, benefits and risks.

Epidural Anesthesia

Epidural anesthesia can provide surgical anesthesia, intraoperative muscle relaxation, and intrapartum and postoperative analgesia. It involves the use of a catheter to inject a drug into the epidural space. This procedure has a slow onset of action of about 10-15 minutes and can last for one to two hours.

* Corresponding Author's Email: agohachika@yahoo.com.

In: Postoperative Pain
Editors: Indraneil Mukherjee et al.
ISBN: 978-1-68507-971-0

Because the medication is administered in the epidural space where the epidural fat is present, fatty tissue absorption competes with neural tissue distribution subsequently affecting its potency and duration of action [1]. Therefore, epidural anesthesia is administered at much higher doses than doses for spinal anesthesia. Epidural anesthesia is commonly used during childbirth because of its long-lasting effects as the catheter allows for repeated or continuous administration of medications. Patients receiving epidural anesthesia are still able to sense pressure but not pain, as it provides a more analgesic effect than complete anesthesia.

Indications

Epidural anesthesia can also be used for many other procedures that require blockade in the lower extremity including orthopedic, vascular, genitourinary, gynecologic, colorectal, and cardiothoracic surgeries. Major orthopedic procedures that can be performed under epidural anesthesia include primary hip or knee arthroplasty, surgery for hip fracture, revision arthroplasty, bilateral total knee arthroplasty, acetabular bone grafting, and insertion of long-stem femoral prostheses. This provides a quicker recovery of motor function, and is associated with better postoperative pain control and a reduction of intraoperative blood loss when compared with general anesthesia.

Examples of vascular procedures performed with epidural blockade include abdominal aortic aneurysm repair, renal artery bypass, aorto-femoral bypass, embolectomy and thrombectomy [2]. Avoiding general anesthesia in these high-risk patient populations possibly enhances graft patency, reducing the need for re exploration and reducing the risk of thromboembolic complications. Because patients undergoing lower limb vascular surgery commonly have multiple major systemic diseases, such as coronary artery disease, cerebrovascular disease, diabetes mellitus, chronic renal insufficiency, chronic HTN, and chronic obstructive pulmonary disease (COPD), placing them at high risk for complications associated with general anesthesia such as pulmonary and cardiac events which in turn lead to longer hospitalization and increased mortality [2]. These patient with multiple comorbidities can benefit from epidural anesthesia. However, because of some of these comorbidities, these patients are most likely on anticoagulants or antithrombotic agents preoperatively which may put them at risk of epidural hematomas and other epidural related complications. Thus further consideration is required.

Both spinal and epidural anesthesia with a lower thoracic sensory level blockage can be used for transurethral resection of the prostate (TURP) [2]. Neuroaxal anesthesia is preferred over general anesthesia as it allows earlier detection of mental status changes associated with local absorption of large volumes of irrigation solution (TURP syndrome). Neuroaxial anesthesia also gives the patient the ability to communicate breakthrough pain which is indicative of capsule and/or bladder perforation, and reduced risk of blood loss and deep vein thrombosis.

Technique

Epidural anesthesia can be administered by the median or paramedian approach. The median approach requires the patient to sit up straight, back bent at the waist and head tucked into the chest. The patient is being administered oxygen and their vital signs are monitored. This is a sterile procedure, therefore proper handwashing, donning of sterile gloves and gown, use of sterile equipment, and maintenance of a sterile work area is required. Standard premade trays are available, after appropriate skin cleansing for sterility, a sterile drape is placed and taped on the patient. The provider then examines for the desired area depending on the procedure, can be anatomically or ultrasonographically performed in preoperative setting, the overlying skin is anesthetized using which is then injected with lidocaine 1% to decrease the amount of discomfort during the procedure.

A Tuohy needle is used for obtaining epidural access. The positioning of the needle is important to ensure the proper location of the epidural catheter. The epidural needle is advanced through skin, soft tissue, and spinal ligaments until the tip of the epidural needle enters the epidural space. This space is determined by the loss of resistance as the needle passes the ligamentum flavum and into the epidural space. Assessment of loss of resistance is done with the use of a syringe filled with air or saline. With the air technique, the needle is advanced while continuous pressure is applied to the plunger of the air-filled syringe, upon which resistance is felt. Compression of the air-filled syringe signals passage through the ligamentum flavum, hence the loss of resistance. With saline, the presence of an air bubble within the saline syringe will disappear on entering the epidural space. Once the epidural space is identified, the catheter is introduced into the space and placed at a desired location [3].

With the paramedian approach, the needle is inserted 2cm lateral to the midline, allowing the needle to bypass the supraspinous and interspinous ligaments thus the ligamentum flavum will be the first and only resistance encountered. The paramedian approach is commonly used in patients with spinal abnormalities and thoracic procedures where the spinous processes are angulated and closely approximated, allowing the needle to bypass bony structures.

Contraindications

Contraindications to epidural anesthesia includes patient refusal, sepsis, elevated intracranial pressure, anticoagulants, thrombocytopenia, coagulopathies, preexisting central nervous system injuries, preexisting neurologic injury and previous back surgery [2].

Complications

Most patients receiving epidural anesthesia complain of shivering, ringing of the ears, backache, headache, soreness around the area of insertion, nausea, vomiting, and/or difficulty urinating [4]. Hypotension, infection, and cardiovascular collapse are anticipated adverse effects that can occur with epidural anesthesia. Hypotension results primarily from vasodilation and increased vascular bed capacitance. This is caused by the direct inhibition of the sympathetic outflow to the nerves innervating the blood vessels causing arterial and venous vasodilation [5]. In rare instances, permanent nerve damage may result in the area where the catheter was inserted. Epidural hematomas may occur and are caused by vascular trauma from the epidural needle and/or catheter into the epidural space [3]. If epidural hematoma/abscess is suspected, a CT or MRI scan is indicated followed by immediate surgical decompression of the hematoma in order to regain motor function. Research shows that epidural anesthesia compared with non-epidural methods is associated with an increased incidence of assisted vaginal birth [6]. Due to its neural blockage, epidural anesthesia makes pushing more difficult and additional medications or interventions may be needed, such as forceps, vacuum or cesarean section.

Although rare and commonly associated with spinal anesthesia, severe headache caused by leakage of spinal fluid may occur. Postdural puncture headache is also a feared complication if the dura is punctured during an epidural catheter placement. The reported incidence of PDPH after unintentional dural puncture (UDP) with an epidural needle (which is larger in diameter than a spinal needle) for labor analgesia in women is about 88 percent [7]. Treatment for PDPH if symptoms persist, is a procedure called a "blood patch", which is an injection of the patient's blood into the epidural space.

Spinal Anesthesia

Spinal anesthesia, also known as a subarachnoid block, is done by injecting an anesthetic of choice into the cerebrospinal fluid. This is done without the use of a catheter and the anesthetic agent is usually given as a single low dose [3]. This procedure has a rapid onset of action of approximately 5 minutes and lasts for hours depending on the agent used. The spinal block provides a much stronger anesthetic effect, leaving the patient with a complete loss of sensation and motor function. Because of the low dose requirements, systemic toxicity is uncommon during spinal anesthesia.

Indications

As with epidural anesthesia, spinal anesthesia is used for surgical procedures involving the lower abdomen, pelvis, perineal and lower extremities. Spinal anesthesia is best for short procedures. This is unlike epidural anesthesia where a catheter is placed to provide extended administration of anesthesia.

Technique

Spinal anesthesia can be performed with the patient in the lateral decubitus or sitting position. The sitting position is preferred over the lateral decubitus as it provides a more symmetric anatomy. The sitting position also allows the dural sac to be distended allowing a larger focus for the spinal needle. With the patient positioned in the sitting position, the leg hanging from the side of the bed, spine flexed with the patient's waist bent and chin brought towards the chest. This position will optimize the interlaminar space between the desired vertebral levels. The desired access site is palpated and the preferred site of entry is usually the space between 2 palpable spinous processes. Sterile technique must be maintained. The area is prepared with chlorhexidine and alcohol solution; the skin is swabbed in an outward circular motion, starting from the desired skin entry. The sterile drape is placed on the patient's back to isolate the access site. The local anesthetic is injected, most commonly 1mL of 1% lidocaine, and a wheal forms which will be used as a marker for the insertion site. The two most common needles used for spinal anesthesia are open-cut beveled needle and a closed tapered tip pencil point needle with a side port. A pencil point needle (Whitacre or Sprotte) is preferred over a beveled tip (Quincke) needle as it has a lower association with post dural puncture headaches [3]. This is because post dural puncture headaches are more common with large bore needles, therefore smaller cutting needles such as 24 or 25-gauge pencil point needles are preferred.

There are two standard approaches for spinal anesthesia: midline and paramedian. For the midline approach, the spinal needle is introduced into the skin and angled slightly cephalad. The needle passes through the skin, followed by the subcutaneous fat. As the needle approaches the supraspinous ligament and the interspinous ligament, increased resistance is felt. Ligamentum favum would present as a "pop" followed by loss of resistance which may not be felt given smaller gauge of needle. The needle is further inserted until the dura and subarachnoid membranes are penetrated which will cause a flow of cerebrospinal fluid. For the paramedian approach, the local anesthetic is placed about 2cm away from the midline and the spinal needle is inserted at an angle towards the midline [3]. With this approach, the supraspinous and interspinous ligaments are bypassed resulting in decreased resistance felt upon reaching the ligamentum flavum.

Continuous Spinal anesthesia can be achieved by advancing a catheter through the needle into the subarachanoid space. The catheter must not exceed 2 – 4cm into the subarachnoid space due to risk of impaling the spinal cord [3]. This method allows for repeated drug administration to maintain the duration of the motor and sensory block.

In comparison to epidural anesthesia, spinal anesthesia must be injected below L2 to avoid injury to the spinal cord. Since spinal anesthesia bypasses surrounding subcutaneous tissue associated with epidural anesthesia, the injected dose is much smaller, and a much rapid onset of action [3]. Spinal anesthesia also gives a more profound neuromuscular block, blocking all motor and sensory function below the level of injection.

Contraindications

Absolute contraindications for spinal anesthesia includes patient refusal, increased intracranial pressure, infection at the injection site and suspicion of sepsis. Relative contraindications include use of anticoagulants, thrombocytopenia, coagulopathies, due to the risk of hematomas, severe hypovolemia and hypotension [2].

Complications

Post-dural puncture headache is the most common complication associated with spinal anesthesia [8]. This is thought to be a result of loss of cerebrospinal fluid that is greater than the rate of cerebrospinal fluid production, causing a decrease in intracranial pressure. Thus, the headache is usually worse when upright, better when lying flat and is often associated with neck stiffness, photophobia, nausea, or auditory disturbances. Risk factors associated with PDPH include prior headaches, younger age, female gender, pregnancy and low body mass index (≤25kg/m2) [9]. Patients more likely to develop PDPH benefit from 24 or 25 gauge pencil-tipped (Whitacre or Sprotte) needles as they have a lower incidence of reported PDPH than beveled (Quincke) tip needles [3]. Epidural blood patch (EBP) is considered the definitive treatment for PDPH. EBP involves the injection of a patient's blood through the epidural needle into the epidural space. The mechanism of action is unclear but is thought to increase lumbar and intracranial cerebrospinal fluid pressure by mass effect and as the blood clots and plugs the cerebrospinal leak. The clotted blood may also facilitate healing at the punctured site by initiating an inflammatory reaction. Blood disorders and anticoagulation use are contraindications for epidural blood patch as well as systemic infections or infection at the site for epidural needle placement. Other complications associated with spinal anesthesia includes nausea, vomiting, spinal hematoma, neurological injury, hypotension and low-frequency hearing loss.

References

[1] Reina MA, Franco CD, López A, Dé Andrés JA, van Zundert A. Clinical implications of epidural fat in the spinal canal. A scanning electron microscopic study. *Acta Anaesthesiol Belg* 2009; 60(1):7-17. PMID: 19459550.

[2] Toledano Roulhac D and Van de Velde Marc. "Chapter 24: Epidural Anesthesia and Analgesia". *Hadzic's Textbook of Regional Anesthesia and Acute Pain Management*, McGraw-Hill Medical, 2017.

[3] Miller RD et al. Miller's Anesthesia, 7th edition, Churchill Livingstone: p 409, 1616-8. 2009.

[4] Crowley LJ, Buggy DJ. Shivering and Neuraxial Anesthesia. *Regional Anesthesia & Pain Medicine* 2008; 33:241-252.

[5] Kathrine Holte, Foss Nicolai B, Svensén Christer, Lund, Madsen Claus Jan L, Kehlet Henrik. Epidural Anesthesia, Hypotension, and Changes in Intravascular Volume. *Anesthesiology* 2004; 100:281-286 doi: https://doi.org/10.1097/00000542-200402000-00016.

[6] Anim-Somuah M, Smyth RM, Jones L. Epidural versus non-epidural or no analgesia in labour. *Cochrane Database Syst Rev* 2011; 12:CD000331. Update 2018.

[7] Sprigge JS, Harper SJ. Accidental dural puncture and post dural puncture headache in obstetric anaesthesia: presentation and management: A 23-year survey in a district general hospital. *Anaesthesia* 2008 Jan; 63(1):36-43. doi: 10.1111/j.1365-2044.2007.05285.x. PMID: 18086069.

[8] Kwak KH. Postdural puncture headache. *Korean J Anesthesiol* 2017; 70(2):136-143. doi:10.4097/kjae.2017.70.2.136.

[9] de Almeida SM, Shumaker SD, LeBlanc SK et al. Incidence of post-dural puncture headache in research volunteers. *Headache* 2011; 51:1503.

Chapter 10

Regional Anesthesia for Truncal Surgery (Thorax + Abdomen)

Fatma Shalan* and Joseph Kennedy, MD
City University of New York School of Medicine, New York, NY, USA

Transversus abdominis plane (TAP) block is an often-used regional anesthetic technique in the perioperative setting for surgeries involving the abdominal wall. With the necessity and growth of multi-modal analgesia methodologies, TAP blocks serve as a useful adjunct in the treatment of somatic incisional pain in the abdominal wall. The block is performed via ultrasound-guided injection of a local anesthetic into the TAP, which anatomically is defined as a plane between the transversus abdominis and internal oblique muscles. The innervation of the anterolateral abdominal wall by the upper and lower TAP plexuses are composed of the thoracoabdominal nerves as well as the ilioinguinal and ilio-hypogastric nerves. Thus, to provide full analgesia for the abdominal wall via the TAP block, several injections are required. Indications for TAP blocks include but are not limited to major abdominal and colorectal surgeries, hernia repairs, Cesarean sections, and other procedures involving the abdominal wall. A major limitation of the TAP block, however, is the lack of analgesia for visceral pain. Other abdominal regional blocks, including the quadratus lumborum block, have the advantage of providing both somatic as well as visceral analgesia whilst also providing analgesia over a larger surface area. However, more literature is needed comparing the different regional blocks modalities to expand their use in the perioperative setting.

* Corresponding Author's Email: fshalan000@citymail.cuny.edu.

In: Postoperative Pain
Editors: Indraneil Mukherjee et al.
ISBN: 978-1-68507-971-0

In this chapter, we go over in more depth the underlying anatomy of the TAP block, as well as the techniques used to perform the procedure. We additionally review the indications, contraindications, limitations, and side effects of the abdominal regional blocks, in addition to reviewing the medications used for these regional techniques. We also examine literature on other related regional anesthetic techniques, including the quadratus lumborum and rectus sheath blocks, in comparison to the TAP block to better understand the role of each regional anesthetic technique in the perioperative setting. Lastly, we discuss the gaps in the literature related to TAP blocks and other regional anesthetic techniques for abdominal surgeries, as well as more recent research and techniques related to these blocks.

TAP Blocks

Anatomy

First described by Dr. Rafi in 2001, the TAP block has become one of, if not the most common truncal anesthesia block used within the perioperative setting (Rafi). The anatomical basis for the block is the potential transversus abdominis plane (TAP), which is a fascial plane superficial to the transversus abdominis muscle, the innermost muscular layer of the anterolateral abdominal wall (Hesham Elsharkawy and Bendtsen 2021). Anteriorly, the transversus abdominis muscle lies posterior to the rectus abdominis muscles and extends to the xiphoid process. Posteriorly, the transversus abdominis forms an aponeurosis with the internal oblique muscle which attaches to the thoracolumbar fascia (TLF). The rectus abdominis, internal oblique, external oblique, and transverses abdominis are the four innervated paired muscles included in the anterolateral abdominal wall.

The anterolateral abdominal wall is innervated by the anterior rami of the spinal nerves T7 to L1, which includes the intercostal nerves (T7-T11), the subcostal nerve (T12) and the ilio-hypogastric and ilioinguinal nerves (L1). The parietal peritoneum, a component of the anterolateral wall, is innervated by somatic and visceral afferent nerves and receives sensitive branches from the lower intercostal nerves as well. (Struller et al. 2017) The branches of anterolateral abdominal wall innervations communicate at multiple locations. One of these communications includes large branch communications on the anterolateral abdominal wall from the intercostal/upper TAP plexus and plexuses that run with the deep circumflex iliac artery DCIA, lower TAP plexus and the deep inferior epigastric artery (DIEA) (rectus sheath plexus) (Rozen et al. 2008). Since these segmental nerves communicate just above the transversus abdominis muscle, the subfascial spread of local anesthetic can provide anterolateral abdominal wall analgesia.

There are several different approaches for guided TAP blocks, such as lateral, posterior, and subcostal approaches. The subcostal approach of a TAP block involves the deposition of local anesthetic in between the transversus abdominis and rectus abdominis, medial to the linea semilunaris which would ideally block T6-T9 (Tsai et al. 2017). The lateral TAP nerve block includes deposition of local anesthetic in the midaxillary line between the thoracic cage and iliac crest as well as between the internal oblique and transversus abdominis muscles and ideally should reach intercostal nerves T10– T11 and the subcostal nerve T12 (Hesham Elsharkawy and Bendtsen 2021). Worthy of remembering is the umbilicus is innervated by T10. Because the L1 segmental nerves are not included in the lateral nerve block an additional anterior TAP nerve medial to the anterior superior iliac spine is required. The posterior approach of TAP consists of depositing local anesthetic in the neurovascular plane between the transverse muscle and the internal oblique muscle in correspondence of Petit's lumbar triangle, anatomic space formed by the margin of the great posterior dorsal, the margin of the external oblique anteriorly, and lower iliac crest (Calixto-Flores and Díaz-Angúlo 2020). The TAP nerve blocks provide somatic analgesia of the abdominal wall and the parietal peritoneum (Hesham Elsharkawy and Bendtsen 2021).

Indications

TAP blocks are mainly indicated for anesthesia and analgesia of the somatic abdominal wall from the pubis to the level of the umbilicus without neuro-axial blockade (Chuan 2014). The Transversus Abdominis Plane (TAP) block provides intraoperative and postoperative analgesia for upper and lower abdominal incisions, where an epidural is contraindicated or considered too invasive for the minor nature of the surgery (Craig 2021b). In the literature, transversus abdominis plane blocks have been used for a multitude of surgical interventions (Tsai et al. 2017). In general, TAP blocks are indicated for abdominal surgeries such as Cesarean delivery, laparoscopic cholecystectomy, hysterectomy, colorectal resection, appendectomy, inguinal hernia repair, prostatectomy, and bariatric surgery (Tran et al. 2019).

Controversy exists in the literature in regard to the spread and level of block achieved with a single TAP injection. Early studies have shown a T7-L1 spread with a single posterior injection making the block suitable for midline abdominal incisions (McDonnell and Laffey 2007) other studies however, failed to demonstrate a spread cephalad to T10 making it far more suitable for lower abdominal surgery (Shibata et al. 2007). Bilateral blocks are required for midline incisions. In conclusion, TAP blocks have been proven to be most reliable for providing postoperative analgesia for abdominal incisions below the umbilicus.

Complications/Contraindications

Complications related to TAP blocks are rare. Some complications have been reported in the literature, including: (Mavarez and Ahmed 2021)

- Bowel perforation
- Hematoma
- Liver/Spleen laceration
- Intrahepatic injection
- Intraperitoneal injection of local anesthetic
- Retroperitoneal hematoma due to vascular injury
- Transient femoral nerve blockage
- Local infection
- Intravascular injection
- Local Anesthetic systemic toxicity

Technique

Landmark Approach

In Rafi's classic description of the TAP block, patients were placed supine with abdomen exposed and surface anatomic landmarks were used to determine the needle insertion site within the lumbar triangle of Petit, and a single "pop" sensation served as an endpoint for appropriate needle depth (Rafi 2001). Using surface landmarks, the practitioner must identify the lumbar triangle of Petit, which is bound medially by the external oblique, inferiorly by the iliac crest, and posteriorly by the latissimus dorsi (Young et al. 2012). The next step is to place a blunt-tipped 80-100mm 22G needle inserted perpendicular to the skin with the appreciation of two gives (loss of resistance) or "pop." The needle passes through the fascial extensions of the internal oblique muscle and fascial plane above transversus abdominis and after negative aspiration, 20–30 ml of local anesthetic (LA) is injected for continuous analgesia.

Ultrasound Guidance Approach

Patients are placed supine with abdomen exposed and using a high-frequency linear or curvilinear ultrasound transducer orientated transversely, the practitioner should begin scanning the abdomen between the iliac crest and the lower costal margin at the mid-axillary line (Hebbard 2009). The most superficial layer on ultrasound is skin and subcutaneous fat. The most superficial of the three muscular layers is the external oblique, followed by the internal oblique, and lastly, the transversus abdominis muscle. Posteriorly scanning the internal oblique and transversus abdominis muscles shows the two layers come together to form the thoracolumbar fascia. Scanning medially, the aponeurosis of the three muscle layers can be seen coming together to form the rectus sheath. Below the transversus abdominis muscle lies parietal peritoneum that can be visualized with loops of bowel sliding underneath. Upon identifying the transversus abdominis plane, numb the patient's skin using lidocaine, then penetrate the skin with the block needle using an 80-100 mm 22G blunt needle 2cm medial to probe at 30-degree angle and in-plane technique, making sure to visualize the needle tip on ultrasound throughout its entire trajectory. Upon entering the transversus abdominis plane (TAP) between the internal oblique and the transversus abdominis muscles, the local anesthetic is slowly and incrementally injected, after aspiration is negative for blood. After negative aspiration, inject 20-30cc of local/thread catheter. This spread can be traced superiorly and inferiorly between the internal oblique muscle and transversus abdominis muscle.

Rectus Sheath Block

Anatomy

The rectus sheath block was first described by Schleich in 1899 when it was used to achieve peri-operative relaxation of the anterior abdominal wall (DL 1899). More recently, the rectus sheath block has been used to achieve post-operative analgesia in a variety of clinical settings, including following laparoscopy (Azemati and Khosravi 2005) umbilical hernia repair (Willschke et al. 2006), abdominoplasty (Anwar et al. 2008), upper abdominal and major gynecological surgery (Yentis, Hills-Wright, and Potparic 1999). The rectus abdominis muscle, also known as the "abdominal muscle," is a paired muscle running vertically on each side of the anterior wall of the human abdomen, as well as that of some other mammals. There are two parallel muscles, separated by a midline band of connective tissue called the linea alba. The rectus abdominis muscle is oval shaped and positioned under the superficial fascia of the abdomen. Laterally, the aponeurosis of the external oblique, internal oblique and transversus abdominis muscles split to form two lamellae that surround the muscle anteriorly and posteriorly (forming the rectus sheath), before rejoining again in the midline to insert on the linea alba (Hesham Elsharkawy and Bendtsen 2021).

The anterior abdominal wall has a multiple segmental nerve supply derived from the anterior divisions of the lower thoracic (T7–12) and first lumbar (L1) nerves. These nerves pass between the internal oblique and transversus abdominis muscles in the transversus abdominis plane, where they branch extensively and communicate widely with each other. These nerves pierce the posterior aspect of the rectus sheath where they branch and communicate in the rectus sheath plexus that runs alongside the deep inferior epigastric artery. The 9th, 10th, and 11th intercostal nerves are located in the space between the rectus abdominis muscle and its posterior rectus sheath (Hesham Elsharkawy and Bendtsen 2021). Muscular and cutaneous branches are given off as the nerves enter the muscle and finally terminate in the skin. Deep to the rectus sheath is the pre-peritoneal fat, peritoneum and abdominal contact with the bowel which can be seen sliding under ultrasound. The rectus sheath block aims to bathe the nerves of the rectus sheath plexus in local anesthetic as they pass through the rectus sheath space between the rectus abdominis muscle and the posterior layer of the sheath.

Indications

A rectus sheath block provides intraoperative and postoperative periumbilical analgesia (T9-T11) for mid-line abdominal incisions. Specifically, it may be useful for the following umbilical hernia repair, paraumbilical hernia repair, epigastric hernia repair, pyloromyotomy, laparoscopic surgery, Abdominoplasty and excision of urachal remnants (Craig 2021a). The rectus sheath nerve block is a useful technique for umbilical surgery, particularly in pediatric patients.

Complications/Contraindications

Complications related to rectus sheath blocks are rare. Some complications have been reported in the literature, including: (Craig 2021a)

- Peritoneal puncture
- Perforation of the bowel
- Visceral puncture
- Major vessel puncture
- Mesenteric vessel puncture
- Inferior epigastric vessel puncture
- Retroperitoneal hematoma.

Technique

Landmark Approach

The most widely described approach for a rectus sheath block is a blind technique. Utilizing this technique, the needle passes through the anterior rectus sheath and through the rectus abdominis muscle and the local anesthetic is injected on the posterior wall of the rectus sheath (Yarwood and Berrill 2010).

With the patient lying supine, a point is identified 2–3 cm from midline, slightly cephalad to the umbilicus at the apex of bulge of the rectus abdominis muscle. An 80-100 mm 22G needle, directed at right angles to the skin, is initially passed through the skin until the resistance of the anterior sheath can be felt. A definitive 'pop' should be felt as it passes through. The needle is advanced further until the firm resistance of the posterior rectus sheath is felt and injection of 10–20 cc of local anesthetic is made in 5 ml aliquots. The procedure is repeated on the opposite side of the midline (Yarwood and Berrill 2010).

Ultrasound Guidance Approach

With the patient lying supine, the ultrasound probe is placed in a transverse plane and positioned where there is optimum ultrasonographic visualization of the posterior rectus sheath. Color Doppler can be used to identify the epigastric arteries so that their puncture can be avoided. The needle is inserted in-plane in a medial to lateral orientation, through the subcutaneous tissue, to pierce through the anterior rectus sheath. The needle is further advanced through the body of the muscle until the tip rests on the posterior rectus sheath.

After negative aspiration, 1 to 2 mL of local anesthetic is injected to verify needle tip location. When injection of the local anesthetic appears to be intramuscular, the needle is advanced 1 to 2 mm and its position is checked by injection of another aliquot of local anesthetic. This is repeated until the correct needle position is achieved (Hesham Elsharkawy and Bendtsen 2021). An out of plane technique may be more suitable for obese patients because the needle tip may not be seen throughout the procedure. In this case, administer small boluses (0.5-1cc) as needle is advanced through the internal abdominal muscle to confirm position of needle tip.

Quadratus Lumborum Block(s)

Anatomy

The Quadratus lumborum muscle is a posterior abdominal wall muscle that originates from the posteromedial iliac crest and inserts into the medial border of the twelfth rib and the transverse processes of the first to fourth lumbar vertebrae. The quadratus lumborum and psoas major muscles traverse posterior to the lateral and medial arcuate ligaments of the diaphragm, respectively. The lateral free border of quadratus lumborum is angled from craniomedial to caudolateral. Posterior to the quadratus lumborum muscle lies the erector spinae muscle group, consisting of the multifidus, longissimus, and iliocostalis (Hesham Elsharkawy, El-Boghdadly, and Barrington 2019).

The thoracolumbar fascia surrounds the quadratus lumborum muscle by a fibrous composite of aponeurotic tissue. The thoracolumbar fascia is part of a myofascial girdle that surrounds the lower torso and is important for posture, load transfer, and stabilization of the lumbar spine. (Hesham Elsharkawy, El-Boghdadly, and Barrington 2019) The two-layered model incorporates a posterior layer surrounding the erector spinae muscles and an anterior layer lying between the erector spinae and the quadratus lumborum muscles (Willard et al. 2012). In the three-layered model, the posterior thoracolumbar fascia layer surrounds the erector spinae muscles, the middle layer passes between the erector spinae muscles and quadratus lumborum, and the anterior layer lies anterior to both quadratus lumborum and psoas muscles. The three-layered model is more commonly used. Regardless of which model is accepted, the fascial planes in the abdominal compartment follow the quadratus lumborum and psoas muscles through the medial and lateral arcuate ligaments and the aortic hiatus of the diaphragm, forming the endothoracic fascia (Hesham Elsharkawy, El-Boghdadly, and Barrington 2019). This provides a potential pathway for spread of injectate, such as local anesthetic, from the abdominal to the thoracic cavity and paravertebral space, thereby achieving clinical effect (Saito et al. 1999; M. K. Karmakar, Gin, and Ho 2001; Dam et al. 2017) the lumbar inter-fascial triangle, situated along the lateral border of the paraspinal muscles from the twelfth rib to the iliac crest, provides a theoretical pathway for injectate spread deep to the thoracolumbar fascia (Hesham Elsharkawy, El-Boghdadly, and Barrington 2019).

Indications

Most of the indications for QL nerve blocks are based on case reports and clinical anecdotal experience. QLB1 and QLB2 indicate different injection areas for quadratus lumborum blocks. QLB1 anesthetic injections are indicated for abdominal surgeries below the umbilicus. QLB2 anesthetic injections are indicated in abdominal surgeries above or below the umbilicus (any type of operation that requires intra-abdominal visceral pain coverage and abdominal wall incisions as high as T6). Trans-muscular quadratus lumborum blocks have been shown to be effective and are indicated in abdominal surgeries above or below the umbilicus (any type of operation that requires intra-abdominal visceral pain coverage and abdominal wall incisions as high as T6) as well. The various QL nerve blocks share the same indications as of the TAP nerve block. They are indicated in surgeries such as large-bowel resections, open/laparoscopic appendectomies, cholecystectomies, cesarean sections, total abdominal hysterectomies, open prostatectomies, renal transplant surgeries, nephrectomies, abdominoplasties, iliac crest bone grafts, Ileostomies, exploratory laparotomies, and bilateral nerve blocks for midline incisions.

Complications/Contraindications

The QLB has similar contraindications to other fascia plane blocks, such as the transversus abdominis plane block (Hutschenreuter 1977; Young et al. 2012). These absolute contraindications include the following:

- Patient refusal
- True local anesthetic allergy

- Risk of local anesthetic toxicity; in other words, the patient has already received the maximum recommended local anesthesia dose.
- Local infection at the procedure site

Technique

In regard to QL blocks, the lateral decubitus position is preferred over the supine position as it gives more exposure to the neuro-axial structures, stability in handling the ultrasound probe and needle, and offers more patient comfort.

Lateral QL Block

A needle insertion lateral (anterior) to the ultrasound transducer with an anterior-to-posterior needle trajectory. Local anesthetic is deposited at the lateral border of quadratus lumborum muscle after the needle tip penetrates the transversus abdominis aponeurosis (Børglum, Gögenür, and Bendtsen 2016). It is important to note that the posterior TAP block is shown to provide longer analgesia and more extensive spread than lateral TAP block, posterior approach should be the preferred approach in clinical practice (Uppal, Sancheti, and Kalagara 2019).

Posterior QL Block

This can be performed using an in-plane approach using an anterior-to-posterior or posterior-to-anterior trajectory. Local anesthetic is injected on the posterior surface of quadratus lumborum muscle, between the quadratus lumborum and erector spinae muscles (Hesham Elsharkawy, El-Boghdadly, and Barrington 2019). The anesthetic is spread mainly along the middle thoracolumbar fascia intertransverse area.

Anterior QL Block

This can be performed using an in-plane approach as well, with a needle insertion medial to the ultrasound transducer, using a posterior-to-anterior trajectory (Dam et al. 2016). Alternatively an in-plane approach, with an anterior-to-posterior trajectory can be used. A further option is with the subcostal oblique anterior approach; the needle insertion is caudal to the transducer, and the trajectory is in-plane, caudal–lateral to cranial–medial. The point of injection of local anesthetic lies in the tissue plane between the quadratus lumborum and psoas muscles (Dam et al. 2016; Hansen et al. 2016; H. Elsharkawy 2016). The anesthetic is spread to lumbar nerve roots and branches and the thoracic paravertebral space.

Thoracic and Lumbar Paravertebral Blocks

Thoracic Anatomy

Thoracic paravertebral block (TPVB) is the technique of injecting local anesthetic alongside the thoracic vertebra close to where the spinal nerves emerge from the intervertebral foramen. This produces unilateral, segmental, somatic, and sympathetic nerve blockade, which is effective for anesthesia and in treating acute and chronic pain of unilateral origin from the chest and abdomen. The thoracic paravertebral space (TPVS) is a wedge-shaped space containing intercostal nerves, dorsal rami, the sympathetic chain, adipose tissue and intercostal vessels. It is located on either side of the vertebral column. The parietal pleura forms the anterolateral boundary. The base is formed by the vertebral body, intervertebral disc, and the intervertebral foramen with its contents (Manoj K. Karmakar et al. 2020). The apex of the wedge is continuous laterally in conjunction with the intercostal space. The left and right paravertebral spaces at specific levels are in continuity with each other medially via the intervertebral foramen and epidural space and anteriorly via the paravertebral space.

Lumbar Anatomy

The lumbar plexus is formed by the union of the anterior primary rami of L1, L2, and L3 and the greater part of L4 within the substance of the psoas muscle. It also receives a variable contribution from T12 (subcostal nerve) and L5. The lumbar plexus is located in an intramuscular fascial plane or "compartment," also referred to as the psoas compartment, within the posterior one-third of the psoas muscle and is very closely related to the lumbar transverse processes. The larger anterior (fleshy) part of the psoas muscle originates from the anterolateral surface of the vertebral body and the intervertebral disc, while the thinner posterior (accessory) part of the psoas muscle originates from the anterior aspect of the transverse processes. The two parts of the muscle fuse to form the main bulk of the psoas muscle, but close to the vertebral bodies, they are separated by a fascia or space that contains the lumbar nerve root, branches of the lumbar artery, and the ascending lumbar vein. This wedge-shaped space close to the intervertebral foramen is called the lumbar paravertebral space (LPVS). After it exits the intervertebral foramen, the lumbar nerve root enters the LPVS after which, instead of entering the psoas muscle at the same vertebral level, it takes a steep caudal course and enters the psoas compartment at the vertebral level below (Manoj K. Karmakar 2020).

Indications

Thoracic paravertebral block offers several technical and clinical advantages and is indicated for anesthesia and analgesia when the afferent pain input is predominantly unilateral from the chest and abdomen (Manoj K. Karmakar 2001). Anesthesia wise, the surgeries indicated for TPVB are breast surgeries, Herniorrhaphy, and chest wound explorations. In terms of postoperative analgesia (as part of a balanced regimen). TPVB is indicated for thoracotomy, thoracoabdominal esophageal surgery, cholecystectomy, renal surgeries, breast surgery, liver resection, appendicectomy, and minimally invasive cardiac surgery. For chronic pain management it is indicated for benign and malignant neuralgia.

Complications/Contraindications

Infection at the site of needle insertion, empyema, allergy to local anesthetic drugs, and tumor occupying the TPVS are some of the few contraindications (Manoj K. Karmakar 2001). A coagulopathy, bleeding disorder or therapeutic anticoagulation are considered as relative contraindications for TPVB (Richardson and Lönnqvist 1998). One must exercise caution in patients with kyphoscoliosis and patients who have had previous thoracotomy. Chest deformity in the former may predispose to thecal or pleural puncture, whereas obliteration of the TPVS by scar tissue and adhesion of the lung to the chest wall (Thomas, Sanders, and Berrisford 1999) in the latter may predispose to pleural and pulmonary puncture.

The main contraindications for TPVB include:

- Patient refusal
- Hypersensitivity reaction or allergy to local anesthetics
- Coagulopathy or systemic anticoagulation (INR > 1.4 or insufficient time since stopping anticoagulant according to ASRA guidelines)
- Infection at the injection site
- Tumor occupying the region

- Respiratory infection, or persistent pleural enlargement: due to the risks of pneumothorax.
- According to some authors, a deformity of the rib cage may predispose to a pleural or intrathecal puncture.

Technique

Landmark

It is preferable to perform TPVB with the patient in the sitting position because the surface anatomy is better visualized, and patients are often more comfortable. However, when this is not possible or practical, TPVB can also be performed with the patient in the lateral, or prone position. Surface landmarks are identified and marked with a skin marker before block placement. Skin markings are also made 2.5 cm lateral to the midline at the thoracic levels that are to be blocked. A 22-gauge Tuohy needle is recommended for TPVB. Advance the Tuohy until contact is made with the transverse process. This usually occurs within 1.0–1.5 cm from the superior edge of the transverse process. Although a subtle "pop" or "give" may be appreciated as the needle traverses the superior costotransverse process, this should not be entirely relied on. Instead, the depth of the needle placement should be guided by the initial bone contact (skin-transverse process + 1.0–1.5 cm). The loss of resistance technique may be used as an alternative. After negative aspiration (checking for CSF, blood, or air), inject 3-5mL of local anesthetic at each level or place catheter. Typically, a single level will block 3 dermatomes.

Ultrasound Guidance

Out of Plane

The transducer is placed transversally at 8 cm lateral to the midline in the sagittal plane. After identification of the rib and the pleura, the transducer is rotated to an oblique transversal position along the long axis of the rib and tilted until the intercostal muscles are visualized. The Tuohy needle is introduced in-plane at the lateral side of the probe and advanced into the space between the internal and innermost intercostal muscles like described above. This technique technically constitutes an intercostal block and relies on spread of local anesthetic fluid toward the contiguous TPV space medially and from there to adjacent ipsilateral TPV spaces (Krediet et al. 2015). Depression of the pleura with local injection should be visualized if the costotransverse ligament is traversed. The utilization of hydro-dissection would aid in confirming position.

In Plane

The transducer is placed transversally at 8 cm lateral to the midline in the sagittal plane. After identification of the rib and the pleura, the transducer is rotated to an oblique transversal position along the long axis of the rib and tilted until the intercostal muscles are visualized. The needle is introduced in-plane at the lateral side of the probe and advanced into the space between the internal and innermost intercostal muscles. This technique technically constitutes an intercostal block and relies on spread of local anesthetic fluid toward the contiguous TPV space medially and from there to adjacent ipsilateral TPV spaces. The TPVS appears as a hypoechoic triangle bounded by the pleura. The hyperechoic innermost intercostal membrane that is contiguous with the costotransverse ligament medially can be visualized above. The Tuohy needle should be advanced medially into the TPVS. 3-5 mL of local anesthesia is then injected at multiple sites.

Iliohypogastric and Ilioinguinal Nerve Blocks

Anatomy

The ilioinguinal and iliohypogastric nerves form part of the lumbar plexus. The lumbar plexus consists of T12-L4. Both the iliohypogastric (IH) and ilioinguinal (II) nerves arise from L1 and emerge from the upper part of the lateral border of the psoas major muscle. The ilioinguinal nerve is a smaller nerve and courses caudad to the iliohypogastric nerve. The iliohypogastric and ilioinguinal nerve come off of the lumbar plexus and are the two most cephalad branches of the plexus. Both nerves cross obliquely anterior to the quadratus lumborum and iliacus muscles and perforate the transverse abdominis muscle near the anterior part of the iliac crest. In the anterior abdominal trunk, the nerves travel between the transverse abdominis and the internal oblique muscles ("Ilioinguinal/Iliohyprogastric Nerve Block").

Indications

The ilioinguinal-iliohypogastric nerve block provides intraoperative and postoperative analgesia for inguinal surgeries. It may be useful for providing analgesia for inguinal hernia repairs, orchidopexies, Hydrocoele repair and varicocoele surgeries. In addition, it has also been used, in combination with T11 and T12 intercostal nerve blocks, to provide post-operative pain relief after renal transplant (Shoeibi, Babakhani, and Mohammadi 2009). Its use in adult patients undergoing laparotomy via a Pfannenstiel incision did not result in a reduction in pain score, length of hospital stay, or postoperative morphine consumption (SA et al. 2008). The block is also used in chronic pain management for patients with persistent inguinal post-herniorrhaphy pain, however, a recent study concluded that the block was not useful for either the diagnosis or management of this condition (Bischoff et al. 2012).

Complications/Contraindications
Contraindications recorded in the literature include:

- Patient refusal
- Infection
- Patient taking anticoagulant or non-aspirin antiplatelet therapy
- Coagulopathy

Technique
The aim of iliohypogastric and ilioinguinal nerve blocks are to provide local anesthetic spread between the transversus abdominis muscle and the internal oblique muscle lying in between the vicinity of the 2 nerves. This will block the hypogastric region, the inguinal crease, mid-upper thigh, mons pubis, part of labia, root of the penis and the anterior part of the scrotum. It is important to consider there is variation in block in between individuals due to anatomical variations.

Landmark
The classical approach uses a landmark technique which blocks the ilioinguinal and iliohypogastric nerves once they have separated into the different fascial layers. The injection is made at a point 2 cm medial and 2 cm cephalad to the anterior superior iliac spine using a 25 mm 22G needle advanced perpendicular to the skin. After an initial pop sensation as the needle

penetrates the external oblique aponeurosis, around 5 ml of local anaesthetic is injected. The needle is then inserted deeper until a second pop is felt penetrating the internal oblique, to lie between it and the transversus abdominis muscle. A further 5 ml of local anesthetic is injected to block the iliohypogastric nerve (van Schoor et al. 2005). A fan-wise subcutaneous injection of 3–5 ml can be made to block any remaining sensory supply from the intercostals and subcostal nerve (Yarwood and Berrill 2010).

U/S Guidance

The ultrasound probe is placed obliquely on a line joining the anterior superior iliac spine and the umbilicus, immediately superior to the anterior superior iliac spine. Identify both the ilioinguinal and the iliohypogastric nerves as 2 hyperechoic structures 1cm apart in fascial plane between the internal oblique muscle and the transverse abdominal muscle. It may not be possible to accurately identify each nerve exactly on ultrasound; therefore, the most important aspect is to ensure that the needle is in the correct fascial layer. However, using the doppler can help identify the deep circumflex iliac artery that lies adjacent to the iliohypogastric and ilioinguinal nerves in the same plane. Insert a 5-8 cm 22 G needle parallel and advance in medial-to-lateral approach in plane and the ultrasound beam until the tip reaches the fascial plane. After negative aspiration (checking for CSF, blood, or air), inject 3-5 mL of local anesthetic.

References

Anwar, M. U., J. Rawlins, P. Baker, M. Fairbrass, and I. T. Foo. 2008. "Per-operative infiltration of the rectus sheath in abdominoplasty." *Aesthetic Plast Surg* 32 (1): 178. https://doi.org/10.1007/s00266-007-9013-x.

Azemati, S., and M. B. Khosravi. 2005. "An assessment of the value of rectus sheath block for postlaparoscopic pain in gynecologic surgery." *J Minim Invasive Gynecol* 12 (1): 12-5. https://doi.org/10.1016/j.jmig.2004.12.013.

Bischoff, J. M., Z. J. Koscielniak-Nielsen, H. Kehlet, and M. U. Werner. 2012. "Ultrasound-guided ilioinguinal/iliohypogastric nerve blocks for persistent inguinal postherniorrhaphy pain: a randomized, double-blind, placebo-controlled, crossover trial." *Anesth Analg* 114 (6): 1323-9. https://doi.org/10.1213/ANE.0b013e31824d6168.

Børglum, J., I. Gögenür, and T. F. Bendtsen. 2016. "Abdominal wall blocks in adults." *Curr Opin Anaesthesiol* 29 (5): 638-43. https://doi.org/10.1097/aco.0000000000000378.

Calixto-Flores, Arnulfo, and Wladimir Díaz-Angúlo. 2020. "Effectiveness and Safety of Continuous Transverse Abdominal Plane Blocks vs Epidural Analgesia in Donor Nephroureterectomy." *Transplantation proceedings* 52 (4): 1081-1086. https://doi.org/10.1016/j.transproceed.2020.02.004.

Chuan, Alwin. 2014. *Regional anesthesia : a pocked guide*. First edition. ed. New York: Oxford University Press.

Craig, Richard. 2021a. "Rectus Sheath." https://www.euroespa.com/science-education/specialized-sections/espa-pain-committee/us-regional-anaesthesia/truncal-blocks/rectus-sheath/.

---. 2021b. "Transversus Abdominus Plane Block." https://www.euroespa.com/science-education/specialized-sections/espa-pain-committee/us-regional-anaesthesia/truncal-blocks/transversus-abdominus-plane-block/.

Dam, M., C. K. Hansen, J. Børglum, V. Chan, and T. F. Bendtsen. 2016. "A transverse oblique approach to the transmuscular Quadratus Lumborum block." *Anaesthesia* 71 (5): 603-4. https://doi.org/10.1111/anae.13453.

Dam, M., B. Moriggl, C. K. Hansen, R. Hoermann, T. F. Bendtsen, and J. Børglum. 2017. "The Pathway of Injectate Spread With the Transmuscular Quadratus Lumborum Block: A Cadaver Study." *Anesth Analg* 125 (1): 303-312. https://doi.org/10.1213/ane.0000000000001922.

DL, Schleich. 1899. In *schmerzlose operationen*, 240.

Elsharkawy, H. 2016. "Quadratus lumborum block with paramedian sagittal oblique (subcostal) approach." *Anaesthesia* 71 (2): 241-2. https://doi.org/10.1111/anae.13371.

Elsharkawy, Hesham, and Thomas F. Bendtsen. 2021. "Ultrasound-Guided Transversus Abdominis Plane and Quadratus Lumborum Nerve Blocks." NYSORA.

Elsharkawy, Hesham, Kariem El-Boghdadly, and Michael Barrington. 2019. "Quadratus Lumborum Block: Anatomical Concepts, Mechanisms, and Techniques." *Anesthesiology* 130 (2): 322-335. https://doi.org/10.1097/aln.0000000000002524. https://doi.org/10.1097/ALN.0000000000002524.

Hansen, C. K., M. Dam, T. F. Bendtsen, and J. Børglum. 2016. "Ultrasound-Guided Quadratus Lumborum Blocks: Definition of the Clinical Relevant Endpoint of Injection and the Safest Approach." *A A Case Rep* 6 (2): 39. https://doi.org/10.1213/xaa.0000000000000270.

Hebbard, P. D. 2009. "Transversalis fascia plane block, a novel ultrasound-guided abdominal wall nerve block." *Can J Anaesth* 56 (8): 618-20. https://doi.org/10.1007/s12630-009-9110-1.

Hutschenreuter, K. 1977. "[Indications and contraindications of regional anesthesia (author's transl)]." *Langenbecks Arch Chir* 345: 487-92. https://doi.org/10.1007/bf01305525.

"Ilioinguinal/Iliohyprogastric Nerve Block." Accessed 2021. http://www.usra.ca/regional-anesthesia/specific-blocks/trunk/ilioinguinalnerve.php.

Karmakar, M. K., T. Gin, and A. M. Ho. 2001. "Ipsilateral thoraco-lumbar anaesthesia and paravertebral spread after low thoracic paravertebral injection." *Br J Anaesth* 87 (2): 312-6. https://doi.org/10.1093/bja/87.2.312.

Karmakar, Manoj K. 2020. "Lumbar Paravertebral Sonography and Considerations for Ultrasound-Guided Lumbar Plexus Block." NYSORA.

Karmakar, Manoj K., Roy A. Greengrass, Malikah Latmore, and Matthew Levin. 2020. "Thoracic and Lumbar Paravertebral Block - Landmarks and Nerve Stimulator Technique." Accessed 2021. https://www.nysora.com/regional-anesthesia-for-specific-surgical-procedures/abdomen/thoracic-lumbar-paravertebral-block/.

Karmakar, Manoj K. 2001. "Thoracic Paravertebral Block." *Anesthesiology* 95 (3): 771-780. https://doi.org/10.1097/00000542-200109000-00033. https://doi.org/10.1097/00000542-200109000-00033.

Krediet, Annelot C., Nizar Moayeri, Geert-Jan van Geffen, Jörgen Bruhn, Steven Renes, Paul E. Bigeleisen, and Gerbrand J. Groen. 2015. "Different Approaches to Ultrasound-guided Thoracic Paravertebral Block: An Illustrated Review." *Anesthesiology* 123 (2): 459-474. https://doi.org/10.1097/aln.0000000000000747. https://doi.org/10.1097/ALN.0000000000000747.

Mavarez, Ana C., and Andaleeb A. Ahmed. 2021. *Transabdominal Plane Block*. StatPearls Publishing LLC.

McDonnell, J. G., and J. G. Laffey. 2007. "Transversus abdominis plane block." *Anesth Analg* 105 (3): 883. https://doi.org/10.1213/01.ane.0000268542.45107.79.

Rafi, A. N. 2001. "Abdominal field block: a new approach via the lumbar triangle." *Anaesthesia* 56 (10): 1024-6. https://doi.org/10.1046/j.1365-2044.2001.02279-40.x.

Richardson, J., and P. A. Lönnqvist. 1998. "Thoracic paravertebral block." *Br J Anaesth* 81 (2): 230-8. https://doi.org/10.1093/bja/81.2.230.

Rozen, W. M., T. M. Tran, M. W. Ashton, M. J. Barrington, J. J. Ivanusic, and G. I. Taylor. 2008. "Refining the course of the thoracolumbar nerves: a new understanding of the innervation of the anterior abdominal wall." *Clin Anat* 21 (4): 325-33. https://doi.org/10.1002/ca.20621. https://www.ncbi.nlm.nih.gov/pubmed/18428988.

SA, Wehbe, Ghulmiyyah LM, Dominique el-KH, Hosford SL, Ehleben CM, Saltzman SL, and Sillis ES. 2008. "Prospective randomized trial of iliohypogastric-ilioinguinal nerve block on post-operative morphine use after inpatient surgery of the female reproductive tract." *Journal of Negative Results in Biomedicine*.

Saito, T., S. Den, K. Tanuma, Y. Tanuma, E. Carney, and C. Carlsson. 1999. "Anatomical bases for paravertebral anesthetic block: fluid communication between the thoracic and lumbar paravertebral regions." *Surg Radiol Anat* 21 (6): 359-63. https://doi.org/10.1007/bf01631341.

Shibata, Y., Y. Sato, Y. Fujiwara, and T. Komatsu. 2007. "Transversus abdominis plane block." *Anesth Analg* 105 (3): 883; author reply 883. https://doi.org/10.1213/01.ane.0000268541.83265.7d.

Shoeibi, G., B. Babakhani, and S. S. Mohammadi. 2009. "The efficacy of ilioinguinal-iliohypogastric and intercostal nerve co-blockade for postoperative pain relief in kidney recipients." *Anesth Analg* 108 (1): 330-3. https://doi.org/10.1213/ane.0b013e31818c1b13.

Struller, F., F. J. Weinreich, P. Horvath, M. K. Kokkalis, S. Beckert, A. Konigsrainer, and M. A. Reymond. 2017. "Peritoneal innervation: embryology and functional anatomy."

Pleura Peritoneum 2 (4): 153-161. https://doi.org/10.1515/pp-2017-0024. https://www.ncbi.nlm.nih.gov/pubmed/30911646.

Thomas, P. W., D. J. Sanders, and R. G. Berrisford. 1999. "Pulmonary haemorrhage after percutaneous paravertebral block." *Br J Anaesth* 83 (4): 668-9. https://doi.org/10.1093/bja/83.4.668.

Tran, De Q., Daniela Bravo, Prangmalee Leurcharusmee, and Joseph M. Neal. 2019. "Transversus Abdominis Plane Block: A Narrative Review." *Anesthesiology* 131 (5): 1166-1190. https://doi.org/10.1097/ALN.0000000000002842. https://doi.org/10.1097/ALN.0000000000002842.

Tsai, Hsiao-Chien, Takayuki Yoshida, Tai-Yuan Chuang, Sheng-Feng Yang, Chuen-Chau Chang, Han-Yun Yao, Yu-Ting Tai, Jui-An Lin, and Kung-Yen Chen. 2017. "Transversus Abdominis Plane Block: An Updated Review of Anatomy and Techniques." *BioMed research international* 2017: 8284363-12. https://doi.org/10.1155/2017/8284363.

Uppal, Vishal, Sushil Sancheti, and Hari Kalagara. 2019. "Transversus Abdominis Plane (TAP) and Rectus Sheath Blocks: aTechnical Description and Evidence Review." *Current Anesthesiology Reports* 9 (4): 479-487. https://doi.org/10.1007/s40140-019-00351-y. https://doi.org/10.1007/s40140-019-00351-y.

van Schoor, A. N., J. M. Boon, A. T. Bosenberg, P. H. Abrahams, and J. H. Meiring. 2005. "Anatomical considerations of the pediatric ilioinguinal/iliohypogastric nerve block." *Paediatr Anaesth* 15 (5): 371-7. https://doi.org/10.1111/j.1460-9592.2005.01464.x.

Willard, F. H., A. Vleeming, M. D. Schuenke, L. Danneels, and R. Schleip. 2012. "The thoracolumbar fascia: anatomy, function and clinical considerations." *J Anat* 221 (6): 507-36. https://doi.org/10.1111/j.1469-7580.2012.01511.x.

Willschke, H., A. Bösenberg, P. Marhofer, S. Johnston, S. C. Kettner, O. Wanzel, and S. Kapral. 2006. "Ultrasonography-guided rectus sheath block in paediatric anaesthesia--a new approach to an old technique." *Br J Anaesth* 97 (2): 244-9. https://doi.org/10.1093/bja/ael143.

Yarwood, J, and A Berrill. 2010. "Nerve blocks of the anterior abdominal wall." *Continuing Education in Anaesthesia Critical Care & Pain* 10 (6): 182-186. https://doi.org/10.1093/bjaceaccp/mkq035. https://doi.org/10.1093/bjaceaccp/mkq035.

Yentis, S. M., P. Hills-Wright, and O. Potparic. 1999. "Development and evaluation of combined rectus sheath and ilioinguinal blocks for abdominal gynaecological surgery." *Anaesthesia* 54 (5): 475-9. https://doi.org/10.1046/j.1365-2044.1999.00805.x.

Young, Mark J., Andrew W. Gorlin, Vicki E. Modest, and Sadeq A. Quraishi. 2012. "Clinical implications of the transversus abdominis plane block in adults." *Anesthesiology research and practice* 2012: 731645-731645. https://doi.org/10.1155/2012/731645. https://pubmed.ncbi.nlm.nih.gov/22312327. https://www.ncbi.nlm.nih.gov/pmc/articles/PMC3270549/.

Chapter 11

Peripheral Nerve Blocks for Orthopedic Surgeries

Rayna Walburger*, **MD**
Icahn School of Medicine at Mount Sinai, New York, NY, USA

Abstract

Approximately 22.3 million orthopedic surgeries were performed in 2017. Orthopedic surgeries can be performed with general or regional anesthesia or a combination of methods. Providing adequate analgesia is important as one of the measures of patient satisfaction with surgical outcomes is postoperative pain management. Previously, oral opioids were the drug of choice for pain management. However, with the current opioid crisis, the approach to postoperative pain management has shifted toward a multimodal regimen, with regional anesthesia being an important component. This multimodal approach has been shown to be effective in treating postoperative pain.

Orthopedic surgeries encompass a wide range of procedures, in which regional anesthesia can be used to target the motor and sensory nerves to the specific part of the body that is being operated on. Peripheral nerve blocks are used in surgical procedures to anesthetize a cluster of peripheral nerves as either a primary anesthetic or to decrease pain and discomfort after the procedure.

* Corresponding Author's Email: rayna3208@gmail.com.

In: Postoperative Pain
Editors: Indraneil Mukherjee et al.
ISBN: 978-1-68507-971-0

Indications

There are no specific set of guidelines outlining the indications for peripheral nerve blocks. However, they can help avoid the side effects associated with general anesthesia and systemic pain medications. Peripheral nerve blocks can be used in combination with general anesthesia or with sedation if general anesthesia is contraindicated, or not desired. Contraindications to general anesthesia can include patients at risk for respiratory depression, difficult airways, those at high risk for postoperative nausea and vomiting (PONV), and patients who desire to remain conscious or avoid systemic medications such as during pregnancy.

Two of the most common orthopedic surgeries performed are total knee replacement and total hip replacement. One concern with these surgeries is the association with significant postoperative pain and its detrimental effects on the recovery of the patient. Patients with uncontrolled postoperative pain can have prolonged recovery time with reduced mobility and delayed rehabilitation. Multiple studies have found that with the administration of peripheral nerve blocks, patients have reported both better pain control and less opioid consumption when compared with opioids alone. This also results in a decrease in hospital stay, with some procedures being performed in an outpatient setting.

Medications

See chapter "Local Anesthetics" for detailed information on the anesthetics that are used for peripheral nerve blocks.

Technique

The location of the nerve block is determined by the procedure that is being performed and which nerve, nerves, or plexuses would provide the best anesthetic coverage. Once the target is chosen, anatomic landmarks can be used to identify the location along with a technique to provide nerve identification. These include ultrasound guidance or nerve stimulation; however, ultrasound guidance is often the preferred method. Several studies have shown that ultrasound guided nerve blocks result in more effective nerve blocks when compared to nerve stimulation. Direct visualization with the ultrasound aids in identifying the nerve and helps to prevent intraneural injection of the anesthetic, which can result in nerve toxicity or direct trauma to the nerve. The peripheral nerve block can be given as a single injection or continuous infusion via a perineural catheter. The limitation of a single injection is the shorter duration of action, typically between 12-24 hours. This may result in rebound pain after discharge. With the continuous peripheral nerve block, patients are able to obtain pain relief for extended periods of time.

For ultrasound guided nerve blocks, the probe used depends on the depth of the nerve. High frequency probes should be used for more superficial nerves as they provide better quality imaging. Low frequency probes should be used for deeper nerves as they provide better penetration than high frequency probes. In-plane needling allows visualization of the entire length of the needle throughout the procedure. Once the needle tip is in the desired location, aspiration should be performed before injection of anesthetic to confirm the needle is not in an intravascular space. If any resistance is met, injection of the anesthetic should be stopped as the needle tip may be intraneural. For all nerve blocks, sterile technique is used and the area is disinfected.

Upper Extremity Blocks

Common upper extremity blocks include brachial plexus blocks using interscalene, supraclavicular, infraclavicular, and axillary nerve blocks and nerve blocks at the wrist and elbows.

Brachial Plexus Nerve Blocks

The brachial plexus nerve block has several approaches including interscalene, supraclavicular, infraclavicular and axillary. The approach used is determined by several factors including desired anesthesia distribution, limiting factors, and contraindications.

Interscalene brachial plexus blocks provide anesthesia to the shoulder and upper arm. Due to the spread of local anesthetic during injection, the supraclavicular branches of the cervical plexus are also blocked resulting in anesthesia to the skin supplying the acromion and clavicle. Injection of 7-15mL is sufficient to provide analgesia for this block. The patient is placed in a supine or semi-lateral decubitus position with the head turned away from the side that is going to be blocked. Anatomic landmarks that are important to identify include the cricoid cartilage, sternocleidomastoid muscle, clavicle, acromion, and carotid artery. The probe is used to identify the carotid artery and then scanned laterally to identify the anterior and middle scalene muscles with the brachial plexus in between. The needle is inserted in a lateral to medial fashion. During injection, you should observe the brachial plexus being moved away from the needle. A potential complication of interscalene brachial plexus block is phrenic nerve block. If this occurs, patients may have compromised respiratory function. To prevent unwanted phrenic nerve block a smaller volume anesthetic can be used or a more distally performed block can be used as an alternative. Another potential complication is intravascular injection as the neck is a highly vascular area; color doppler can be used to minimize this complication.

Supraclavicular blocks are indicated for surgeries of the arm, elbow, forearm, hand, and may be possible for shoulder surgery. Injection of 20-25mL in the target area would provide analgesia. Anatomic landmarks on ultrasound that are important include the subclavian artery, first rib, and parietal pleura. The first rib and parietal pleura are located just lateral and deep to the subclavian artery. The brachial plexus can be visualized as round, hypoechoic structures immediately posterior and superficial to the artery. The individual trunks of the brachial plexus can be seen at the costoclavicular area where they join together. Patients are often placed in supine position with their heads turned away from the side that will be blocked. The probe is initially placed just above the clavicle at its midpoint with the probe titled caudally. To avoid intravascular injection, color doppler should routinely be used for this block. With proper positioning, injection of the anesthetic results in displacement of the plexus away from the needle. Needle advancement during injection may be required for successful block. Although it has a lower frequency of phrenic nerve block, it remains a potential complication.

Infraclavicular brachial plexus blocks provide anesthesia to the upper limb below the shoulder. They are indicated for arm, elbow, forearm, and hand surgery. To achieve a successful block, 20-30mL of local anesthetic should be injected. The major anatomic landmark on ultrasound is the axillary artery. The patient is placed in a supine position with head tilted away from the side that will be blocked. To improve visualization of the plexus, the patient's arm can be abducted 90° and the elbow flexed. The probe is placed in a parasagittal plane just inferior to the clavicle and medial to the coracoid process to identify the axillary artery, pectoralis major muscle, and the pectoralis minor muscle.

The brachial plexus does not need to be identified on ultrasound; identification of the axillary artery is sufficient. The needle is inserted in-plane toward the posterior aspect of the axillary artery, advancing through the pectoralis major and minor muscles. Injection in a U-shaped pattern around the axillary artery should result in an effective nerve block.

Axillary brachial plexus blocks provide anesthesia to the midarm through the hand making surgery of the elbow, forearm, and hand indications for its use. Local anesthetic injection of 15-20mL should be adequate for the block. The axillary artery is the landmark that will be used to identify the brachial plexus, although the individual nerves are usually identifiable. The patient is placed in supine position with the arm abducted to 90°. The probe is placed in the short axis of the arm. Once the axillary artery is identified, the branches of the brachial plexus should try to be identified, though they are not always visible. The needle is inserted in-plane and carefully advanced to first inject anesthetic posterior to the axillary artery to anesthetize the radial nerve. The needle is then repositioned to anesthetize the median and ulnar nerves. The musculocutaneous nerve should be identified and also anesthetized to complete the block.

Elbow Blocks

The three main nerves that can be blocked at the elbow are the median, ulnar, and radial nerves. Blocks performed at the elbow are used for hand and wrist surgery and may be used to supplement brachial plexus blocks. The patient is placed in supine position for all three of these nerve blocks with arm location differing depending on the target nerve. For median and ulnar nerve blocks, the arm is abducted and for radial nerve block the arm is flexed with the patient's palm resting on the patient's abdomen. In-plane needling is typically used for all three of these blocks. For most adults injection of 4-5mL around each nerve is sufficient to provide a successful block at the elbow.

The distribution of anesthesia for ulnar nerve blockade at the elbow includes sensory blockade to the medial aspect of the hand, fifth digit, and medial aspect of the fourth digit. Blocking the median nerve at the elbow provides anesthesia to the anterolateral aspect of the hand, the first through third digit, and lateral aspect of the fourth digit. For radial nerve blocks, the distribution of anesthesia is to the dorsolateral aspect of the hand including the thumb to the lateral aspect of the fourth digit up to the distal interphalangeal joints.

The lateral aspect of the forearm is innervated by the lateral cutaneous nerve of the forearm, a branch of the musculocutaneous nerve. If lateral wrist surgery is planned, a separate block of this nerve may need to be performed. This can be accomplished by injecting the anesthetic laterally from the biceps tendon to the brachioradialis muscle. The use of a tourniquet on either the arm or forearm requires additional anesthesia with sedation or additional analgesia.

The landmark for a radial nerve block is the biceps tendon. The probe is placed anterolaterally about 3cm from the elbow crease. The radial nerve lies in the fascial plane between the brachioradialis and brachialis muscles. The radial nerve can be traced more proximally and be seen in the spiral groove of the humerus. Although it may be easier to identify at the mid humerus level, injection at the level of the elbow is preferred as it reduces the chances of intravascular injection. If nerve stimulation is used, proper placement of the needle would result in finger or wrist extension.

For a median nerve block the probe is placed in the anterior cubital fossa. The landmark is the brachial artery which can be palpated. The median nerve lies medially to the brachial artery. A medial to lateral approach is preferred as to avoid the artery. If nerve stimulation is used, finger or wrist flexion or hand pronation will occur.

The ulnar nerve has the anatomic landmarks of the ulnar groove which lies in between the medial epicondyle and the olecranon process. The probe is placed posteromedially with the ulnar nerve visualized under the brachial fascia and superficial to the triceps muscle. The ulnar nerve is confined in a small space and caution must be used when injecting the anesthetic. Avoid over-flexing the elbow which would compress the nerve into the fossa. It is also important to limit the injection dose to 5mL.

Wrist Nerve Block

Blocks of the nerves at the wrist are indicated for wrist and finger surgery. Similar to the nerve blocks at the elbow, three separate blocks are required. Wrist nerve blocks provide the desired anesthesia without the immobility that may result from more proximal blocks of the upper extremity. If all three nerves are blocked, the entire hand will be anesthetized except for the distribution of the deep branch of the radial nerve. These nerves are located very superficial in the distal forearm. The patient is placed in supine position for all three nerve blocks. Due to the limited space in the wrist, the nerve blocks are often performed approximately 5-10cm proximal to the wrist.

Injection of 3-4mL of anesthetic is often enough for a successful block at the wrist.

The landmarks used to identify the median nerve are the flexor palmaris longus and the flexor carpi radialis. These tendons are made more prominent by flexing the wrist. The probe is placed at the wrist crease to visualize the median nerve. Several tendons may also be visualized at this level making identification of the median nerve difficult. By moving the probe proximally, the nerve will be better visualized without the tendons in the ultrasound image. Performing this block more proximally in the forearm, results in easier identification of the nerve.

The ulnar nerve lies medially to the ulnar artery making it easily identified on ultrasound. The probe is placed at the wrist and moved medially to visualize the ulnar nerve and artery. They can be traced more proximally to distinguish the ulnar nerve from the flexor carpi ulnaris tendon.

The radial nerve divides into its terminal branches at the wrist, making it difficult to use the ultrasound to identify the nerve. For this reason, the block may be performed at the level of the forearm where the radial nerve is seen lateral to the radial artery and superficial to the radius. Another method may be used that does not require ultrasound. Anesthetic injection around the radial styloid process often results in successful radial nerve blockade.

Lower Extremity Blocks

Common lower extremity blocks include lumbar plexus, femoral, fascia iliaca, sciatic, adductor canal, obturator, popliteal and ankle blocks.

Lumbar Plexus Block

A lumbar plexus block is usually performed using anatomic landmarks and nerve stimulation techniques. Lumbar plexus blocks are difficult to perform and are performed by trained individuals. The difficulty lies in the depth of the nerves, with small movements resulting in the needle tip being in a location that will not result in a successful block. Due to the precision and difficulty of this nerve block, many resort to epidural and spinal blocks. However, ultrasound guided lumbar plexus blocks may aid in successful blocks as it will provide direct visualization of the needle tip.

Lumbar plexus blocks are indicated for a variety of lower extremity surgeries including femoral shaft and neck fractures, knee surgeries, and surgeries of the anterior thigh. Anesthesia of the entire lower extremity would result from blocking five nerves: the femoral, sciatic, obturator, lateral femoral cutaneous, and genitofemoral nerve. The sciatic nerve is not part of the lumbar plexus and provides innervation to the lower leg making a lumbar plexus block alone not adequate for major lower extremity surgery. The lumbar plexus is made up of anterior primary rami of L1-L4 with variable contributions from T12 and L5.

The lumbar plexus lies within the psoas major muscle and is anterior to the transverse processes of the lumbar vertebrae. The locations of the femoral nerve and lateral femoral cutaneous nerves are fairly consistent with the location of the obturator nerve being variable.

The patient is placed in a lateral decubitus position with the "operative leg" up and flexed at the hip and knee. Due to the depth of the lumbar plexus, a low frequency curved probe should be used for better penetration. Anatomic landmarks of the posterior superior iliac spine, iliac crest, lumbar spinous processes, and the intercristal line are identified. The probe can be placed either transverse or sagittal. For a sagittal scan, the probe is placed 4cm medial to the lumbar spinous processes with the orientation marker pointing cranially. For a transverse scan, the probe is positioned 4 cm medial to the lumbar spinous processes along the intercristal line. The orientation marker is directed laterally and the probe is directed medially to produce a transverse oblique view. Three techniques have been described to perform ultrasound guided lumbar plexus block including trident view, paramedian transverse scan, and the shamrock method.

As stated earlier this is a difficult block to perform and has some risks associated with it. Due to the high vascularity of the lumbar paravertebral region, intravascular injections have been described. However, color doppler can help decrease the chance of intravascular injections. Lumbar plexus blocks are more difficult to perform in the elderly, even with ultrasound. On ultrasound, the echo intensity of skeletal muscle is increased in the elderly, which results in imaging appearing whiter. This makes it difficult to delineate structures on ultrasound. It is also difficult to perform in the obese, as imaging is difficult with excess fat.

Lateral Femoral Cutaneous Nerve Block

The lateral cutaneous nerve block provides anesthesia to the anterolateral thigh. Lateral femoral cutaneous nerve blocks may be used for analgesia postoperatively for hip surgery, meralgia paresthetica, and muscle biopsy of the proximal lateral thigh. The actual area that is anesthetized varies from patient to patient as the anatomic course of the nerve varies in each patient. Injection of 5mL for adults should be sufficient to provide adequate analgesia. The patient may be placed in supine or lateral position and sterile technique used. The anatomic landmark used for transducer placement is the anterior superior iliac spine (ASIS). The probe should be placed inferiorly and medially to the ASIS. On ultrasound, the lateral femoral cutaneous nerve should be visualized between the tensor fasciae latae muscle (TFLM) laterally and the sartorius muscle medially. The needle is inserted in-plane, lateral to medial until in the fascial plane between the TFLM and sartorius muscles. The anesthetic should be seen spreading around the lateral femoral cutaneous nerve or in the plane between the TFLM and the sartorius muscle. If nerve stimulation is used, paresthesia over the anterolateral thigh should be felt with nerve stimulation.

Femoral Nerve Block

A femoral nerve block provides anesthesia to the anterior and medial thigh, the knee, medial leg and foot and hip, knee, and ankle joints. Due to this distribution, femoral nerve blocks can be used for surgeries of the femur, patella, quadriceps tendon, and knee or for analgesia for hip fracture. Injection of 10-15mL of anesthetic should provide analgesia.

The patient should be placed in a supine position. The femoral artery is identified by palpation in the femoral crease and the ultrasound used to identify the femoral artery. The femoral nerve should be visible lateral to the femoral artery. If not visible, the probe can be titled cranially and caudally, and pressure can be applied to the probe. However, before injecting the anesthetic pressure should be released as it can obscure the view of veins and can prevent proper spread of the anesthetic in the appropriate planes. Once the femoral nerve is identified, local anesthetic should be injected superficially under the skin, approximately 1cm lateral to the probe, to anesthetize the area prior to inserting the block needle.

The block needle should then be inserted laterally in-plane to the probe, advancing medially until the needle tip is above, below, or lateral to the femoral nerve. The needle tip should either be below the fascia iliaca or between the two fascial layers to ensure success of the nerve block. Once in the desired location, aspirate then inject the local anesthetic. The femoral nerve should be pushed away from the injection site as the anesthetic is injected. If nerve stimulation is used, motor response from the quadriceps muscles should be elicited by needle contact with the femoral nerve.

Fascia Iliaca Nerve Block

A fascia iliaca nerve block can anesthetize both the femoral nerve and lateral femoral cutaneous nerve which both lie beneath the iliacus muscle fascia. The femoral nerve block provides anesthesia to the anterior and medial thigh, the knee, medial leg and foot and hip, knee, and ankle joints. The lateral cutaneous nerve block provides anesthesia to the anterolateral thigh. The extent of the area anesthetized depends on the quantity of anesthetic injected and the distribution of the anesthetic under the fascia iliaca. A fascia iliaca block may be used for surgery of the anterior thigh or knee, or for analgesia for hip or knee procedures. For adult patients 20-40mL of dilute local anesthetic should be used.

The technique is similar to performing a femoral nerve block. The patient is placed in a supine position. The landmark of the femoral artery may be used to aid in placement of the ultrasound probe. The probe is placed in the transverse position in the femoral crease. The identification of the sartorius muscle can be made with lateral movement of the probe. Movement medially will show the iliopsoas muscle with the fascia iliaca above the iliopsoas muscle, femoral nerve and femoral artery. Once the probe is in proper position local anesthetic is injected lateral to the probe. The needle is then inserted in-plane and advanced medially. The needle is then passed through the fascia iliaca. A "pop" can usually be heard indicating the needle has pierced the fascia. Direct visualization with the ultrasound, should show the anesthetic separating the fascia iliaca from the iliopsoas muscle toward the femoral nerve medially and sartorius muscle laterally. If the anesthetic is visualized being injected above the fascia iliaca or within the muscle fibers, repositioning of the needle should be performed.

Obturator Nerve Block

An obturator nerve block provides anesthesia to the medial thigh. However, the adductor muscles are also innervated by the sciatic nerve and the femoral nerve. Due to the multiple nerves that provide innervation to the medial thigh, an obturator nerve block may not result in complete weakness of the adductor muscles. To assess the success of the block, the patient's leg is placed in abduction and the patient is told to adduct the leg against resistance. If the patient has weakness or is unable to adduct the leg, it is considered a successful block. An obturator nerve block can be used for relief of painful adductor muscle contractions, to prevent adduction of the thigh during transurethral bladder surgery, additional analgesia after knee surgery, and may provide postoperative analgesia after hamstring tendon harvest for anterior cruciate ligament reconstruction surgery. Injection of 5-10mL of local anesthetic into both fascial planes or around both nerves should result in a successful block.

The obturator nerve originates from the lumbar plexus from the anterior fibers of L2-L4. The obturator nerve runs medially over the psoas muscle and exits the pelvis by passing through the obturator canal and dividing into the anterior and posterior divisions. The anterior division descends between the adductor longus and adductor brevis and the posterior division descends through the obturator externus muscle and courses anteriorly to the adductor magnus muscle.

The patient is placed in supine position with the thigh adducted and externally rotated. There are two different techniques that can be used to perform this block. The first is an interfascial block where the anesthetic is injected into the interfascial plane and the second is identifying the anterior and posterior branches and injecting anesthetic around the nerves. The transducer is placed medially in the inguinal crease identifying the femoral vein and moving medially to identify the adductor muscles. For the interfascial plane approach, placement of the needle tip between the pectineus and adductor brevis targets the anterior branch and placement of the needle tip between the adductor brevis and adductor magnus targets the posterior division. Correct injection is confirmed by visualizing the separation of the muscle. For the approach identifying the two branches of the nerves, the probe is scanned approximately 3cm distally from the inguinal crease. The anterior branch can be seen between the adductor longus and adductor brevis and the posterior branch can be seen between the adductor brevis and adductor magnus.

Popliteal Sciatic Nerve Block

The popliteal sciatic nerve block provides motor and sensory anesthesia to the leg and foot below the knee, except for the medial leg and foot. This nerve block may be used for foot, ankle, or achilles tendon surgery. The sciatic nerve is formed from the spinal nerves L4 to S3. The sciatic nerve splits into 2 branches in the popliteal fossa, the common peroneal and the tibial nerve. This division is variable in patients and may occur more proximally or distally depending on the anatomic variation in each patient. A successful block should result from injection of 15-20mL of local anesthetic around the sciatic nerve. There is more than one approach when performing the popliteal sciatic nerve block. If the posterior approach is used, the patient is placed in either prone or lateral position. A footrest may be used to decrease muscle tension. If the lateral approach is used, the patient is placed in either supine or lateral position. The patient's foot can be placed on a footrest or the patient's knee flexed with stabilization of the ankle on the bed.

First, the approach being used is chosen and the patient is placed in the correct positioning. The transducer can be placed at the popliteal crease and the popliteal artery identified. The popliteal vein should be seen posterior to the artery. The tibial nerve should be visualized superficial and lateral to the artery and vein. On ultrasound, the biceps femoris can be seen lateral to the popliteal artery and the semitendinosus and semimembranosus muscles medially. The probe should be moved cranially to follow the tibial nerve until it combines with the common peroneal nerve to form the sciatic nerve. At the point where the nerves combine to form the sciatic nerve, the sheath surrounding the sciatic should be identified. Injection of the sheath surrounding the sciatic nerve, called Vloka's sheath, will result in a successful sciatic nerve block.

For the lateral approach, a local anesthetic is injected 2-3cm above the edge of the probe. The needle is inserted in-plane and advanced toward the sciatic nerve. For the posterior approach, the lateral to medial in-plane or out of plane approach can be used. Once the needle tip is in the appropriate location, injection of the anesthetic should result in separation of the common peroneal and tibial nerves within Vloka's sheath. For nerve stimulation, contact of the needle with either branch of the sciatic nerve should result in motor response of either the calf or foot.

Saphenous (Adductor Canal) Nerve Block

A saphenous nerve block provides anesthesia to the medial leg and foot. This block can be used in addition to a sciatic nerve block during ankle surgeries, saphenous vein stripping or harvesting, and analgesia for knee surgery in addition to other pain management modalities. The adductor canal is bordered laterally by the vastus medialis, anteriorly by the sartorius muscle, and medially by the adductor longus. The saphenous nerve lies anterior to the femoral artery. The proximal saphenous nerve block is performed in supine position with the leg abducted and externally rotated for access to the medial thigh. For saphenous nerve block, the artery should be followed distally to where the artery still lies deep to the sartorius muscle, while an adductor canal block is performed more proximally. The patient should be injected with 5-10mL of local anesthetic for a successful block.

The transducer is placed on the anteromedial aspect of the thigh in the distal third of the thigh. After identification of the femoral artery, it is followed distally through the adductor canal where it becomes the popliteal artery. The needle is inserted in-plane lateral to medial, advancing toward the femoral artery. Once the needle tip is visualized anterior to the femoral artery, aspiration should be performed to confirm the needle is not intravascular. If in the correct location, injection of the anesthetic results in spread around the femoral artery. The saphenous nerve does not have a motor supply, allowing for lower concentrations of anesthetic. If a large amount of anesthetic is used, the spread of the local anesthetic to one of the motor branches of the femoral nerve may result and cause a delay in ambulation of the patient.

Ankle Nerve Block

Ankle nerve blocks are used for distal foot and toe surgery. There are five separate nerves to be anesthetized in an ankle nerve block and 3-5mL of local anesthetic should be administered around each nerve for a successful block. Two of the nerves are deep, the tibial and deep peroneal nerves, and three of the nerves are superficial, the superficial peroneal, sural, and saphenous nerves. The saphenous nerve is the only one of the five that is a branch of the femoral nerve and not the sciatic nerve. The patient is placed in supine position for all five blocks, a footrest placed under the calf, and internal or external rotation of the leg depending on the block.

The tibial nerve is the largest of the five. A block of the tibial nerve provides anesthesia over the posterolateral aspect of the leg, the lateral foot, and the sole of the foot. The tibial nerve courses down the leg posterior to the tibia and passes posterior and lateral to the medial malleolus. The probe is placed just proximal to the medial malleolus and the tibial nerve will be posterior to the posterior tibial artery. Several tendons will also be visualized at this location, following the nerve proximally will help in its identification as the tendons will turn into their muscle bellies.

The deep peroneal nerve innervates the triangular area between the first and second toes, the ankle joint, and the extensor muscles of the ankle. It is a branch of the common peroneal nerve and it courses down the anterior compartment of the leg lateral to the anterior tibial artery. As the deep peroneal nerve continues distally it becomes anterior to and then medial to the anterior tibial artery and passes under the extensor retinaculum as it enters the ankle.

A superficial peroneal nerve block provides anesthesia to the dorsum of the foot. It is a branch of the common peroneal nerve that arises at the neck of the fibula and courses down the anterolateral surface of the leg. The superficial peroneal nerve divides into its terminal branches approximately 15cm above the level of the ankle. The probe can be placed 10cm above the lateral malleolus and the branches visualized. Movement of the probe more proximal will show the branches coming together to form the superficial peroneal nerve.

The sural nerve provides sensory innervation to the lateral ankle and foot. It travels midline in the posterior leg anterior to the gastrocnemius muscle and courses toward the lateral malleolus as it approaches the ankle. The small saphenous vein can be used as a landmark as the sural nerve is often close to it.

A saphenous nerve block provides anesthesia to the medial surface of the leg and foot below the knee. It courses down the medial side of the leg alongside the great saphenous vein. Due to its size, it is easier to visualize the nerve more proximal from the ankle using the great saphenous vein as a landmark.

Contraindications

There are several contraindications to using peripheral nerve blocks. Absolute contraindications include allergy to the local anesthetic and patient refusal. However, there are also some instances where peripheral nerve blocks should potentially be avoided or postponed. In the case of an active infection in the area of the injection site, peripheral nerve blocks should be avoided. Caution should also be used in patients with a history of coagulopathy and those currently on antithrombotic agents.

Adverse Effects

There are associated adverse effects of both single and continuous peripheral nerve blocks that should be considered. Some of these adverse effects include vascular puncture and bleeding, nerve damage, and local anesthetic systemic toxicity (LAST). With visualization using an ultrasound, the risk of vascular puncture is decreased. Nerve damage does remain a concern. If resistance is met during administration of anesthetic, the needle should be repositioned as you may be injecting intraneural. The side effects of tingling, pins and needles, and pain with pressure may occur for weeks to months after the surgery. The incidence of nerve damage has been reported to be as high as 8.2%. The signs and symptoms of LAST range from local to systemic effects and are dose dependent. They include metallic taste, tinnitus, perioral numbness, seizures, cardiac arrest and death. However, the use of ultrasound during block performance has been found to decrease the incidence of LAST.

Continuous nerve blocks have several other adverse effects that may occur. These complications include catheter dislodgement, obstruction, fluid leakage at the catheter site, bacterial colonization, and infection. All of these potential complications must be considered and explained to the patient prior to performing.

Conclusion

Peripheral nerve blocks serve as primary anesthetic or adjunct to postoperative pain management regimens. They have shown benefit in decreasing opioid use and increasing recovery time. There are several upper and lower extremity nerve blocks that can be performed depending on the targeted nerve and distribution of desired sensory and motor anesthesia. Despite the benefits, there are also adverse effects that need to be considered before performing the procedure. The most common adverse effect is nerve damage with resultant tingling and pins and needle sensation. Overall, peripheral nerve blocks should be considered before performing orthopedic procedures.

References

Abrahams M. S., Aziz M. F., Fu R. F., Horn J. L. Ultrasound guidance compared with electrical neurostimulation for peripheral nerve block: a systematic review and meta-analysis of randomized controlled trials. *Br J Anaesth.* 2009;102(3):408-417. doi:10.1093/bja/aen384.

Abrahams M. S., Aziz M. F., Fu, R. F., Horn J. L. Ultrasound guidance compared with electrical neurostimulation for peripheral nerve block: a systematic review and meta-analysis of randomized controlled trials. *Br J Anaesth.* 2009;102(3):408-417. doi:10.1093/bja/aen384.

Abrahams, M. S., M. F. Aziz, R. F. Fu, and J. L. Horn. 2009. "Ultrasound Guidance Compared with Electrical Neurostimulation for Peripheral Nerve Block: A Systematic Review and Meta-Analysis of Randomized Controlled Trials." *British Journal of Anaesthesia* 102 (3): 408–17. https://doi.org/10.1093/bja/aen384.

Chan E. Y., Fransen M., Parker D. A., Assam P. N., Chua N. Femoral nerve blocks for acute postoperative pain after knee replacement surgery. *Cochrane Database Syst Rev.* 2014;2014(5):CD009941. Published 2014 May 13. doi:10.1002/14651858.CD009941.pub2.

Chan V. W., Perlas A., McCartney C. J., Brull R., Xu D., Abbas S. Ultrasound guidance improves success rate of axillary brachial plexus block. *Can J Anaesth.* 2007;54(7):176-182. doi:10.1007/BF03022637.

Chan V. W., Perlas A., Rawson R., Odukoya O. Ultrasound-guided supraclavicular brachial plexus block. *Anesth Analg.* 2003;97(5):1514-1517. doi:10.1213/01.ane.0000062519.61520.14.

Chan, Ee Yuee, Marlene Fransen, David A. Parker, Pryseley N. Assam, and Nelson Chua. 2014. "Femoral Nerve Blocks for Acute Postoperative Pain after Knee Replacement Surgery." *Cochrane Database of Systematic Reviews* 2014 (5). https://doi.org/10.1002/14651858.CD009941.pub2.

Chan, Vincent W. S., Anahi Perlas, Colin J. L. McCartney, Richard Brull, Daquan Xu, and Sherif Abbas. 2007. "Ultrasounds Guidance Improves Success Rate of Axillary Brachial Plexus Block." *Canadian Journal of Anesthesia* 54 (3): 176–82. https://doi.org/10.1007/BF03022637.

Chan, Vincent W. S., Anahi Perlas, Regan Rawson, and Olusegun Odukoya. 2003. "Ultrasound-Guided Supraclavicular Brachial Plexus Block." *Anesthesia and Analgesia* 97 (5): 1514–17. https://doi.org/10.1213/01.ANE.0000062519.61520.14.

Danelli G., Fanelli A., Ghisi D., et al. Ultrasound vs nerve stimulation multiple injection technique for posterior popliteal sciatic nerve block. *Anesthesia.* 2009;64(6):638-642. doi:10.1111/j.1365-2044.2009.05915.x.

Danelli, Ghisi, A. Fanelli, D. Ghisi, E. Moschini, M. Rossi, A. Ortu, M. Baciarello, and G. Fanelli. 2009. "Ultrasound vs Nerve Stimulation Multiple Injection Technique for Posterior Popliteal Sciatic Nerve Block." *Anaesthesia* 64 (6): 638–42. https://doi.org/10.1111/j.1365-2044.2009.05915.x.

Garimella V., Cellini C. Postoperative pain control. *Clin Colon Rectal Surg.* 2013;26(3):191-196. doi:10.1055/s-0033-1351138.

Garimella, Veerabhadram, and Christina Cellini. 2013. "Postoperative Pain Control." *Clinics in Colon and Rectal Surgery*. https://doi.org/10.1055/s-0033-1351138.

Liu F. C., Liou J. T., Tsai Y. F., et al. Efficacy of ultrasound-guided axillary brachial plexus block: a comparative study with nerve stimulator-guided method. *Chang Gung Med J*. 2005;28(6):396-402.

Liu, Fu Chao, Jiin Tarng Liou, Yung Fong Tsai, Allen H. Li, Yuan Yi Day, Yu Ling Hui, and Ping Wing Lui. 2005. "Efficacy of Ultrasound-Guided Axillary Brachial Plexus Block: A Comparative Study with Nerve Stimulator-Guided Method." *Chang Gung Medical Journal* 28 (6): 396–402.

Morrison R. S., Dickman E., Hwang U., et al. Regional Nerve Blocks Improve Pain and Functional Outcomes in Hip Fracture: A Randomized Controlled Trial. *J Am Geriatr Soc*. 2016;64(12):2433-2439. doi:10.1111/jgs.14386.

Morrison, R. Sean, Eitan Dickman, Ula Hwang, Saadia Akhtar, Taja Ferguson, Jennifer Huang, Christina L. Jeng, et al. 2016. "Regional Nerve Blocks Improve Pain and Functional Outcomes in Hip Fracture: A Randomized Controlled Trial." *Journal of the American Geriatrics Society* 64 (12): 2433–39. https://doi.org/10.1111/jgs.14386.

Nguyen, James T. 2018. "Post-Operative Pain Control." *Global Reconstructive Surgery* 26 (3): 50–55. https://doi.org/10.1016/B978-0-323-52377-6.00008-2.

Qin Q., Yang D., Xie H., Zhang L., Wang C. Ultrasound guidance improves the success rate of axillary plexus block: a meta-analysis. *Braz J Anesthesiol*. 2016;66(2):115-119. doi:10.1016/j.bjane.2015.01.002.

Qin, Qin, Debao Yang, Hong Xie, Liyuan Zhang, and Chen Wang. 2016. "Ultrasound Guidance Improves the Success Rate of Axillary Plexus Block: A Meta-Analysis." *Brazilian Journal of Anesthesiology (English Edition)*. https://doi.org/10.1016/j.bjane.2015.01.002.

Touray S. T., de Leeuw M. A., Zuurmond W. W., Perez R. S. Psoas compartment block for lower extremity surgery: a meta-analysis. *Br J Anaesth*. 2008;101(6):750-760. doi:10.1093/bja/aen298.

Touray, S. T., M. A. De Leeuw, W. W. A. Zuurmond, and R. S. G. M. Perez. 2008. "Psoas Compartment Block for Lower Extremity Surgery: A Meta-Analysis." *British Journal of Anaesthesia* 101 (6): 750–60. https://doi.org/10.1093/bja/aen298.

Trasolini N. A. The Opioid Crisis and the Orthopedic Surgeon. *The journal of arthroplasty*. 2018;33(11):3379-3382.e1. doi:10.1016/j.arth.2018.07.002.

Trasolini, Nicholas A., Braden M. McKnight, and Lawrence D. Dorr. 2018. "The Opioid Crisis and the Orthopedic Surgeon." *Journal of Arthroplasty* 33 (11): 3379-3382.e1. https://doi.org/10.1016/j.arth.2018.07.002.

Widmer B., Lustig S., Scholes C. J., et al. Incidence and severity of complications due to femoral nerve blocks performed for knee surgery. *Knee*. 2013;20(3):181-185. doi:10.1016/j.knee.2012.11.002.

Widmer, Benjamin, Sébastien Lustig, Corey J. Scholes, Allen Molloy, Sean P. M. Leo, Myles R. J. Coolican, and David A. Parker. 2013. "Incidence and Severity of Complications Due to Femoral Nerve Blocks Performed for Knee Surgery." *Knee* 20 (3): 181–85. https://doi.org/10.1016/j.knee.2012.11.002.

Zhao J., Davis S. P. An integrative review of multimodal pain management on patient recovery after total hip and knee arthroplasty. *Int J Nurs Stud*. 2019;98:94-106.doi:10.1016/j.ijnurstu.2019.06.010.

Zhao, J., and Suja P. Davis. 2019. "An Integrative Review of Multimodal Pain Management on Patient Recovery after Total Hip and Knee Arthroplasty." *International Journal of Nursing Studies* 98: 94–106. https://doi.org/10.1016/j.ijnurstu.2019.06.010.

Chapter 12

Patient-Controlled Anesthesia Pump

Alice Lee*

City University of New York School of Medicine, New York, NY, USA

Abstract

Traditionally, opioids were given as an intramuscular injection as needed. However, this led to inadequate pain relief in many patients after surgery. In 1963, Roe et al. published a study that showed that smaller doses of analgesics given intravenously were more effective at pain control than traditional intramuscular injections [1].

In 1973, Marks et al. published a paper that documented the large proportion of patients with inadequately managed pain with traditional analgesics and exposed the lack of sophistication and misinformation many health care professionals had regarding opioid analgesics [2, 3]. This led to increased interest and research in developing better opioid pharmacologic and finding novel ways of delivery [2].

The true pioneer of the PCA pump can be credited to Sechzer, who, in 1968, published a paper on a study where patients were given analgesia on demand through IV by the nursing staff [4]. Because postoperative pain is cyclical and varies depending on the surgery type and patient characteristics, analgesia on demand is an excellent way to treat postoperative pain.

In 1971, Sechzer delivered pain medication through a machine on a patient demand schedule, achieving pain relief and patient satisfaction at a relatively low drug dosage [5].

The first prototypic PCA pumps were developed by Sechzer, Forest, et al., and Keeri-Szanto [5-7]. The first commercially available PCA

* Corresponding Author's Email: alee003@citymail.cuny.edu.

In: Postoperative Pain
Editors: Indraneil Mukherjee et al.
ISBN: 978-1-68507-971-0

pump was developed by the Welsh National School of Medicine in 1976 [8].

PCA Paradigm

A study done by Austin et al. looked at the relationship between meperidine blood concentrations and pain [9]. Previously, it was believed that the variable response to intramuscular narcotics was due to the unpredictability of blood concentrations resulting from variable absorption [9]. The PCA pump works by administering a pre-determined dose of analgesic through an infusion pump when patients push the demand button. The lowest concentration at which analgesia is achieved is the minimal effective analgesic concentration (MEAC). This concentration varies amongst individuals. Pharmacokinetics did not correlate with the dose required to achieve analgesia, but opioid blood concentration did [9, 10]. In order to have continuous, successful analgesia, an individual's MEAC must be met, and that concentration must be kept continuous without too much variability [11]. Achieving this is impossible with intramuscular injections, whereas with a PCA pump, titration to achieve MEAC followed by having patients self-dose maintains the plasma opioid dose [2].

PCA Modes

The initial loading or breakthrough dose is the first dose given to reach MEAC. The provider, not the patient, does this. The demand dose is the dose given after it is activated by the patient when they push the button to maintain the MEAC. Lockdown interval is the delay after a patient has self-administered their dose to prevent over-dosing. The PCA pump will not administer another dose during this period no matter how many times the patient pushes the button. Depending on the programming or type of PCA pump, there could be a background infusion rate that gives doses of analgesia regardless of whether the patient presses the demand button. Some have a 1-hour or 4-hour limit, limiting the dose given in that timeframe. This is less than the highest dose possible if the patient presses the button at every possible interval. Also, if the patient reaches the maximum dose set by the program, they may need more analgesia to reach MEAC. Those in favor believe this is an additional safety measure, whereas those against it argue that no data suggests increased safety.

Owen et al. hypothesize that patients would continually press, without limit, the demand button until their pain was managed [12]. However, if the dose is too small, patients will become frustrated and stop pressing the button even if the pain is not managed. This leads to poor pain management and frustration on the patient's part. Therefore, each demand dose must be significant enough to provide appreciable pain relief but not be too large in that concentrations are at toxic levels [13]. Also, patients should be coached to increase the frequency of demand dosing.

The lockout period aims to prevent overdosing by administering a dose of analgesia before enough of it has cleared from the blood. The lockout period will depend on the analgesia used. There are many rationales for how long the lockout period should be. One suggests that when the movement of the drug between plasma and brain becomes negative (i.e., the drug is leaving the brain instead of entering the brain), the next dose should be administered [14]. The onset of analgesia varies from ~1 minute for alfentanil to ~6 minutes for morphine, and the durations are between ~2 minutes for alfentanil to ~96 minutes for morphine. Due to the long duration of morphine, it is a good choice for a gradual titration [2].

Indications

Patient-controlled analgesia (PCA) pump allows patients to deliver analgesia at their preferred schedule and dose [15]. Indications for PCA pump include acute or acute over chronic pain and postoperative and labor pain, especially in patients who cannot tolerate oral medications [15]. The use of PCA pumps also decreases the burden on hospital staff as patients are delivering analgesia themselves. Post-surgical patients with indwelling nerve or epidural catheters are ideal for PCA pumps [15]. Patients can titrate and administer medication on their schedule, which allows for better pain control compared to pain management on a nursing schedule [15]. PCA pumps are less cost-effective than traditional dosing, do not affect hospital length of stay, and have a higher opioid consumption; however, there is no significant difference in opioid-related side effects.

Whether PCA is more cost-effective than conventional intramuscular opioid administration is unresolved. Conventional therapy requires more nursing time, but the PCA pump has the cost of equipment [16].

Equipment

The equipment for the PCA pump will differ depending on what route the analgesia is administered [15]. However, all PCA pumps contain a locking device, medication chamber, programming screen, and the patient button [15]. Electronic PCA pumps have settings for both continuous infusion and patient-controlled boluses. The reservoir that holds the medication and the patient-controlled button is designed to prevent access to the drug or program without a key or code. An anti-reflux and anti-siphon valve is added to prevent complications [16].

Complications

Complications of PCA pump can arise from the problems in the mechanism of the procedure or from the analgesia itself [15]. One complication is "run-away" pumps which describe an error in which a dose is delivered at an incorrect dose or interval. Although rare, this requires monitoring patients to prevent overdose[15]. Another complication is a failure of the anti-reflux valve, which is when analgesia flows into the IV fluid infusion line instead of the line meant to go into the patient. When the IV line is flushed, a higher than intended dose can be administered to the patient, causing an overdose [15]. A third complication is if the syringe is damaged or incorrectly placed into the PCA machine. This can lead to all the analgesia in the syringe emptying the patient by gravity, leading to an overdose. This complication can be prevented by cross-clamping the IV line when changing the syringe and keeping the PCA pump at or below the level of the IV catheter in the patient. Some devices have an anti-siphon valve to prevent this complication. A fourth complication is PCA by proxy when someone else pushes the PCA patient button for the patient as they believe the patient is in pain. A fifth complication is PCA machine tampering. To prevent this, health care workers should keep the medications locked, and programming should only be allowed to health care professionals with a code. Also, the devices should be checked regularly for evidence of any tampering [15]. Additional complications are associated with having a peripheral line, central line, or indwelling nerve catheter, including infection, catheter dislodgement, skin irritation, allergic reaction, and nerve damage. Other complications are the side effects of opioid medications:

vomiting, constipation, nausea, urinary retention, pruritus, and respiratory depression [15].

Respiratory depression is the most dangerous complication of opioid use. The risk of respiratory depression can be separated as caused by patient or disease factors and apply to all forms of opioid administration. This includes the side effects of opioid medications mentioned above. The other category can be characterized as PCA-specific errors. This includes accidental bolus administration, inappropriate dose prescription, inappropriate lockout interval, drug errors, inappropriate drug selection, and misconnection of the machinery [2].

Although mishaps with IV-PCA from human error are minor, they can have fatal consequences[17]. A case report by Vicente et al. described a case in which a 19-year-old female who, after undergoing a cesarean section, had a morphine IV-PCA. 1mg/mL was ordered but was unavailable, so the nurse substituted with a 5mg/mL, and the patient was found dead from respiratory depression.

Safety

There is an inherent safety to the PCA pump in those patients who will become too sedated to press and administer more opioids. The idea is that this will occur before severe respiratory depression. However, the use of a basal infusion bypasses this inherent safety feedback. Studies have shown that basal infusions did not lead to better pain control, nor did they increase sleep quality. There is an increased risk of severe respiratory depression, especially in opioid naïve patients, and increased side effects like vomiting and excessive sedation. There is good evidence that there is little risk of respiratory depression with PCA alone and without the basal infusion. Although there are reports of mild desaturation, patients are less likely to severe decompensate when compared with intermittent IM injection of opioids. The recommendation by the Anesthesia Patient Safety Foundation is that patients on PCA pumps should continuously be monitored with a pulse oximeter [18].

Limitations

Patients experience opioid side effects such as nausea, vomiting, pruritus, sedation, and confusion. Although PCA is safe, there have been documented cases of life-threatening mishaps. Also, according to a study by Provenzano et al., PCA is inferior to epidural analgesia and nerve block techniques after significant surgery. Also, in the case of IV-PCA, patients are connected to an IV pole which may impede postoperative mobilization [2, 19]. Children under the age of 5 are not suitable candidates for PCA as using the pump requires a basic understanding.

Initial Dosing and Adjustment

Other pharmacologic agents should be used to reduce the potential for opioid-related side effects. The initial loading dose should be administered every 5-10 minutes until the patient's self-reported pain scale is <4/10 or respiratory rate is <12 breaths/minute.

If the patient does not have adequate analgesia, an increased demand dose should be discussed. If there is still no adequate pain relief after an increased demand dose, a basal infusion should be considered for 4 hours after an increased demand dose.

Basal infusions in opioid-naïve patients should be done cautiously as there is an increased risk of respiratory depression. Once a patient's baseline daily opioid consumption is determined, it should be divided by 24 to calculate the hourly dose.

If a larger demand dose is required to achieve analgesia, there should be a more extended lockout period [2].

Opioid Tolerance and Chronic Pain

In contrast to patients who are opioid naïve, patients with opioid tolerance and chronic pain require a higher opioid dose. Although PCA has been used for acute pain management postoperatively, other therapies such as regional analgesia techniques should be considered.

Psychological Factors

The reason for the success of the PCA pump is that the patients are in control of their pain and pain relief. Many factors such as fear, confusion, or other psychological or cognitive factors may get in the way of patients using the PCA pump correctly [2].

Prior to giving patients the PCA pump, a cognitive assessment must be given to ensure they thoroughly understand the concept of the PCA pump and how it is to be used.

Also, a baseline pain sensation, touch, and motor function should be established. Other variables that must be investigated prior include opioid tolerance, pain assessment, and respiratory assessment.

Multimodal Approach

PCA should not be the only therapy used for pain management postoperatively. It should be used in conjunction with NSAIDs, local wound infiltration, and peripheral nerve blocks, to name a few. NSAIDs have been shown to improve analgesia and decrease the number of opioids needed. Further studies have been done with the addition of various other drugs such as lidocaine and ketamine to see if pain relief and various side effects were improved. Many considerations, including costs and potential for error, should be considered before adding other medications to the PCA pump [2].

Route of Administration

Analgesia can be administered through an intravenous (IV) line, central line, peripheral nerve catheters, or trans-dermally [15]. Any peripheral vein can be used for the IV line. The internal jugular, subclavian, or femoral vein can be used for the central line. The epidural catheter is placed between the dura and ligamentum flavum [15]. Peripheral nerve catheters are placed near a nerve or nerve plexus, and transdermal delivery is placed on the epidermis [15].

Transdermal Delivery

The ideal drug for transdermal delivery should have low molecular weight (<600 Da) and high lipid solubility. This makes fentanyl HCl an ideal opioid as its molecular weight is 372.93Da and is higher lipophilic. Also, fentanyl is more potent than morphine but metabolizes to an inactive metabolite. Iontophoretic technology (ITS) delivers a charge to the fentanyl forcing it out. Positively charged fentanyl has deficient passive transport across the skin but will readily pass through if an electrical potential gradient is applied [2]. The electrical current is activated when the patient presses the button, and the fentanyl then moves into the skin [16]. The fentanyl ITS consists of a drug unit containing the drug and a controller containing the electronics, which must be assembled immediately prior to application. An advantage of the transdermal device compared to other PCA pumps is that it does not require IV lines and tubing, and the pre-programmed system decreases the chances of error [20]. Another advantage is that the delivery system is a small, self-contained unit without a needle allowing greater patient mobility. A disadvantage is that the single, pre-programmed dose cannot be adjusted to add a continuous basal infusion or changed to meet specific patient pain needs [2].

A study done by Chelly et al. gave 205 patients 40 μg of fentanyl over 10-minutes is given transdermally. The results showed that this method was influential in managing acute postoperative pain [21].

Epidural Delivery

After IV-PCA, epidural delivery is the following most common route of delivery. As opposed to the IV-PCA, a continuous infusion should be used [2]. Over administration could lead to motor block or hypotension. If the epidural catheter is displaced, continued self-administration could lead to systemic toxicity [22].

A combination of an opioid and a local anesthetic such as bupivacaine, levobupivacaine, or ropivacaine, should be used to get superior analgesia [2]. The optimal opioid should be lipid-soluble such as fentanyl or sufentanil; however, hydrophilic opioids such as morphic and hydromorphone have been used. The demand dose is most commonly set at 2-4mL with a lockout of 10-20 minutes. 3-10mL/hr is the standard dose for continuous infusions.

Continuous infusion or intermittent bolus epidural analgesia is labor-intensive and requires health care personnel intervention. When compared with the continuous epidural infusions, patient-controlled epidural anesthesia offers superior patient satisfaction and results in a need for fewer interventions by nursing staff [2].

There is a risk of neurologic injury with the use of epidural catheters. The optimal analgesic combination of local anesthetic and opioid needs to be further studied. Fentanyl is preferred over morphine because it is faster acting, and there is a decreased risk of respiratory depression [22].

Peripheral Nerve Catheter PCA

Like epidural delivery, the most used technique is a continuous local anesthetic infusion. However, patient-controlled regional analgesia allows the patient to control the intensity and duration of the pain while minimizing motor and sensory blockade side effects. Pain management by brachial plexus blockade after shoulder or hand surgery has been documented in the literature [23, 24].

After ambulatory surgery to the hand or shoulder, oral NSAIDs and other analgesics safe to take at home may not be adequate for sufficient pain relief. A catheter technique that uses disposable, inexpensive pumps can allow patients to self-administer local anesthetic at home. Common side effects are numbness of fingers, poor arm control, dizziness, and nausea. Technical problems can include the catheter falling out [23]. There is a concern of infection risk with using a catheter at home. Also, adequate patient education is necessary as there is a risk of accidental delivery of all the anesthetic if the patient does not close the clamp. There is a risk of systemic delivery because of the proximity of blood vessels to the brachial sheath. Luckily, even if the entire contents of the balloon, which can be up to 80mL of local anesthetic, enter the systemic system, it is below the safe large doses reported in the literature.

Choice of Opioid

Morphine is the "gold standard" for IV-PCA as it has been the most studied and most commonly used opioid in the United States. Morphine is eliminated by glucuronidation; its active metabolite, morphine-6-glucuronide, is excreted by the kidneys. Patients with impaired renal function have the potential for prolonged side effects and delayed onset of respiratory depression. If serum creatinine is >2.0mg/dL, it is recommended that morphine should be avoided. The liver excretes hydromorphone, which is a good alternative for patients with impaired renal function. It is more potent than morphine, so 0.2mg is considered equivalent to 1.0mg of morphine. It is commonly used at 0.5-1mg/mL and is ideal for opioid-tolerant patients. Fentanyl is 80-100 times more potent than morphine and has a short duration of action. 25-30µg is equivalent to 1mg of morphine. Fentanyl is highly lipophilic, which is the reason for its quicker onset. It can be used in patients with impaired renal function as it is not eliminated renally.

Meperidine traditionally was the 2nd most common opioid used in PCA. It is 1/10th as potent as morphine, so 10mg is equivalent to 1 mg of morphine. However, its use is discouraged as its metabolite normeperidine is neurotoxic and has no analgesic properties. Normeperidine accumulation can cause side effects from anxiety and tremors to seizures. It is also excreted renally. It is contraindicated in patients with renal failure, seizure disorder, or those taking monoamine oxidase inhibitors. The recommended dose is 10mg/kg per day for three days. However, some patients may require a higher dose to achieve MEAC. Sufentanil requires a 4-6µg demand dose, and in contrast to other opioids, a background infusion may be necessary [2].

Pediatric Population

PCA is now regarded as the standard for the delivery of postoperative analgesia in patients over the age of 5 [25]. In a study by Shin et al., patients randomized into the PCA group had significantly lower pain scores than patients in the conventional intramuscular group. Both groups had the exact incidence of side effects. The conclusion was that PCA is safe and effective postoperatively in pediatric patients with significant surgeries such as rib cartilage graft, iliac bone graft, and extensive flap surgeries [26]. The correct dose of opioids should be calculated based on weight and must be programmed into the PCA device.

Pediatric patients should be carefully screened both physically and cognitively. The pediatric patient must have a basic understanding of the principle of the PCA pump and understand that if they feel pain, they should push the button, and there will be pain relief, albeit delayed. Also, the patient should understand that there may not be a complete elimination of pain. At times, the patient's caretakers will decline to have the patient self-administer pain medication but will want to do so themselves. However, this comes with similar risks described above [27]. Parents are also concerned about the addiction potential. The risk of dependence is very low in patients without a preexisting substance abuse history. Also, a history of substance abuse is not a contraindication. All patients should have the appropriate analgesia [27].

Compared to the adult population, the number of adverse events is not well documented, and it is believed that they are grossly underreported. As in the adult population, there is a risk of respiratory depression. Because vital signs are different in the pediatric population, the child's clinical condition must be evaluated prior to and during the analgesia administration [27].

Conclusion

Patient-controlled analgesia (PCA) pumps allow patients to self-control the administration of opioids in response to pain. The indication for the usage of PCA pumps is pain management, which includes acute, chronic, postoperative, and labor management. They are especially useful for patients who cannot tolerate oral intake of medications. Post-surgical patients are ideal candidates, especially those with indwelling nerve or epidural catheters. Multiple studies have shown superior patient satisfaction when compared with traditional intramuscular administration. Although there are complications and risks of severe respiratory depression, adequate patient education, correct machine setup, and clinically checking on the patient should decrease those risks.

References

[1] Roe BB. Are postoperative narcotics necessary? *Archives of Surgery*, 1963. 87(6): p. 912-915.

[2] Grass JA. Patient-controlled analgesia. *Anesthesia and Analgesia*, 2005. 101(5S): p. S44-S61.

[3] Marks RM and Sachar EJ. Undertreatment of medical inpatients with narcotic analgesics. *Annals of internal medicine*, 1973. 78(2): p. 173-181.

[4] Sechzer PH. Objective measurement of pain. in *The Journal of the American Society of Anesthesiologists*, 1968. The American Society of Anesthesiologists.

[5] Sechzer PH. Studies in pain with the analgesic-demand system. *Anesthesia and Analgesia,* 1971. 50(1): p. 1-10.
[6] Forrest Jr WH, Smethurst PW and Kienitz ME. Self-administration of intravenous analgesics. *The Journal of the American Society of Anesthesiologists,* 1970. 33(3): p. 363-364.
[7] Keeri-Szanto M. Apparatus for demand analgesia. *Canadian Anaesthetists' Society Journal,* 1971. 18(5): p. 581-582.
[8] Evans J et al. Apparatus for patient-controlled administration of intravenous narcotics during labour. *The Lancet,* 1976. 307(7949): p. 17-18.
[9] Austin K, Stapleton J and Mather L. Relationship between blood meperidine concentrations and analgesic response: A preliminary report. in *The Journal of the American Society of Anesthesiologists*, 1980. The American Society of Anesthesiologists.
[10] Tamsen A et al. Patient-controlled analgesic therapy, Part II: Individual analgesic demand and analgesic plasma concentrations of pethidine in postoperative pain. *Clinical Pharmacokinetics*, 1982. 7(2): p. 164-175.
[11] Ferrante FM, Ostheimer GW and Covino BG. *Patient-controlled analgesia*, Vol. 1. 1990: Blackwell scientific publications Boston.
[12] Owen H, Mather L and Rowley K. The development and clinical use of patient-controlled analgesia. *Anaesthesia and Intensive Care,* 1988. 16(4): p. 437-447.
[13] Owen H et al. Variables of patient-controlled analgesia 1. bolus size. *Anaesthesia,* 1989. 44(1): p. 7-10.
[14] Mather L and Owen H. The pharmacology of patient-administered opioids. *Patient-controlled analgesia,* Boston: Blackwell Scientific Publications, 1990: p. 27-50.
[15] Pastino A and Lakra A. *Patient Controlled Analgesia (PCA).* 2019.
[16] Mann C, Ouro-Bang'na F and Eledjam J-J. Patient-controlled analgesia. *Current drug targets,* 2005. 6(7): p. 815-819.
[17] Vicente KJ et al. Programming errors contribute to death from patient-controlled analgesia: Case report and estimate of probability. *Canadian Journal of Anesthesia,* 2003. 50(4): p. 328-332.
[18] Vorenkamp KE and Durieux ME. Patient-controlled analgesia. *Journal of neurosurgery,* 2009. 111(2): p. 340-341.
[19] Provenzano D and Grass J. Is epidural analgesia superior to IV-PCA. *Evidence-based practice of anesthesiology*, Philadelphia: WB Saunders, 2004: p. 441-8.
[20] Fanelli A, Sorella MC and Chelly JE. Iontophoretic transdermal fentanyl for the management of acute perioperative pain in hospitalized patients. *Expert opinion on pharmacotherapy*, 2016. 17(4): p. 571-577.
[21] Chelly JE et al. The safety and efficacy of a fentanyl patient-controlled transdermal system for acute postoperative analgesia: a multicenter, placebo-controlled trial. *Anesthesia and Analgesia*, 2004. 98(2): p. 427-433.
[22] Liu SS, Allen HW and Olsson GL. Patient-controlled epidural analgesia with bupivacaine and fentanyl on hospital wards: Prospective experience with 1,030 surgical patients. *The Journal of the American Society of Anesthesiologists,* 1998. 88(3): p. 688-695.

[23] Rawal N et al. Patient-controlled regional analgesia (PCRA) at home: controlled comparison between bupivacaine and ropivacaine brachial plexus analgesia. *The Journal of the American Society of Anesthesiologists,* 2002. 96(6): p. 1290-1296.

[24] Ilfeld BM, Morey TE and Enneking FK. Continuous infraclavicular brachial plexus block for postoperative pain control at home: A randomized, double-blinded, placebo-controlled study. *The Journal of the American Society of Anesthesiologists,* 2002. 96(6): p. 1297-1304.

[25] McDonald AJ and Cooper MG. Patient-controlled analgesia. *Pediatric drugs,* 2001. 3(4): p. 273-284.

[26] Shin D et al. Postoperative pain management using intravenous patient-controlled analgesia for pediatric patients. *Journal of Craniofacial Surgery,* 2001. 12(2): p. 129-133.

[27] Lehr VT and BeVier P. Patient-controlled analgesia for the pediatric patient. *Orthopaedic Nursing,* 2003. 22(4): p. 298-304.

Chapter 13

Oral Analgesia for Intubated Patients

Fatma Shalan[*] and Joseph Kennedy, MD
City University of New York School of Medicine, New York, NY, USA

Abstract

Pain is a frequent occurrence and an even more difficult ailment to treat in the critically ill patient. Not only is pain a complex pathology, as it is a truly individual experience with many potential sources, but it can also be hard to elucidate in the noncommunicative patient, such as in those who are intubated or obtunded. It is crucial to remember that simply because a patient cannot articulate their pain does not mean that the patient is not experiencing pain. Moreover, pain must be distinguished from two other very frequent pathologies within the critically ill: anxiety and delirium. Improper identification of pain in the critically ill, especially those who are noncommunicative, can ultimately lead to improper therapeutic management of such patients, which, in turn, can lead to poor outcomes for patients. Thus, it is important to have assessment-driven and standardized protocols for the management of pain in such patients. Literature has consistently shown that implementation of pain management algorithms in ICUs not only increases assessment of critically ill patient's pain but also significantly decreased length of stay in the ICU and duration of ventilation. As pain in critically ill patients is frequently both overtreated with opioids as well as undertreated due to lack of standardized protocols and noncommunicative patients, validated assessment and treatment algorithms for pain, delirium and agitation are needed to assure the best possible care in this at-risk population.

---

[*] Corresponding Author's Email: fshalan000@citymail.cuny.edu.

In: Postoperative Pain
Editors: Indraneil Mukherjee et al.
ISBN: 978-1-68507-971-0

In this chapter, we review the epidemiology and background of pain within the critical care settings with a specific focus on noncommunicative patients. Furthermore, we examine standardized approaches to the diagnosis of pain by focusing on the validated behavioral pain scales specifically designed for noncommunicative critically ill patients. Additionally, we review treatment approaches for pain in the critically ill, with a particular focus on application of multi-modal analgesia in this setting. We also explore nonpharmacological therapeutic interventions and what their roles are for the noncommunicative critically ill patient in pain. Lastly, we assess the gaps in the literature on this topic and discuss possible areas for new investigations.

Background

Pain is the most common reason people seek medical care (Fishman 2007). Pain is a vulnerable topic to discuss as a patient. Every pain discomfort is subjective and unique to a patient's experience. The International Association for the Study of Pain's (IASP) definition of pain is "An unpleasant sensory and emotional experience associated with actual or potential tissue damage or described in terms of such damage ("International Association for the Study of Pain (IASP) " 1994). Pain has been proven to be especially a significant problem in critically ill patients who cannot communicate. Since pain is multidimensional and subjective, (van Boekel et al. 2017) the patient's self-report is the gold standard for assessment; however, in ICU's, patient related factors and the patient's condition, including endotracheal intubation, reduced level of consciousness, sedation, and administration of paralyzing drugs can alter verbal communication and make pain assessment difficult (Gélinas 2016). Therefore, moderate to severe pain is a common phenomenon experienced by patients in the Intensive Care Units (ICUs) (K. A. Puntillo et al. 2001). Multiple intrinsic and extrinsic sources contributing to this pain include underlying health conditions or disease, trauma, and routine care procedures (Li, Puntillo, and Miaskowski 2008). As practitioners in healthcare, it is imperative and our responsibly to ease a patients discomforts and pain, especially if they're unable to self-report or communicate their sufferings.

Epidemiology

Different studies have indicated that between 10% and 50% of adult hospitalized critically ill noncommunicative patients experience moderate-to-severe pain, and this has a negative impact on different levels. When critical care nurses were asked to assess pain intensity by using a visual analog scale, 35% to 55% of nurses underrated the patient's pain (Hamill-Ruth and Marohn 1999) In critically ill patients, pain is a significant problem – particularly for patients who are unable to communicate. The exact prevalence of pain among critically ill patients is unknown, but available literature shows that as many as 70% of these patients suffer moderate intensity pain during their stay in the hospital (Gélinas 2016). In one study conducted by Puntillo et al. about 30%-50% of patients in the intensive care units (ICUs) experienced moderate-to-severe pain (K. A. Puntillo 1990). In addition, reports show that more than 75% of critically ill patients receive ineffective analgesia during admission in critical care units as well (Haonga et al. 2011). Untreated pain can result in negative consequences, including multisystem complications and development of chronic disabling pain (Sigakis and Bittner 2015). Besides the physical suffering, acute pain elicits psychological responses such as fear, anxiety, demoralization and feelings of helplessness, fatigue and loss of control (Wells, Pasero, and McCaffery 2008). As a result, pain is one of the major causes of impaired sleep among critically ill patients and contributes to the development of delirium, depression and post-traumatic stress disorder. In some cases, inadequately managed acute pain can also progress to chronic pain syndrome (Dunwoody et al. 2008). Adequate assessment, analgesia and other management practices can assure patients' comfort by removing or reducing all the aforementioned complications (Kizza and Muliira 2015).

Pain Pathophysiology

Critical care practitioners need to have an understanding of pain and pain management because, despite growing evidence of pain and its long-term consequences, there has been little progress in improving the treatment of acute pain in the last 20 years (Correll, Vlassakov, and Kissin 2014). Pain has been shown to be a major stressor in the ICU, and chronic pain is a major sequela of critical illness, as reported by nearly half of the survivors of an ICU episode (Novaes et al. 1999; Battle, Lovett, and Hutchings 2013). Optimal management of pain in critically ill patients requires knowledge of pain physiology and etiology, appropriate assessment tools for different patient populations, and pharmacologic and nonpharmacologic treatment strategies.

Pain and its severity do not necessarily reflect tissue damage or its extent, and tissue damage may occur in the absence of pain (Battle, Lovett, and Hutchings 2013). Most commonly, acute pain is the physiologic and psychological response to nociception. Nociception is the transfer of information from a location of tissue damage to the central nervous system. Nociceptors are primarily nonspecific free endings of afferent nerve fibers that act as sensory receptors specializing in perceiving tissue trauma from chemical, thermal, and mechanical sources (N. and F. 1999). On exposure to a noxious stimulus, a nerve impulse is generated (a process called transduction) and transmitted to the spinal cord and brain from the point of transduction or tissue injury. The signal is then perceived in higher structures, such as the cortical and limbic systems, to be pain. After perception, modulation (the inhibition or facilitation of input from the brain) influences further nociception.

During transduction, tissue damage and breakdown cause the release of inflammatory intracellular mediators such as prostaglandins, substance P, bradykinin, histamine, serotonin, and other cytokines (Millecamps M). This release is responsible for the generation of a nerve impulse and the sensitization of other nociceptors, which increases their excitability. Nerve impulses travel along nerve axons to the dorsal horn of the spinal cord, where they cause the release of excitatory and inhibitory neurotransmitters such as glutamate, aspartate, and g-aminobutyric acid (GABA) and neuropeptides such as substance P and endogenous opioids. Excitatory neurotransmitters and substance P forward the nociceptive impulse to the brain, while the inhibitory neurotransmitters and endogenous opioids are responsible for inhibition of nociceptive transmission. In the setting of peripheral inflammation, there is upregulation of dorsal horn neuronal receptor expression in transmitters of primary sensory or nociceptive neurons as well as a decrease in transmission inhibition, which may facilitate further pain transmission (Woolf and Salter 2000).

Standardized Approaches to Pain Diagnoses in Uncommunicative Critically Ill Patients

Assessment and management of pain in critically ill patients have recently received increased attention (Carroll et al. 1999; K. Puntillo 2003; Erdek and Pronovost 2004). Scientific advances in understanding pain mechanisms, multidimensional methods of pain assessment, and analgesic pharmacology have improved pain management practices. However, pain assessment for critically ill patients, especially for nonverbal patients, continues to present a challenge for clinicians and researchers. Pain experts agree that a patient's self-report of pain intensity is the most valid measure (Hamill-Ruth and Marohn 1999). Unfortunately, most of the existing scales are designed for use with patients who can respond verbally to assessment commands. Consequently, pain management in nonverbal patients, such as elderly patients with cognitive impairment, is often guided by less precise and wholly untested methods.

Thus far, two pain scales comprising behavioral indicators has been validated in the intensive care unit (ICU), the critical care pain observation tool and the behavioral pain scale developed by Payen et al.(Payen et al. 2001) The behavioral pain scale (BPS), is used to assess pain in patients who had undergone thoracic or abdominal surgery or who had been admitted for management of multiple trauma (Aïssaoui et al. 2005). The behavioral pain scale is composed of 3 subscales: facial expression, (Miner and Krauss 2007; Chanques et al. 2006; K. A. Puntillo 1990) movement of the upper limbs, (K. A. Puntillo 1990; Miner and Krauss 2007) and compliance with mechanical ventilation. The BPS reflects objective visible behavior at 1 specific time point, whereas the NRS (Numerical pain rate scale) represents a global impression of pain, including several contextual factors during a longer time period.(Ahlers et al. 2008) Gélinas et al. (Gélinas et al. 2006) developed the Critical Care Pain Observation Tool (range 0–8). Various studies have proved the validity of the BPS. One study in Morocco performed a validation study and showed that the BPS had good psychometric properties when used with critically ill patients. And in particular, the BPS showed a high inter-rater reliability (ICC = 0.95) and a satisfactory internal consistency. The behavioral pain scale has proven to be a reliable tool in the use of ICU's.

The Critical-Care Pain Observation Tool (CPOT), developed in French, has 4 sections, each with different behavioral categories: facial expression, body movements, muscle tension, and compliance with the ventilator for intubated patients or vocalization for extubated patients. Items in each section are scored from 0 to 2, with a possible total score ranging from 0 to 8. The CPOT was developed as follows. Some items and their operational definitions were derived from previously described instruments for pain assessment (Mateo and Krenzischek 1992; Payen et al. 2001; K. A. Puntillo et al. 1997; Ambuel et al. 1992). In addition, pain indicators were described by using findings from a chart review of the medical files of 52 critically ill patients (Gélinas et al. 2004) and from 9 focus groups with 48 critical care nurses and interviews of 12 physicians. In one study, (Gélinas et al. 2006) content validity of the CPOT was established with 4 physicians and 13 critical care nurses. Their findings in total validated the CPOT, which was developed specifically to assess pain in ICU patients, especially in noncommunicative patients. The Currently, the Critical-Care Pain Observation Tool and Behavioral Pain Scale are both considered the gold standard for pain evaluation in non-communicant ICU patients due to their high reliability, ease of use and relatively high sensitivity and specificity.

Treatment Approaches for Pain

Pain management for the critically ill patient in the intensive care unit (ICU) provides physicians with the challenge of maximizing patient comfort while avoiding the risks of over-sedation. Adequate pain control for patients has been a long-standing goal for physicians. However, preventing iatrogenic over-sedation has become increasingly important as we better understand the negative impact it has on patients' experiences and outcomes. Pain control in the critically ill patient is further complicated by the fact that their disease pathologies can be numerous and ever changing with associated effects on multiple organ functions (Park et al. 2001) The constantly evolving and complicated nature of these patients makes balancing analgesia and sedation a dynamic process that is unique for every patient. Titrating sedative and analgesic medications to maximize the patient's tolerance of pain while avoiding excessive sedation can, therefore, be a challenging task for caregivers [2].

Opioids

The primary class of medications utilized for pain control in ICU settings are the opioid-based analgesics (Kohler et al. 2016). Opioids are considered the first-line drug class of choice to treat non-neuropathic pain in critically ill patients, according to The American College of Critical Care Medicine (Barr et al. 2013). Despite the large side-effect profile of opioids, they remain the mainstay of pain control as the most effective modality to treat moderate-to severe pain. Morphine, hydromorphone, fentanyl and remifentanil are the primary opioids used to manage pain in critically ill patients (Payen et al. 2007). Intravenous (iv.) is the most common route of opioid delivery in the ICU. Enteral administration of opioids (and other pain medications) should be limited to those patients with adequate absorptive capacity and motility of the GI tract. Other routes of administration such as intramuscular, subcutaneous and transdermal are discouraged due to unpredictable absorption.

Intravenous opioids, when titrated to similar pain intensity endpoints, are stated to be equally effective, although the level of evidence for this is weak – grade C (Barr et al. 2013). Opioids do vary in regard to their lipid solubility, volume of distribution and metabolism. The choice of opioid is often determined by pharmacokinetics. For example, morphine should be avoided in patients with renal insufficiency due to accumulation of the active metabolite morphine-6-glucuronide which has agonism for both the μ- and δ-opioid receptors. Additionally, morphine-3-glucuronide has been associated with neurotoxicity which manifests clinically as acute delirium, myoclonus, seizures, hallucinations and hyperalgesia. The lipophilic opioid fentanyl has a rapid onset and short duration from redistribution, but with prolonged administration elimination is delayed due to a large volume of distribution. Unfortunately, robust clinical trials comparing various opioids in the ICU setting are lacking. Furthermore, opioids are frequently administered concurrently with sedative-hypnotic agents (called 'cosedation' or 'analgosedation'). Experts do, however, recommend addressing pain and using opioids first, followed by sedatives (Jacobi et al. 2002; Sessler and Varney 2008). Opioid analgesia has unique considerations in the critically ill patient: lack of high-level evidence for clinical decision-making, the inability of many patients to communicate their pain, difficulty in distinguishing adverse drug events from other medical problems and bioavailability concerns.

Nonopioid Analgesia

Acetaminophen is a centrally acting COX inhibitor commonly used as an analgesia adjunct. Multiple meta-analyses have concluded that 24-h consumption of morphine significantly decreases with acetaminophen; however, no significant reduction in pain scores was apparent and, most importantly, the addition of acetaminophen did not significantly decrease the incidence of respiratory depression or sedation (Elia, Lysakowski, and Tramèr 2005; Remy, Marret, and Bonnet 2005; Maund et al. 2011). Studies using both oral and IV forms of acetaminophen were included in the meta-analyses perhaps masking the effect of one form over the other. Memis et al. found that using iv. acetaminophen (4 g/day) in the intubated patient after major surgery significantly decreased meperidine consumption (76.75 ± 18.2 mg vs 198 ± 66.4 mg; $p < 0.01$) and extubation time (64.3 ± 40.6 min vs 204.5 ± 112.7 min; $p < 0.01$), as well as postoperative nausea and sedation scores (one of 20 patients vs eight of 20 patients; $p < 0.05$) (Memis et al. 2010). Given the low side-effect profile of acetaminophen and its potential benefits, particularly in iv. form, it seems reasonable to continue acetaminophen as an adjunct in patients' multi-modal analgesia. Doses of acetaminophen should be decreased (up to 2600–3200 mg/day) and possibly avoided in patients with an acute hepatitis/ hepatic insufficiency or in cases of cachexia due to decreased levels of glutathione (Bertin, Keddad, and Jolivet-Landreau 2004).

NSAIDs and COX-2 inhibitors were also found to significantly decrease 24-h morphine consumption, and better than acetaminophen (mean reduction of 6.34 mg for acetaminophen to 10.92 mg for COX-2 inhibitors) (Maund et al. 2011). Pain intensity reduction was also statistically significant with continuous and multiple-dose regimens of NSAIDs, not single-dose (Elia, Lysakowski, and Tramèr 2005). Although NSAIDs were found to reduce sedation, like acetaminophen, there was no statistically significant difference as compared with placebo. Potential adverse effects of NSAIDs include gastrointestinal bleeding, renal injury, colorectal anastomotic leakage and cardiovascular events (Mathiesen et al. 2014) Nevertheless, if given to the appropriate patient without a major risk of bleeding or underlying renal failure, NSAIDs would be a reasonable analgesic adjunct to help minimize the utilization of other more sedating medications such as opioids.

Neuropathic Agents

Many critically ill patients are inflicted by neuropathy whether inherent (i.e., diabetic neuropathy or radiculopathy) or iatrogenic (ICU neuropathy or medication related). Few studies have looked into neuropathic pain management in the ICU population specifically (Pandey et al. 2005). However, systematic reviews and meta-analysis for the general population are robust and continually revised. Earlier this year, the Special Interest Group on Neuropathic Pain (NeuPSIG) of the IASP updated their Recommendations for Pharmacotherapy of Neuropathic Pain. After considering new treatments, clinical trials and standards of quality evidence assessment, first-line treatment for neuropathic pain now includes gabapentinoids (pregabalin, gabapentin), serotonin-norepinephrine reuptake inhibitors (SNRIs; duloxetine, venlafaxine, milnacipran) and tricyclic antidepressants (TCAs; amitriptyline, imipramine, clomipramine) only (Finnerup et al. 2015). Number needed to treat for 50% pain relief were 7.7 (95% CI: 6.5–9.4) for pregabalin; 7.2 (95% CI: 5.9–9.21) for gabapentin; 6.4 (95% CI: 5.2–8.4) for SNRIs; and 3.6 (95% CI: 3.0–4.4) for amitriptyline; overall all treatments showed a moderate positive effect. Lidocaine patches are no longer a first line treatment due to weak quality evidence, but remain a second-line treatment due to its excellent safety profile (Dworkin et al. 2007). This new update also places strong opioids like oxycodone or morphine as third-line treatments primarily due to their safety profile and risk for abuse and misuse (Finnerup et al. 2015).

Ketamine

Unlike other sedative-analgesic agents, ketamine can provide its effects while maintaining hemodynamic stability via sympathomimetic stimulation and respiratory drive. Ketamine infusions are commonly used for post-operative analgesia, but are increasingly described as useful adjuncts for analgesia in critical illness. Moitra et al. recently published a case series reporting a decrease in morphine equivalents and decreased lethargy with use of a low-dose ketamine (0.5–4 μg/kg/min) infusion in a palliative patient who was previously suffering from over sedation secondary to receiving 30 mg of morphine equivalents per day (Moitra et al. 2016). In a double-blind RCT assessing morphine consumption in surgical ICU patients after major abdominal surgery, the authors also found that a low-dose ketamine (1–2 μg/kg/min) infusion significantly decreased the cumulative consumption of morphine over 48 h compared with placebo, although the side-effect profiles were comparable (Guillou et al. 2003)Recent reviews report that there is Oxford level 2b, GRADE C evidence suggesting that ketamine does not increase ICP but may even lower ICP in certain cases (Zeiler et al. 2014; Wang et al. 2014). Although only limited data exists for the critically ill patients, low-dose ketamine infusions may be a good complement to pure opioid analgesia, given some evidence of opioid-sparing effects. Further research needs to be done to further elucidate its role in analgesia and sedation in the ICU setting; however, in low doses it may have the ability to decrease levels of sedation while contributing to improved pain control in this population (Kohler et al. 2016).

Regional Anesthesia

Regional anesthesia is an excellent alternative to pharmacologic pain management. Bolus and infusion methods of administering regional anesthesia have repeatedly been shown to improve pain scores, decrease opioid use, decrease opioid related side effects (i.e., nausea, sedation, pruritus) and increase patient satisfaction particularly in the perioperative period (Bingham et al. 2012; Chan et al. 2014). However, the usefulness of regional anesthesia in the ICU setting has been less established due to a lack of clinical trials. Moreover, critically ill patients often have underlying medical issues (i.e., coagulopathy, sepsis) or are receiving aggressive treatment (i.e., anticoagulants like heparin or warfarin) that may be contraindications. Unlike postoperative pain management, which focuses on acute pain immediately after surgery, critically ill patients often have subacute or chronic pain issues that require long-standing pain control. Thus, there are several issues to consider before utilizing regional anesthesia on the critically ill patient but, if no contraindications exist, it can be an excellent form of pain management (Kohler et al. 2016).

Non-Pharmacological Therapeutic Interventions

Music Therapy

Music therapy is a non-pharmacologic modality that can be utilized to manage anxiety and stress and is a therapeutic modality provided by a board certified music therapist (Heiderscheit, Chlan, and Donley 2011). In the music therapy process, patient strengths and needs are assessed in order to develop an appropriate plan of care. Patients in a variety of clinical settings receiving music therapy have shown significant decreases in heart rate, systolic and diastolic pressure, respiratory rates and anxiety.(Wong, Lopez-Nahas, and Molassiotis 2001; Almerud and Petersson 2003) Recent research explored the use of music therapy as a means of managing stress for mechanically ventilated patients being weaned from the ventilator. Hunter et al. reported high satisfaction rates for patients and nurses and that music therapy was successful in treating anxiety associated with weaning from mechanical ventilation (Hunter et al. 2010).

Massage Therapy

The effects of massage explored thus far on critically ill patients' sleep were addressed in two studies. In line with findings in patients with breast cancer (Kashani and Kashani 2014) and congestive heart failure (Sable, Sivabalan, and Shetti 2017), massage was found to be effective in improving the quality of sleep in critical illness in one post-test only RCT (Richards 1998)and in one non-randomized pre- and post-test study (Shinde and Anjum 2014). There was no mention of adverse effects in the identified studies. Although no firm conclusions can be drawn because of the large heterogeneity among studies, massage interventions appear to have several positive impacts for critically ill patients that can be observed with small sample sizes, which implies a rather large size of massage effects (Jagan, Park, and Papathanassoglou 2019).

Cold Therapy

Cold application is a non-pharmacological pain-relieving method. It has been utilized for years (Singh and Gopinath 2005; Houston and Jesurum 1999). Regarding the activity of inflammatory enzymes rises with increasing temperatures, ice is believed to help control pain by inducing local anesthesia around the treatment area. Investigators have also shown that it decreases edema, cellular metabolism, and local blood flow (Modabber et al. 2013). The main beneficial effect of cold during recovery is the cold-related vasoconstriction that may limit vessel permeability and thus inflammatory processes, reducing muscle pain (Dykstra et al. 2009). According to various studies cold therapy has been shown to relieve pain in critically ill patients (Mohammadi et al. 2018; Hsieh, Chen, and Lu 2017). However, the literature indicates more research needs to be implicated for critically ill patients in the future.

Conclusion

Largely, pain in the critically ill noncommunicative patient is still a very complex issue that requires appropriate diagnosis, assessment, and management of the pain itself and treating all the underlying co-morbidities as well. Many different factors make it challenging, especially the difficulty in communicating with an ICU patient. However, by looking at the patient as a whole, treating pain early with the multimodal approach, there seems to be some promising results in improving outcomes. It has shown that the improved outcomes in critically ill patients in the perioperative period seen with optimized pain management and ICU can shorten hospital stays, decreased inpatient costs, and limit the use of limited resources (Czernicki et al. 2019).

The latest research has found that the development of standardized mechanisms and protocols to optimize the diagnosis, assessment, and management of pain in the critically ill can provide the best outcomes. The numerical rating scale, critical care pain observation criteria, and behavior pain scale has shown higher reliability to accurately assess pain in the critically ill. Most importantly, preemptive analgesia and the emphasis on early pain control—in the perioperative setting, ICU, and post-discharge—are crucial in minimizing chronic post-discharge pain. Finally, the multimodal approach is still found to be the most effective. This includes pharmacological treatments, regional nerve blocks, as well as alternative methods that are cheap, safe, and easily available. More research needs to be conducted on non-pharmacological techniques as not many studies exist on music therapy, massage therapy and cold therapy. However, all these aspects of analgesia together have shown to help control pain, provide psychological support, and prevent long-term co-morbidities in the critically ill.

References

Ahlers, S. J., L. van Gulik, A. M. van der Veen, H. P. van Dongen, P. Bruins, S. V. Belitser, A. de Boer, D. Tibboel, and C. A. Knibbe. 2008. "Comparison of different pain scoring systems in critically ill patients in a general ICU." *Crit Care* 12 (1): R15. https://doi.org/10.1186/cc6789.

Aïssaoui, Younès, Amine Ali Zeggwagh, Aïcha Zekraoui, Khalid Abidi, and Redouane Abouqal. 2005. "Validation of a Behavioral Pain Scale in Critically Ill, Sedated, and Mechanically Ventilated Patients." *Anesthesia & Analgesia* 101 (5): 1470-1476. https://doi.org/10.1213/01.Ane.0000182331.68722.Ff. https://journals.lww.com/anesthesia-analgesia/Fulltext/2005/11000/Validation_of_a_Behavioral_Pain_Scale_in.37.aspx.

Almerud, S., and K. Petersson. 2003. "Music therapy--a complementary treatment for mechanically ventilated intensive care patients." *Intensive Crit Care Nurs* 19 (1): 21-30. https://doi.org/10.1016/s0964-3397(02)00118-0.

Ambuel, B., K. W. Hamlett, C. M. Marx, and J. L. Blumer. 1992. "Assessing distress in pediatric intensive care environments: the COMFORT scale." *J Pediatr Psychol* 17 (1): 95-109. https://doi.org/10.1093/jpepsy/17.1.95.

Barr, J., G. L. Fraser, K. Puntillo, E. W. Ely, C. Gélinas, J. F. Dasta, J. E. Davidson, J. W. Devlin, J. P. Kress, A. M. Joffe, D. B. Coursin, D. L. Herr, A. Tung, B. R. Robinson, D. K. Fontaine, M. A. Ramsay, R. R. Riker, C. N. Sessler, B. Pun, Y. Skrobik, and R. Jaeschke. 2013. "Clinical practice guidelines for the management of pain, agitation, and delirium in adult patients in the intensive care unit." *Crit Care Med* 41 (1): 263-306. https://doi.org/10.1097/CCM.0b013e3182783b72.

Battle, C. E., S. Lovett, and H. Hutchings. 2013. "Chronic pain in survivors of critical illness: a retrospective analysis of incidence and risk factors." *Crit Care* 17 (3): R101. https://doi.org/10.1186/cc12746.

Bertin, P., K. Keddad, and I. Jolivet-Landreau. 2004. "Acetaminophen as symptomatic treatment of pain from osteoarthritis." *Joint Bone Spine* 71 (4): 266-74. https://doi.org/10.1016/j.jbspin.2003.09.010.

Bingham, A. E., R. Fu, J. L. Horn, and M. S. Abrahams. 2012. "Continuous peripheral nerve block compared with single-injection peripheral nerve block: a systematic review and meta-analysis of randomized controlled trials." *Reg Anesth Pain Med* 37 (6): 583-94. https://doi.org/10.1097/AAP.0b013e31826c351b.

Carroll, K. C., P. J. Atkins, G. R. Herold, C. A. Mlcek, M. Shively, P. Clopton, and D. N. Glaser. 1999. "Pain assessment and management in critically ill postoperative and trauma patients: a multisite study." *Am J Crit Care* 8 (2): 105-17.

Chan, E. Y., M. Fransen, D. A. Parker, P. N. Assam, and N. Chua. 2014. "Femoral nerve blocks for acute postoperative pain after knee replacement surgery." *Cochrane Database Syst Rev* 2014 (5): Cd009941. https://doi.org/10.1002/14651858.CD009941.pub2.

Chanques, G., S. Jaber, E. Barbotte, S. Violet, M. Sebbane, P. F. Perrigault, C. Mann, J. Y. Lefrant, and J. J. Eledjam. 2006. "Impact of systematic evaluation of pain and agitation in an intensive care unit." *Crit Care Med* 34 (6): 1691-9. https://doi.org/10.1097/01.Ccm.0000218416.62457.56.

Correll, D. J., K. V. Vlassakov, and I. Kissin. 2014. "No evidence of real progress in treatment of acute pain, 1993-2012: scientometric analysis." *J Pain Res* 7: 199-210. https://doi.org/10.2147/jpr.S60842.

Czernicki, Michal, Sreekumar Kunnumpurath, William Park, Anamika Kunnumpurath, Gopal Kodumudi, Jing Tao, Vijay Kodumudi, Nalini Vadivelu, and Richard D. Urman. 2019. "Perioperative Pain Management in the Critically Ill Patient." *Current Pain and Headache Reports* 23 (5): 34. https://doi.org/10.1007/s11916-019-0771-3. https://doi.org/10.1007/s11916-019-0771-3.

Dunwoody, C. J., D. A. Krenzischek, C. Pasero, J. P. Rathmell, and R. C. Polomano. 2008. "Assessment, physiological monitoring, and consequences of inadequately treated acute pain." *J Perianesth Nurs* 23 (1 Suppl): S15-27. https://doi.org/10.1016/j.jopan.2007.11.007.

Dworkin, R. H., A. B. O'Connor, M. Backonja, J. T. Farrar, N. B. Finnerup, T. S. Jensen, E. A. Kalso, J. D. Loeser, C. Miaskowski, T. J. Nurmikko, R. K. Portenoy, A. S. C. Rice, B. R. Stacey, R. D. Treede, D. C. Turk, and M. S. Wallace. 2007. "Pharmacologic management of neuropathic pain: evidence-based recommendations." *Pain* 132 (3): 237-251. https://doi.org/10.1016/j.pain.2007.08.033.

Dykstra, J. H., H. M. Hill, M. G. Miller, C. C. Cheatham, T. J. Michael, and R. J. Baker. 2009. "Comparisons of cubed ice, crushed ice, and wetted ice on intramuscular and surface temperature changes." *J Athl Train* 44 (2): 136-41. https://doi.org/10.4085/1062-6050-44.2.136.

Elia, N., C. Lysakowski, and M. R. Tramèr. 2005. "Does multimodal analgesia with acetaminophen, nonsteroidal antiinflammatory drugs, or selective cyclooxygenase-2 inhibitors and patient-controlled analgesia morphine offer advantages over morphine alone? Meta-analyses of randomized trials." *Anesthesiology* 103 (6): 1296-304. https://doi.org/10.1097/00000542-200512000-00025.

Erdek, M. A., and P. J. Pronovost. 2004. "Improving assessment and treatment of pain in the critically ill." *Int J Qual Health Care* 16 (1): 59-64. https://doi.org/10.1093/intqhc/mzh010.

Finnerup, N. B., N. Attal, S. Haroutounian, E. McNicol, R. Baron, R. H. Dworkin, I. Gilron, M. Haanpää, P. Hansson, T. S. Jensen, P. R. Kamerman, K. Lund, A. Moore, S. N. Raja, A. S. Rice, M. Rowbotham, E. Sena, P. Siddall, B. H. Smith, and M. Wallace. 2015. "Pharmacotherapy for neuropathic pain in adults: a systematic review and meta-analysis." *Lancet Neurol* 14 (2): 162-73. https://doi.org/10.1016/s1474-4422(14)70251-0.

Fishman, S. M. 2007. "Recognizing pain management as a human right: a first step." *Anesth Analg* 105 (1): 8-9. https://doi.org/10.1213/01.ane.0000267526.37663.41.

Gélinas, C. 2016. "Pain assessment in the critically ill adult: Recent evidence and new trends." *Intensive Crit Care Nurs* 34: 1-11. https://doi.org/10.1016/j.iccn.2016.03.001.

Gélinas, C., L. Fillion, K. A. Puntillo, C. Viens, and M. Fortier. 2006. "Validation of the critical-care pain observation tool in adult patients." *Am J Crit Care* 15 (4): 420-7.

Gélinas, C., M. Fortier, C. Viens, L. Fillion, and K. Puntillo. 2004. "Pain assessment and management in critically ill intubated patients: a retrospective study." *Am J Crit Care* 13 (2): 126-35.

Guillou, N., M. Tanguy, P. Seguin, B. Branger, J. P. Campion, and Y. Mallédant. 2003. "The effects of small-dose ketamine on morphine consumption in surgical intensive care unit patients after major abdominal surgery." *Anesth Analg* 97 (3): 843-847. https://doi.org/10.1213/01.Ane.0000075837.67275.36.

Hamill-Ruth, R. J., and M. L. Marohn. 1999. "Evaluation of pain in the critically ill patient." *Crit Care Clin* 15 (1): 35-54, v-vi. https://doi.org/10.1016/s0749-0704(05)70038-5.

Haonga, B. T., J. E. Makupa, R. I. Muhina, and K. S. Nungu. 2011. "Pain management among adult patients with fractures of long bones at Muhimbili Orthopaedic Institute in Dar es Salaam, Tanzania." *Tanzan J Health Res* 13 (4): 107-11. https://doi.org/10.4314/thrb.v13i4.56959.

Heiderscheit, A., L. Chlan, and K. Donley. 2011. "Instituting a music listening intervention for critically ill patients receiving mechanical ventilation: Exemplars from two patient cases." *Music Med* 3 (4): 239-246. https://doi.org/10.1177/ 1943862111410981.

Houston, S., and J. Jesurum. 1999. "The quick relaxation technique: effect on pain associated with chest tube removal." *Appl Nurs Res* 12 (4): 196-205. https://doi.org/10.1016/s0897-1897(99)80261-4.

Hsieh, L. Y., Y. R. Chen, and M. C. Lu. 2017. "Efficacy of cold application on pain during chest tube removal: a randomized controlled trial: A CONSORT-compliant article." *Medicine (Baltimore)* 96 (46): e8642. https://doi.org/10.1097/md.00000 00000008642.

Hunter, B. C., R. Oliva, O. J. Sahler, D. Gaisser, D. M. Salipante, and C. H. Arezina. 2010. "Music therapy as an adjunctive treatment in the management of stress for patients being weaned from mechanical ventilation." *J Music Ther* 47 (3): 198-219. https://doi.org/10.1093/jmt/47.3.198.

"International Association for the Study of Pain (IASP)." 1994. *IASP Taxonomy*. Accessed 09/04.

Jacobi, J., G. L. Fraser, D. B. Coursin, R. R. Riker, D. Fontaine, E. T. Wittbrodt, D. B. Chalfin, M. F. Masica, H. S. Bjerke, W. M. Coplin, D. W. Crippen, B. D. Fuchs, R. M. Kelleher, P. E. Marik, S. A. Nasraway, Jr., M. J. Murray, W. T. Peruzzi, and P. D. Lumb. 2002. "Clinical practice guidelines for the sustained use of sedatives and analgesics in the critically ill adult." *Crit Care Med* 30 (1): 119-41. https://doi.org/10.1097/00003246-200201000-00020.

Jagan, Sameera, Tanya Park, and Elizabeth Papathanassoglou. 2019. "Effects of massage on outcomes of adult intensive care unit patients: a systematic review." *Nursing in Critical Care* 24 (6): 414-429. https://doi.org/https://doi.org/10.1111/nicc.12417. https://onlinelibrary.wiley.com/doi/abs/10.1111/nicc.12417.

Kashani, F., and P. Kashani. 2014. "The effect of massage therapy on the quality of sleep in breast cancer patients." *Iran J Nurs Midwifery Res* 19 (2): 113-8.

Kizza, I. B., and J. K. Muliira. 2015. "Nurses' pain assessment practices with critically ill adult patients." *Int Nurs Rev* 62 (4): 573-82. https://doi.org/10.1111/inr.12218.

Kohler, M., F. Chiu, K. M. Gelber, C. A. Webb, and P. D. Weyker. 2016. "Pain management in critically ill patients: a review of multimodal treatment options." *Pain Manag* 6 (6): 591-602. https://doi.org/10.2217/pmt-2016-0002.

Li, D., K. Puntillo, and C. Miaskowski. 2008. "A review of objective pain measures for use with critical care adult patients unable to self-report." *J Pain* 9 (1): 2-10. https://doi.org/10.1016/j.jpain.2007.08.009.

Mateo, O. M., and D. A. Krenzischek. 1992. "A pilot study to assess the relationship between behavioral manifestations and self-report of pain in postanesthesia care unit patients." *J Post Anesth Nurs* 7 (1): 15-21.

Mathiesen, O., J. Wetterslev, V. K. Kontinen, H. C. Pommergaard, L. Nikolajsen, J. Rosenberg, M. S. Hansen, K. Hamunen, J. J. Kjer, and J. B. Dahl. 2014. "Adverse effects of perioperative paracetamol, NSAIDs, glucocorticoids, gabapentinoids and their combinations: a topical review." *Acta Anaesthesiol Scand* 58 (10): 1182-98. https://doi.org/10.1111/aas.12380.

Maund, E., C. McDaid, S. Rice, K. Wright, B. Jenkins, and N. Woolacott. 2011. "Paracetamol and selective and non-selective non-steroidal anti-inflammatory drugs for the reduction in morphine-related side-effects after major surgery: a systematic review." *Br J Anaesth* 106 (3): 292-7. https://doi.org/10.1093/bja/aeq406.

Memis, D., M. T. Inal, G. Kavalci, A. Sezer, and N. Sut. 2010. "Intravenous paracetamol reduced the use of opioids, extubation time, and opioid-related adverse effects after major surgery in intensive care unit." *J Crit Care* 25 (3): 458-62. https://doi.org/10.1016/j.jcrc.2009.12.012.

Millecamps M, Seminowicz DA, Bushnell MC et al. The biopsychology of pain. In: Weiner IB, ed. Handbook of psychology, Vol. 3: behavioral neuroscience. Hoboken, NJ: John Wiley; 2013:240-71.

Miner, J. R., and B. Krauss. 2007. "Procedural sedation and analgesia research: state of the art." *Acad Emerg Med* 14 (2): 170-8. https://doi.org/10.1197/j.aem.2006.10.101.

Modabber, A., M. Rana, A. Ghassemi, M. Gerressen, N. C. Gellrich, F. Hölzle, and M. Rana. 2013. "Three-dimensional evaluation of postoperative swelling in treatment of zygomatic bone fractures using two different cooling therapy methods: a randomized, observer-blind, prospective study." *Trials* 14: 238. https://doi. org/10.1186/1745-6215-14-238.

Mohammadi, N., A. Pooria, S. Yarahmadi, M. J. Tarrahi, H. Najafizadeh, P. Abbasi, and B. Moradi. 2018. "Effects of Cold Application on Chest Tube Removal Pain in Heart Surgery Patients." *Tanaffos* 17 (1): 29-36.

Moitra, V. K., M. K. Patel, D. Darrah, A. Moitra, and H. Wunsch. 2016. "Low-Dose Ketamine in Chronic Critical Illness." *J Intensive Care Med* 31 (3): 216-20. https://doi.org/10.1177/0885066615587868.

N., Garret, and McShane F. 1999. " The Pathophysiology of Pain." *AANA J.*

Novaes, M. A., E. Knobel, A. M. Bork, O. F. Pavão, L. A. Nogueira-Martins, and M. B. Ferraz. 1999. "Stressors in ICU: perception of the patient, relatives and health care team." *Intensive Care Med* 25 (12): 1421-6. https://doi.org/10.1007/s001340051091.

Pandey, C. K., M. Raza, M. Tripathi, D. V. Navkar, A. Kumar, and U. K. Singh. 2005. "The comparative evaluation of gabapentin and carbamazepine for pain management in Guillain-Barré syndrome patients in the intensive care unit." *Anesth Analg* 101 (1): 220-5, table of contents. https://doi.org/10.1213/01.Ane.0000152186.89020.36.

Park, Gilbert, Douglas Coursin, E. Wesley Ely, Michael England, Gilles L. Fraser, Jean Mantz, Sharon McKinley, Michael Ramsay, Jens Scholz, Mervyn Singer, Robert Sladen, Jeffery S. Vender, and Lorie Wild. 2001. "COMMENTARY: Balancing Sedation and Analgesia in the Critically Ill." *Critical Care Clinics* 17 (4): 1015-1027.

https://doi.org/10.1016/S0749-0704(05)70192-5. https://doi.org/10.1016/S07 49-0704(05)70192-5.

Payen, J. F., O. Bru, J. L. Bosson, A. Lagrasta, E. Novel, I. Deschaux, P. Lavagne, and C. Jacquot. 2001. "Assessing pain in critically ill sedated patients by using a behavioral pain scale." *Crit Care Med* 29 (12): 2258-63. https://doi.org/10.1097/00003246-200112000-00004.

Payen, J. F., G. Chanques, J. Mantz, C. Hercule, I. Auriant, J. L. Leguillou, M. Binhas, C. Genty, C. Rolland, and J. L. Bosson. 2007. "Current practices in sedation and analgesia for mechanically ventilated critically ill patients: a prospective multicenter patient-based study." *Anesthesiology* 106 (4): 687-95; quiz 891-2. https://doi.org/10.1097/01.anes.0000264747.09017.da.

Puntillo, K. 2003. "Pain assessment and management in the critically ill: wizardry or science?" *Am J Crit Care* 12 (4): 310-6.

Puntillo, K. A. 1990. "Pain experiences of intensive care unit patients." *Heart Lung* 19 (5 Pt 1): 526-33.

Puntillo, K. A., C. Miaskowski, K. Kehrle, D. Stannard, S. Gleeson, and P. Nye. 1997. "Relationship between behavioral and physiological indicators of pain, critical care patients' self-reports of pain, and opioid administration." *Crit Care Med* 25 (7): 1159-66. https://doi.org/10.1097/00003246-199707000-00017.

Puntillo, K. A., C. White, A. B. Morris, S. T. Perdue, J. Stanik-Hutt, C. L. Thompson, and L. R. Wild. 2001. "Patients' perceptions and responses to procedural pain: results from Thunder Project II." *Am J Crit Care* 10 (4): 238-51.

Remy, C., E. Marret, and F. Bonnet. 2005. "Effects of acetaminophen on morphine side-effects and consumption after major surgery: meta-analysis of randomized controlled trials." *Br J Anaesth* 94 (4): 505-13. https://doi.org/10.1093/bja/aei085.

Richards, K. C. 1998. "Effect of a back massage and relaxation intervention on sleep in critically ill patients." *Am J Crit Care* 7 (4): 288-99.

Sable, A., T. Sivabalan, and A. N. Shetti. 2017. "Effectiveness of Back Massage on Sleep Pattern among Patients with Congestive Cardiac Failure." *Iran J Nurs Midwifery Res* 22 (5): 359-362. https://doi.org/10.4103/ijnmr.IJNMR_142_16.

Sessler, C. N., and K. Varney. 2008. "Patient-focused sedation and analgesia in the ICU." *Chest* 133 (2): 552-65. https://doi.org/10.1378/chest.07-2026.

Shinde, MB, and S Anjum. 2014. "Effectiveness of Slow Back Massage on Quality of Sleep Among ICU Patient's." *International Journal of Science and Research 3*: 292-298.

Sigakis, M. J., and E. A. Bittner. 2015. "Ten Myths and Misconceptions Regarding Pain Management in the ICU." *Crit Care Med* 43 (11): 2468-78. https://doi.org/10.1097/ccm.0000000000001256.

Singh, M., and R. Gopinath. 2005. "Topical analgesia for chest tube removal in cardiac patients." *J Cardiothorac Vasc Anesth* 19 (6): 719-22. https://doi.org/10.1053/j.jvca.2005.07.024.

van Boekel, Regina L. M., Kris C. P. Vissers, Rob van der Sande, Ewald Bronkhorst, Jos G. C. Lerou, and Monique A. H. Steegers. 2017. "Moving beyond pain scores: Multidimensional pain assessment is essential for adequate pain management after surgery." *PLOS ONE* 12 (5): e0177345. https://doi.org/10.1371/journal.pone.0177345. https://doi.org/10.1371/journal.pone.0177345.

Wang, X., X. Ding, Y. Tong, J. Zong, X. Zhao, H. Ren, and Q. Li. 2014. "Ketamine does not increase intracranial pressure compared with opioids: meta-analysis of randomized controlled trials." *J Anesth* 28 (6): 821-7. https://doi.org/10.1007/ s00540-014-1845-3.

Wells, N., C. Pasero, and M. McCaffery. 2008. "*Advances in Patient Safety.*

Improving the Quality of Care Through Pain Assessment and Management." In *Patient Safety and Quality: An Evidence-Based Handbook for Nurses*, edited by R. G. Hughes. Rockville (MD): Agency for Healthcare Research and Quality (US).

Wong, H. L., V. Lopez-Nahas, and A. Molassiotis. 2001. "Effects of music therapy on anxiety in ventilator-dependent patients." *Heart Lung* 30 (5): 376-87. https://doi.org/ 10.1067/mhl.2001.118302.

Woolf, C. J., and M. W. Salter. 2000. "Neuronal plasticity: increasing the gain in pain." *Science* 288 (5472): 1765-9. https://doi.org/10.1126/science.288.5472.1765.

Zeiler, F. A., J. Teitelbaum, M. West, and L. M. Gillman. 2014. "The ketamine effect on ICP in traumatic brain injury." *Neurocrit Care* 21 (1): 163-73. https://doi.org/10. 1007/s12028-013-9950-y.

Chapter 14

Postoperative Pain in Patients Who Are on Chronic Opioids

Alice Lee*

City University of New York School of Medicine, New York, NY, USA

Nearly 25% of patients who present for surgery are current opioid users [1]. Patients on long-term opioids and have developed a tolerance or dependence present a distinct challenge when managing postoperative pain [1]. Opioid tolerance can occur in patients with cancer or other pathologies that cause pain who are prescribed opioids for long-term management of their pain. It can also occur in patients who misuse opioids illicitly or not as intended [2]. Adverse effects due to opioid misuse have led to a 90% increase in the emergency department from 2004 to 2009 [3]. Because there has been an increase in prescription rates and opioid-related fatalities, there is concern that they may be related.

Opioids are a significant component of postoperative analgesia. Although tolerance to side effects of opioids is expected in patients who are chronic opioid users, they are not immune to respiratory depression. In a study by Rapp et al., moderate to severe sedation was seen in 50% of chronic opioid patients and 19% of opioid-naïve patients [4]. Also, postoperative pain scores were higher in patients who use chronic opioids. The narrowing may explain the ratio of analgesia-to-respiratory depression in response to opioids. Therefore, it is essential to note that, although pain scales are significant, changes in opioid dosing based on sedation take precedence [4, 5].

* Corresponding Author's Email: alee003@citymail.cuny.edu.

In: Postoperative Pain
Editors: Indraneil Mukherjee et al.
ISBN: 978-1-68507-971-0

Treating the acute postoperative pain as effectively as possible is the main objective in opioid-tolerant patients so they can be discharged from the hospital and return to the care of the provider who primarily cares for their chronic pain [6].

Tolerance and Opioid-Induced Hyperalgesia

Tolerance occurs when the medication's effect decreases with multiple uses requiring an increase in dosage to achieve the same effect. Tolerance will cause an increase in the effective dose (ED50), whereas opioid-induced hyperalgesia leads to a decrease in response at dose zero [7]. It is also hypothesized that opioid use can lead to opioid-induced hyperalgesia, which would also reduce the analgesic effect. The mechanism in which tolerance and opioid-induced hyperalgesia are complex and multifactorial [8].

If pain relief is not adequate and is thought to be due to opioid-induced hyperalgesia, pain relief may be achieved by reducing the opioid dose. However, other causes should be excluded with a thorough assessment. If pain increases, the initial response should increase the opioid dose until adequate analgesia is reached without adverse effects [9].

Acute Pain Management

In opioid-tolerant patients, pain management is multifactorial and aims to adequately manage postoperative pain, prevent withdrawal symptoms perioperatively, and assist with social and socioeconomic issues. In order to adequately manage these patients, detailed preoperative assessments, which include the plan from admission to appropriate discharge planning, should be completed [2]. A collaborative, interdisciplinary approach should be taken, including all clinicians who are and will be involved in acute care and long-term management [10].

Opioids are the gold-standard treatment for moderate to severe acute pain after operations. Patients on chronic opioids usually require much higher levels of opioids; a study by Rapp et al., averaged an opioid need of three times as much as opioid-naïve patients [4]. Patient-controlled analgesia (PCA) pumps are helpful for patients to self-administer additional opioids and minimize the risk of under-dosing. In opioid- naïve patients, a background infusion is not recommended as there is an increased risk of respiratory depression. On the other hand, in patients who are on chronic opioids, a background infusion that is equivalent to the dose of the long-term opioid may be appropriate [11, 12].

Preoperative Management

It is imperative to identify patients who are opioid-tolerant prior to surgery. It is often overlooked and will only become known when it is difficult to manage postoperatively. A thorough history and important information should be taken to elicit questions about current opioid and non-opioid medications, over-the-counter medications, illicit drugs, and alcohol use. Opioid substitution therapies, including methadone or buprenorphine use, should also be asked. Experience and expectations of pain management, diagnosis, and usual pain scores should also be documented. It is also essential to ask about social support, prognosis, mental health diagnoses, and functional status [2].

Patient preferences and long-term management are important when determining a plan [13]. A nonjudgmental approach and reassurance that adequate analgesia is a priority are important. All regular medications, including opioids and other analgesic medications, should be administered on the day of surgery. Patients who are on methadone or other opioid substitution programs and require admission on the day of surgery may be able to arrange a dose that they can administer themselves prior to the surgery [2].

Intraoperative Management

Patients on chronic opioids should be given intraoperative doses if they have not taken their dose preoperatively or if the procedure is prolonged. Assessment of adequate opioids in patients breathing spontaneously can be titrated to respiratory rate. When trying to reestablish spontaneous ventilation, opioid titration to achieve a respiratory rate of eight to ten breaths per minute is a reasonable guide [2]. There is an increased risk of awareness in opioid-tolerant patients under anesthesia, so careful monitoring is necessary [14]. Care should be taken for patients with transdermal drug delivery systems, as other factors such as warming devices can accelerate the drug release [15].

Postoperative Management

Managing postoperative pain is usually more complex in opioid-tolerant patients as there are other factors to consider. Distinguishing between new acute pain from the operation and existing pain is essential. Postoperative pain scores may be higher and may remain elevated in patients who are opioid dependent [4, 16]. If pain scores increase or remain elevated, other reasons for pain should be considered. As pain scores may be difficult to assess, other measures of pain, such as dynamic measures of pain, should also be assessed. Dynamic measures of pain measure the ability to deep breathe, cough, and ambulate [17]. Other measures of pain can also be quantified using the Functional Activity Score [18]. Misperceptions about patients on chronic opioids and "addicts" can lead to biased assessments and hinder adequate pain management.

There are times that good history cannot be taken; chronic opioid use should be suspected as a triad of elevated pain scores, high opioid use, and low incidence of side effects present postoperatively [4]. Identifying patients on chronic opioids may be complex in cases of urgent admissions, patients' inability to communicate, or in the setting of trauma [19]. Obtaining a history from family, friends, or the patient's primary care physicians can help.

Patients should be monitored for side effects even though tolerance to side effects, including sedation, nausea, and respiratory depression, occurs relatively quickly. However, these patients could have significant opioid-related side effects, especially respiratory depression, if opioid doses are increased above baseline [20]. In a study by Rapp et al., opioid-tolerant patients were less likely to report nausea, vomiting, and pruritis than their opioid-naïve counterparts. However, the incidence of sedation was higher in opioid-tolerant patients [4]. This is thought to be due to more commonly prescribed to opioid-tolerant patients. Combining opioids with CNS depressants such as benzodiazepines and clonidine is associated with CNS depression.

Close monitoring is necessary to ensure that the patient has adequate pain control while ensuring the patient does not have respiratory depression. After the immediate postoperative phase, IV opioids should be converted to oral slow-release medications. Short-acting oral agents may also be necessary [6].

Specific Analgesia

Although tramadol is a good choice for opioid-tolerant patients because it has lower abuse potential, it should be combined with another analgesia as it will not provide sufficient analgesia or prevent opioid withdrawal if taken alone. Non-opioid analgesic agents such as paracetamol, non-selective NSAIDs, and COX-2 selective NSAIDs should be used. Although there is limited data on the use in opioid-tolerant patients, it should be included in the treatment regimen unless there is a contraindication. Regional analgesia may also help decrease the need for additional systemic analgesia, although it will not prevent opioid withdrawal. Ketamine use with opioids has been shown to improve postoperative pain [21]. However, it should be used with caution as there is a higher incidence of side effects. Therefore, it is recommended that a fixed rate of ketamine be administered rather than be included in the PCA opioid solution [12]. Some studies have shown a decreased incidence of nausea and pruritis when naloxone is given with opioids at ultra-low doses, [22]. However, it can increase pain at higher doses, and currently, there is no evidence to support the use of naloxone.

Epidural analgesia can provide excellent pain relief in various surgical procedures. Studies have shown that peripheral nerve blocks are superior to opioid analgesia. It is important to note that even if patients receive epidural analgesia, they should receive supplemental opioids to prevent withdrawal symptoms [5]. An initial dose of 40-50% of baseline should be adequate to avoid symptoms of withdrawal and can be tapered at 10-15% daily as tolerated [23].

Opioid Rotation

Changing or rotating one opioid with another has been widely used and documented for palliative care. This improves analgesia and reduces opioid-related side effects [24, 25]. It is believed that rotating opioids is efficacious because of incomplete opioid cross-tolerance, differing receptor activity, and the presence of active metabolites. Using different opioids postoperatively from one used preoperatively may be helpful in pain management [26]. Because other opioids have additional dosage requirements, bioavailability, and active metabolites, careful conversion must ensure adequate analgesia [27, 28].

Addiction

Patients with opioid addiction add an additional layer of complexity to care because of the stigma permeating care. Patients may have concerns about withdrawal and inadequate pain relief. It is important to have specific strategies to prepare for potentially complex interactions. A respectful approach should be taken and acknowledging that opioid addiction is a complicated disease, responding to particular requests while setting reasonable limits on how much and how often analgesic medication will be prescribed [10].

"Drug-seeking" behavior concerns clinicians, especially when patients need to be treated for pain. The approach should include careful clinical judgment, assessing physiologic causes of pain, acknowledging one's biases and stereotypes, and practicing rational prescribing policies [29]. Patients in recovery or an addiction treatment program may not want to receive opioids as they are concerned about their progress. In cases like those, non-opioid strategies should be optimized, and patients should be given reassurance and follow-up support. It is essential to understand that there is no evidence that the use of opioids to treat acute, postoperative pain increases the relapse rate and that, on the contrary, unrelieved pain may trigger a relapse [30].

Chronic Pain

Chronic pain is multifactorial and has a robust psychosocial component. Patients on antidepressants, anti-anxiety medications, and anti-neuropathic pain should continue their treatment. This may be a challenge as some medications are not available parenterally [10]. Methadone can be used to manage patients with chronic pain, especially if there is a neuropathic component [31]. Sleep problems are common in patients with chronic pain and should be considered when creating a treatment plan. Antidepressants such as tricyclic antidepressants should be used over benzodiazepines as they can lead to tolerance and addiction [32].

Risk of Additional Opioids

In general, prescribing additional opioids to patients who are opioid-tolerant in the acute post-operative setting presents little risk. However, if there is suspicion of risk of misuse or diversion, extra care needs to be taken. In the USA, more than 50% of nonmedical users of opioids or other prescription medications are obtained from friends or relatives who received them from a health care professional rather than a drug dealer or stranger [33]. It has been shown that predicting who may be at risk of misuse or abuse, especially by clinicians, is poor [34]. Several tools are available to screen patients for potential opioid addiction or drug-seeking behavior [35-38].

Consequences of Inadequate Postoperative Pain Relief

Evidence shows that inadequate postoperative analgesia may result in physiologic and psychological consequences. It can delay recovery and the return to daily life. If postoperative pain is inadequately treated, it may lead to chronic pain [39]. Anxiety is the psychological factor related most to high levels of pain. This can cause behavioral changes such as increased sensitivity to light and sound and withdrawal from interpersonal contact. This can lead to feelings of helplessness, depression, and resentment, especially if the patient perceives care is being withheld. Interestingly, inadequate pain relief on the day of surgery was believed to predict behavioral problems long after the duration of the pain itself [40].

Insufficient pain control has also been shown to prolong a patient's length of stay in the post-anesthesia care unit and the hospital [40]. Pavlin et al. showed that the most common causes of delayed discharge after ambulatory surgery were pain, drowsiness, nausea, and vomiting [41]. Once patients are discharged, home pain management, especially for patients discharged to nursing homes, is commonly ignored [42]. Postoperative delirium and cognitive dysfunction increase if the pain is not adequately controlled [43]. Also, inadequate pain control is the most common reason patients contact their primary practitioner after leaving the hospital [44].

Multidisciplinary Team

A multidisciplinary team must be in place to address the complex needs of opioid-tolerant patients. Members of the team include the medical team and social workers, psychologists, and spiritual counselors. It is essential to realize that detoxing or rehabilitating patients immediately postoperatively is not an appropriate time to do so. Withholding, decreasing or delaying the administration of opioids can lead to withdrawal and mistrust, fear, and anxiety towards the medical community [45].

References

[1] Jackman, C., Perioperative pain management for the chronic pain patient with long-term opioid use. *Orthopaedic Nursing*, 2019. 38(2): p. 159-163.

[2] Huxtable, C., et al., Acute pain management in opioid-tolerant patients: a growing challenge. *Anesthesia and intensive care*, 2011. 39(5): p. 804-823.

[3] (DAWN), H.o.t.D.A.W.N., *Substance Abuse and Mental Health Services Administration.*

[4] Rapp, S. E., L. B. Ready, and M. L. Nessly, Acute pain management in patients with prior opioid consumption: a case-controlled retrospective review. *Pain,* 1995. 61(2): p. 195-201.

[5] Swenson, J. D., J. J. Davis, and K. B. Johnson, *Postoperative care of the chronic opioid-consuming patient.* Anesthesiology Clinics of North America, 2005. 23(1): p. 37-48.

[6] Cooney, M. F., Management of postoperative pain in opioid-tolerant patients. *Journal of PeriAnesthesia Nursing*, 2015. 30(5): p. 436-443.

[7] Angst, M. S. and J. D. Clark, Opioid-induced hyperalgesia: a qualitative systematic review. *The Journal of the American Society of Anesthesiologists,* 2006. 104(3): p. 570-587.

[8] Chu, L. F., M. S. Angst, and D. Clark, Opioid-induced hyperalgesia in humans: molecular mechanisms and clinical considerations. *The Clinical journal of pain*, 2008. 24(6): p. 479-496.

[9] Macintyre, P. E., et al., *Acute pain management: scientific evidence*. 2010: Australian and New Zealand College of Anaesthetists.

[10] Roberts, L. J., *The opioid-tolerant patient, including those with a substance abuse disorder, in Clinical Pain Management*. 2008, CRC Press. p. 539-557.

[11] George, J. A., et al., The effect of intravenous opioid patient-controlled analgesia with and without background infusion on respiratory depression: a meta-analysis. *Journal of opioid management,* 2010. 6(1): p. 47-54.

[12] Macintyre, P. and S. Schug, Adverse effects of undertreated severe acute pain. *Acute pain management: a practical guide*. 3rd ed. Edinburgh, London, New York, Oxford, Philadelphia, St Louis, Sydney, Toronto, Saunders: Elsevier, 2007: p. 1-7.

[13] Hansson, K. S., et al., The meaning of the experiences of persons with chronic pain in their encounters with the health service. Scandinavian *journal of caring sciences*, 2011. 25(3): p. 444-450.

[14] Myles, P. S., et al., Bispectral index monitoring to prevent awareness during anaesthesia: the B-Aware randomised controlled trial. *The lancet*, 2004. 363(9423): p. 1757-1763.

[15] Prodduturi, S., et al., Transdermal delivery of fentanyl from matrix and reservoir systems: effect of heat and compromised skin. *Journal of pharmaceutical sciences,* 2010. 99(5): p. 2357-2366.
[16] Chapman, C. R., et al., Postoperative pain patterns in chronic pain patients: a pilot study. *Pain Medicine*, 2009. 10(3): p. 481-487.
[17] Rapp, S., et al., Acute pain management of the chronic pain patient on opiates: A survey of caregivers at University of Washington Medical Center. *The Clinical journal of pain*, 1994. 10(2): p. 133-138.
[18] Council, V. Q., Acute pain management measurement toolkit
[19] Broyles, L.M., et al., Clinicians' evaluation and management of mental health, substance abuse, and chronic pain conditions in the intensive care unit. *Critical care medicine*, 2008. 36(1): p. 87-93.
[20] Chang, G., L. Chen, and J. Mao, Opioid tolerance and hyperalgesia. *Medical Clinics*, 2007. 91(2): p. 199-211.
[21] Urban, M. K., et al., Ketamine as an adjunct to postoperative pain management in opioid tolerant patients after spinal fusions: a prospective randomized trial. *HSS Journal®*, 2008. 4(1): p. 62-65.
[22] Cepeda, M. S., et al., Addition of ultralow dose naloxone to postoperative morphine PCA: unchanged analgesia and opioid requirement but decreased incidence of opioid side effects. *Pain,* 2004. 107(1-2): p. 41-46.
[23] Miyoshi, R., Systemic non-opioid analgesics. *Bonica's management of pain*, 2001.
[24] Quigley, C., Opioid switching to improve pain relief and drug tolerability. *Cochrane Database of Systematic Reviews*, 2004(3).
[25] Fine, P. G., R. K. Portenoy, and A.H.E.P. on Evidence, Establishing "best practices" for opioid rotation: conclusions of an expert panel. *Journal of pain and symptom management*, 2009. 38(3): p. 418-425.
[26] Hadi, I., et al., Brief review: perioperative management of the patient with chronic non-cancer pain. *Canadian Journal of Anesthesia*, 2006. 53(12): p. 1190-1199.
[27] Patanwala, A. E., et al., Opioid conversions in acute care. *Annals of Pharmacotherapy*, 2007. 41(2): p. 255-267.
[28] Pereira, J., et al., Equianalgesic dose ratios for opioids: a critical review and proposals for long-term dosing. *Journal of pain and symptom management*, 2001. 22(2): p. 672-687.
[29] Hulse, G., E. Khong, and M. Sim, Acute pain and opioid seeking behaviour. *Australian family physician*, 2004. 33(12).
[30] Alford, D. P., P. Compton, and J. H. Samet, Acute pain management for patients receiving maintenance methadone or buprenorphine therapy. *Annals of internal medicine*, 2006. 144(2): p. 127-134.
[31] Brown, R., et al., Methadone: applied pharmacology and use as adjunctive treatment in chronic pain. *Postgraduate medical journal*, 2004. 80(949): p. 654-659.
[32] Hutchinson, M. R., et al., Evidence that tricyclic small molecules may possess toll-like receptor and myeloid differentiation protein 2 activity. *Neuroscience*, 2010. 168(2): p. 551-563.

[33] U.S. Department of Health and Human Services, S., O. *Abuse and Mental Health Services Administration, and o.A. Studies., Results from the 2009 National. Survey on Drug Use and Health: Volume I.* Summary of National Findings.

[34] Jung, B. and M. M. Reidenberg, Physicians being deceived. *Pain Medicine*, 2007. 8(5): p. 433-437.

[35] Chou, R., et al., Clinical guidelines for the use of chronic opioid therapy in chronic noncancer pain. *The Journal of Pain*, 2009. 10(2): p. 113-130. e22.

[36] Smith, H. S., K. L. Kirsh, and S. D. Passik, Chronic opioid therapy issues associated with opioid abuse potential. *Journal of opioid management*, 2009. 5(5): p. 287-300.

[37] Passik, S. and K. Kirsh, Screening for opioid abuse potential. *Clin. Updates IASP*, 2008. 26(7): p. 1-4.

[38] Meltzer, E. C., et al., Identifying prescription opioid use disorder in primary care: diagnostic characteristics of the Current Opioid Misuse Measure (COMM). *PAIN®*, 2011. 152(2): p. 397-402.

[39] Perkins, F. M. and H. Kehlet, Chronic pain as an outcome of surgery: a review of predictive factors. *The Journal of the American Society of Anesthesiologists*, 2000. 93(4): p. 1123-1133.

[40] Joshi, G. P. and B. O. Ogunnaike, *Consequences of inadequate postoperative pain relief and chronic persistent postoperative pain*. Anesthesiology Clinics of North America, 2005. 23(1): p. 21-36.

[41] Pavlin, D. J., et al., *Pain as a factor complicating recovery and discharge after ambulatory surgery*. Anesthesia & Analgesia, 2002. 95(3): p. 627-634.

[42] Marley, R. A. and J. Swanson, Patient care after discharge from the ambulatory surgical center. *Journal of PeriAnesthesia Nursing*, 2001. 16(6): p. 399-419.

[43] Morrison, R. S. and A. L. Siu, A comparison of pain and its treatment in advanced dementia and cognitively intact patients with hip fracture. *Journal of pain and symptom management*, 2000. 19(4): p. 240-248.

[44] Ghosh, S. and S. Sallam, Patient satisfaction and postoperative demands on hospital and community services after day surgery. *Journal of British Surgery*, 1994. 81(11): p. 1635-1638.

[45] Mitra, S., R. S. Sinatra, and D. C. Warltier, Perioperative management of acute pain in the opioid-dependent patient. *The Journal of the American Society of Anesthesiologists*, 2004. 101(1): p. 212-227.

Chapter 15

Perioperative Considerations and Anesthetic Management of the Geriatric Population

Shreya Reddy*
City University of New York School of Medicine, New York, NY, USA

Adults aged 65 and older are the fastest growing portion of the United States population. In the first decade of this century, the total population increased by 9.7%. This growth was even faster, at 15.1%, for the population aged 65 years and older.

This trend has been persistent throughout the current decade as the "baby boomer" generation continues to age. With the rise of the aging population, there is an expected concurrent rise in surgical procedures conducted on them. The increase in procedures demands a need for safe anesthetic techniques specific to this demographic. Perioperative management and anesthetic considerations of this population are particularly difficult due to significant comorbidities, medication usage, decreased functional capacity, as well as age-related physiological and pharmacodynamic changes [2]. This population is also at increased risk of postoperative complications and inadequate pain management due to diminished cognitive ability [3, 4]. This chapter will focus on the various physiological changes that occur with aging and also discuss current guidelines and considerations related to geriatric patients perioperatively.

* Corresponding Author's Email: sreddy000@citymail.cuny.edu.

In: Postoperative Pain
Editors: Indraneil Mukherjee et al.
ISBN: 978-1-68507-971-0

Preoperative Assessment

Current guidelines for the anesthetic and perioperative management of geriatric patients are separated into preoperative consultation, intraoperative induction techniques and maintenance, and postoperative pain management. There is an increased risk of perioperative complications in this demographic for various reasons, making it imperative to assess specific criteria in geriatric patients preoperatively. The first consideration in the preoperative assessment is to understand treatment goals, establish advanced directives, and weigh the efficacy of the procedure to achieve the patient's goals against any risks. In these discussions, the practitioner must simultaneously assess the patient's cognitive function, decision-making capacity, and functional status.

Functional status is important as patients who are dependent or partially dependent on others to assist with activities of daily living are at increased risk of having adverse events during surgery. Additionally, factors such as depression, malnutrition, dehydration, and immobility should be assessed. Cognitive dysfunction and dementia are common in the elderly population. Having these conditions preoperatively is a strong indicator for postoperative delirium, and cognitive decline. General anesthesia exposure has been shown to be associated with increased cognitive decline in the elderly population. In this particular population, the history of falls is also vital information as it has been shown that patients who have fallen three or more times in the 6 month period preceding surgery have a 100% chance of a complication [6].

Surgical outcomes are also heavily influenced by the patient's overall health status and life expectancy. Thus, the preoperative assessment must also evaluate the patient's medical comorbidities, current medications, and frailty. The presence of comorbidities increases the risk of postoperative complications, so it is necessary to evaluate and optimize all pre-existing conditions. Common comorbidities seen in the geriatric population include diabetes mellitus, cardiovascular disease, and pulmonary complications. Pulmonary diseases are a leading cause of postoperative complications, so pulmonary optimization is essential for these patients. Standard preoperative tests for patients over 65 years include CBC, BMP, and LFT to assess for common disorders such as anemia, renal dysfunction, liver dysfunction, and malnutrition. The presence of these disorders directly correlates to the patient's tolerance and reaction to anesthesia. Other tests should be considered based on the patient's individual comorbidities as well as the type of procedure proposed. Medication reconciliation prior to surgery is necessary to identify any possible drug interactions or adverse effects and adjust accordingly to ensure the patient is properly premedicated prior to surgery.

Physiological & Pharmacological Changes

Aging results in the decreased ability of organs to maintain homeostasis during physiological stress. This phenomenon, although progressive, can be exacerbated by severe health conditions and the significant stress afflicted by surgery. Aging also results in several pharmacodynamic and pharmacokinetic changes in the body. With aging, the level of circulating albumin decreases while the level of α-1 acid glycoprotein increases. Albumin is the main plasma binding protein for acidic drugs, and α-1 acid glycoprotein is the main binding protein for basic drugs. Therefore, the effect of aging varies for different drugs. Another effect of aging is a decrease in total body water and increase in body fat. The decrease in water results in increased serum concentrations of drugs after bolus administration, and the increase in body fat allows for a greater volume of distribution of the drug, resulting in prolonged drug action. Metabolism of the drugs is also affected by decreased hepatic and renal functioning. For these reasons, the elderly are generally more sensitive to anesthetics and require lower dosages of the medications.

Aging leads to several vascular, structural, and autonomic changes in the heart. Blood pressure is commonly labile in older patients due to vascular stiffening and chronic atherosclerotic disease. Many anesthetic medications exacerbate blood pressure changes through vasodilatory and sympatholytic effects. Structurally, decreased ventricular compliance results in diastolic dysfunction, and the elderly heart is unable to compensate for hypovolemia that may occur during surgery. Diastolic dysfunction can also lead to significant pulmonary edema during fluid administration. Additionally, there is a decrease in cardiac output by around 1% each year after the age of 30. Thus, small changes in intravascular volume or venous return during surgery in combination with non-complaint vessels can result in cardiovascular instability. Aging can also result in fibrotic changes in the conduction system of the heart, making these patients more susceptible to arrhythmias [11]. Due to their dependence on atrial filling during diastole, possible atrial arrhythmias further increase the patient's risk of hypotension. The cardiovascular system has several beta-adrenergic receptors which work together with baroreceptors to maintain homeostasis. Dysautonomia of aging includes the diminishing of beta-adrenergic response. Therefore, the elderly patient has an increased reliance on baroreflexes which can be compromised by volume changes and ventricular dysfunction. For these reasons, transfusions in this population also pose a challenge and blood pressure must be carefully monitored throughout the procedure.

There are many pulmonary changes seen with aging, including decreased pulmonary reserve, decreased lung compliance, decreased muscle strength, and diminished response to hypercapnia and hypoxia. The decrease in lung compliance results in a decrease of alveolar surface area, decreased functional residual volume, V/Q mismatch, and decreased PaO_2. Decreased muscle strength and altered pharyngeal function diminishes the cough reflex which increases the risk for aspiration. Additionally, common co-existing conditions such as emphysema, chronic bronchitis, and pneumonia further exacerbate these physiologic changes. Thoracic and upper abdominal surgeries have the highest pulmonary complication rates. Pain after these types of surgeries is most responsible for impaired ventilation and deep breathing, which result in postoperative pulmonary complications such as atelectasis, hypoxemia, infection, and respiratory failure. Adequate pain control is important in these situations to reduce to the risk of pulmonary complications.

Aging affects kidney function as well, and results in a decrease in glomerular filtration rate, renal blood flow, and kidney mass. These changes lead to decreased renal metabolism and slower clearance of medications and metabolites. Additionally, the kidney in an aging patient is slower to maintain homeostasis given the diminished response to vasodilatory stimuli, increasing the risk of acute renal failure in the postoperative period. Given that many anesthetic medications are renally metabolized, higher dosages and prolonged exposure to these medications cause significant strain to the aging kidneys.

The nervous system is the target for majority of the anesthetic drugs used in surgery, therefore, the age-related changes of the nervous system play a significant role in anesthetic management. Age-related changes include a decrease in tissue mass, neuronal density, and concentration of neurotransmitters and neurotransmitter receptors. Another neurological consideration for elderly patients is the increased incidence of delirium. Due to this, the dosage requirements for various anesthetic drugs are reduced as elderly patients require more time for recovery from general anesthesia.

Intraoperative Maintenance

Aging is not a contraindication for anesthesia; however, there are many drugs used commonly for anesthesia during surgery, and various properties of these drugs are important to consider in an elderly patient. Minimum alveolar concentration (MAC) is the concentration of the agent at which 50% of patients will be sufficiently sedated to prevent response to surgical stimulus. MAC for an inhaled drug decreases by approximately 6% every decade of life. It is theorized that this change in MAC is due to alterations in neurotransmitter levels and neurotransmitter receptors in the aging brain. The sensitivity to these inhaled agents is increased in the elderly population and therefore the dosage must be decreased. Brain sensitivity to opioids is also increased with age, therefore, fentanyl, remifentanil, and morphine are more potent in geriatric patients. Clearance of these drugs is decreased as well, so infusion rates should be titrated, and short acting drugs should be used when possible. For neuromuscular blocker medications, duration of drug action may be prolonged if the drug's metabolism is dependent on renal or hepatic excretion. Patients who are paralyzed must be closely monitored and given a reversal agent. Rocuronium and Vecuronium have a potent reversal agent: Sugammadex. Cisatracurium is one neuromuscular blocking agent that is not metabolized renally or hepatically, and thus is unaffected by age. General anesthesia is also associated with hypothermia. Temperature is important to monitor because hypothermia is associated with increased rates of myocardial ischemia and hypoxemia in the postoperative period.

Regional anesthesia with peripheral nerve blocks is a promising alternative to general anesthesia. Regional anesthesia has been shown to decrease the incidence of deep vein thrombosis in the elderly. Additionally, avoiding general anesthesia allows for the patient breathe spontaneously and maintain pulmonary function. Although regional anesthesia has been shown to have more favorable outcomes in the geriatric population, anatomic changes in these patients and duration of action of the drugs used should be kept in mind.

Postoperative Management

Common causes of postoperative morbidity and mortality include atelectasis, pneumonia, neurological disease, myocardial infarction, heart failure, and delirium. Proper preoperative assessment and intraoperative management that is specific to the patient's health status and comorbidities have been shown to decrease the incidence of these problems in the postoperative period. In general, shorter hospitalization time leads to better outcomes for the patient [2]. Minimally invasive procedures as well as regional anesthesia as opposed to general anesthesia have been shown to lead to more favorable outcomes for this specific patient population. Management of pain postoperatively is complex in this population because many of the patients have co-existent diseases and take concurrent medications. This puts them at high risk for drug-drug interactions. Additionally, it is difficult to assess pain in this population due to increased rates of cognitive dysfunction and delirium. Titration methods are widely used for pain management in these types of cases to minimize the adverse side effects of these medications. Patient controlled analgesia setups have also proven to be efficacious for adequate pain management, although the patient must be closely monitored to reduce the incidence of misuse [2]. The effects of surgery and anesthesia in the highly vulnerable geriatric population is still only partly understood, and further research regarding the long-term effects of anesthetic exposure is still needed to determine the risks and benefits for this population.

References

[1] Peters, Ruth. 2006. "Ageing and the Brain." *Postgraduate Medical Journal* 82 (964): 84-88. https://doi.org/10.1136/pgmj.2005.036665.

[2] Esposito, Ciro, Anna Rita Plati, Tiziana Mazzullo, Gianluca Fasoli, Andreana De Mauri, Fabrizio Grosjean, Filippo Mangione, et al., 2007. "Renal Function and Functional Reserve in Healthy Elderly Individuals." *Journal of Nephrology* 20 (5): 617-25.

[3] Irwin, Michael G., Kam Y. Ip, and Yuet M. Hui. 2019. "Anaesthetic Considerations in Nonagenarians and Centenarians." *Current Opinion in Anaesthesiology* 32 (6): 776-82. https://doi.org/10.1097/ACO.0000000000000793.

[4] Bruno, Rosa Maria, Emiliano Duranti, Chiara Ippolito, Cristina Segnani, Nunzia Bernardini, Giulio Di Candio, Massimo Chiarugi, Stefano Taddei, and Agostino Virdis. 2017. "Different Impact of Essential Hypertension on Structural and Functional Age-Related Vascular Changes." *Hypertension* 69 (1): 71-78. https://doi.org/10.1161/HYPERTENSIONAHA.116.08041.

[5] Rooke, G. Alec. 2003. "Cardiovascular Aging and Anesthetic Implications." *Journal of Cardiothoracic and Vascular Anesthesia* 17 (4): 512-23. https://doi.org/10.1016/S1053-0770(03)00161-7.

[6] Das, Sangeeta, Kirsty Forrest, and Simon Howell. 2010. "General Anaesthesia in Elderly Patients with Cardiovascular Disorders: Choice of Anaesthetic Agent." *Drugs and Aging* 27 (4): 265-82. https://doi.org/10.2165/11534990-000000000-00000.

[7] Muravchick, Stanley. 2003. "Anesthesia for the Elderly." *Wylie and Churchill-Davidsons: A Practice of Anesthesia, Seventh Edition* 11 (4): 981-93. https://doi.org/10.1093/med/9780199584048.003.0031.

[8] Teplan, Vladimír. 2020. "Preoperative Assessment in Older Adults." *Casopis Lekaru Ceskych* 159 (1): 4-12.

[9] Visnjevac, Ognjen, Sina Davari-Farid, Jun Lee, Leili Pourafkari, Pradeep Arora, Hasan H. Dosluoglu, and Nader D. Nader. 2015. "The Effect of Adding Functional Classification to ASA Status for Predicting 30-Day Mortality." *Anesthesia and Analgesia* 121 (1): 110-16. https://doi.org/10.1213/ANE.0000000000000740.

[10] Jones, Teresa S., Christina L. Dunn, Daniel S. Wu, Joseph C. Joseph, Deidre Kile, and Thomas N. Robinson. 2013. "Relationship between Asking an Older Adult about Falls and Surgical Outcomes." *JAMA Surgery* 148 (12): 1132-38. https://doi.org/10.1001/jamasurg.2013.2741.

[11] Bettelli, Gabriella. 2010. "Anaesthesia for the Elderly Outpatient: Preoperative Assessment and Evaluation, Anaesthetic Technique and Postoperative Pain Management." *Current Opinion in Anaesthesiology* 23 (6): 726-31. https://doi.org/10.1097/ACO.0b013e3283400b6c.

[12] Halaszynski, Thomas. 2013. "Influences of the Aging Process on Acute Perioperative Pain Management in Elderly and Cognitively Impaired Patients." *Ochsner Journal* 13 (2): 228-47.

[13] Devick, Katrina L., Juraj Sprung, Michelle Mielke, Ronald C. Petersen, and Phillip J. Schulte. 2021. "Association between Surgery with Anesthesia and Cognitive Decline in Older Adults: Analysis Using Shared Parameter Models for Informative Dropout." *Journal of Clinical and Translational Science* 5 (1). https://doi.org/10.1017/cts.2020.519.

[14] Aubrun, Frédéric, and Frédéric Marmion. 2007. "The Elderly Patient and Postoperative Pain Treatment." *Best Practice and Research: Clinical Anaesthesiology* 21 (1): 109-27. https://doi.org/10.1016/j.bpa.2006.12.005.

[15] LARO111. 2005. "*The Older Population Hawaii*." https://www.census.gov/library/publications/2011/dec/c2010br-09.html.

Chapter 16

Postoperative Pain in Head and Neck Procedures

Nikhilesh Chitibomma[1], Juan Garces[1] and Alice Lee[2*]
[1]Staten Island University Hospital – Northwell Health, New York, NY, USA
[2]City University of New York School of Medicine, New York, NY, USA

During the last decades, Head and Neck surgical procedures (HNSPs) have become standard procedures in the United States. An estimated 366,050 HNSPs (142.397 inpatients vs. 223.653 outpatient) were performed in 2006, and over 420,000 HNSPs were performed in 2020. Perioperative management of the head and neck pathologies has also undergone extensive changes. It is well known that postoperative pain is a specific entity that results from an inflammatory response after tissue trauma (surgical incision, dissection, tissue retraction) and direct nerve damage. A wide range of pathophysiologic responses is activated due to tissue injury leading to the release of inflammatory mediators with subsequent nociceptor stimulation and activation of the pain pathway.

Significant progress in managing postoperative pain has been made since the 1990s. Increased awareness of the under-treatment of postoperative pain, improved analgesic techniques, and new analgesic agents have contributed to improvements in postoperative pain management.

[*] Corresponding Author's Email: alee003@citymail.cuny.edu.

In: Postoperative Pain
Editors: Indraneil Mukherjee et al.
ISBN: 978-1-68507-971-0

Source of Postoperative Pain

Postoperative pain after HNSPs is derived primarily from 3 sources: 1. Sore throat from laryngeal or tracheal trauma from intubation, endotracheal or nasogastric tube presence; 2. Posterior neck discomfort from an extended cervical positioning during surgery typical for head and neck procedures; 3. Anterior neck pain from the skin incision or trauma from dissection, retraction, or muscle division.

Postoperative sore throat (POST) secondary to endotracheal intubation is a common problem following surgery and affects the quality and speed of recovery. Jaensson et al. studied using a smaller diameter endotracheal tube (ETT) and the association with a decrease in POST. They found a higher proportion of patients with sore throats when a larger ETT (size 7.0) was used in comparison to a smaller ETT (6.0) (51.1% vs. 27.1%). Benzydamine hydrochloride (BH) has also been used to reduce the incidence and severity of POST. Kim et al. found that BH spray on the ETT cuff reduced POST at 12 hours after total thyroidectomies.

Additionally, nasogastric tubes intraoperatively have been associated as a strong risk factor for POST. Using methods to decrease laryngeal or oropharyngeal trauma associated with intubation is key to minimizing POST. These practices should include small-sized endotracheal tubes and eliminate routine use of nasogastric tubes or esophageal temperature probes if possible.

Neck extension is helpful for exposure to the neck, mediastinum, or substernal area for dissection. Care must be taken to support the neck in patients with limited cervical mobility or cervical degenerative joint disease to avoid postoperative pain from traction. The use of warm and cold pads and alternative therapies such as kinesio taping and electroacupuncture have shown promising results in reducing postoperative pain and analgesic use.

Cervical nerve blocks and local anesthesia to the incision also effectively manage perioperative pain after a surgical procedure. The injection of lidocaine, bupivacaine, or ropivacaine into the skin before incision effectively manages postoperative pain, decreases pain scores, and improves overall patient satisfaction. In addition to subdermal injection at the operative site, bilateral superficial cervical plexus block (BSCPB) seems to improve postoperative pain control. BSCPBs are local anesthetic blocks to the emerging branches of the superficial cervical plexus (lesser occipital, greater auricular, transverse cervical, and supraclavicular nerves). Complication rates with this technique are low, with little risk to deeper structures. A recent meta-analysis demonstrated that BSCPB offers greater analgesic efficacy after surgery, reducing subjective pain scores and longer time to the first postoperative dose of narcotic medications than patients who did not receive BSCPB. Interestingly, studies show that a preoperative block is more efficacious than a postoperative block.

HNSP Procedures

HNSPs procedures are incredibly diverse with a wide range of complexity. In complex surgical procedures, such as those that require larger resections and reconstructions, a more extensive postoperative pain regimen will be required. As mentioned above, pain control should be multimodal, and a combination of local blocks with oral analgesics should be used. The longer operation time associated with some HNSPs is a challenge for postoperative pain management, and often, these patients may require a patient-controlled analgesia pump. In low complexity procedures such as myringotomy, simple excisions, or biopsies, patients will only require analgesia for a shorter time without opioid medications. Uniquely, tonsillectomies are associated with higher pain scores and consumption of analgesic medications. Many HNSPs are performed on pediatric patients, and historically, pain in the pediatric population has been undertreated and under-researched. A contributing factor is that the parents are responsible for pain management at home. Postoperative pain can lead to unplanned visits to healthcare services; therefore, effective pain management is essential.

Pharmacologic Treatments

Postoperative pain management should begin before the patient undergoes surgery. This includes educating patients about the pain they will experience and setting realistic expectations. Patients should also be taught the simple non-pharmacologic measures to reduce pain, such as comfortable positioning, heat/ice pads, and the benefits of distraction. Prevention goes a long way in pain management. However, often most patients require post-operative pain medications. Medications are the mainstay for postoperative pain control for head and neck surgery. Multimodal analgesia is extremely effective for pain control and minimizing side effects. It relies on the additive or synergistic combination of drugs acting on the pain pathway at various points. Typical combinations include local anesthetic wound infiltration, routine NSAIDs, and opioids at low doses added as needed. The benefits of reducing the opioid dose include decreasing the incidence of nausea/vomiting, sedation, sleep disturbance, urinary retention, constipation, and respiratory depression. Various drugs have been used, including N-acetyl-p-amino-phenol (paracetamol, acetaminophen), NSAIDs, Toradol, Tramadol, and opioids.

Opioids (oxycodone, hydrocodone, morphine, tramadol) have long been the mainstay of postoperative analgesia regimens for head and neck endocrine procedures. They are potent drugs with a quick onset of action. However, due to their addictive potential and side effects, there has been a downtrend in their prescription. Lou et al. found that 93% of patients undergoing thyroidectomy or parathyroidectomy required 20 or fewer oral morphine equivalents at the first postoperative visit. Furthermore, Tharakan et al. found that 80% of thyroidectomy and parathyroidectomy patients needed 15 or fewer oral morphine equivalents, with half of the patients not requiring opioid use. Similarly, Sada et al. found that more than half of parathyroidectomy patients did not require opioids postoperatively.

Acetaminophen plays a significant role in the multimodal drug regimen. It decreases the postoperative pain score, the need for opioids, and the incidence of nausea and vomiting. A Kaiser Permanente study found in 469 thyroid and parathyroid surgeries that a postoperative analgesic regimen of oral acetaminophen alone was sufficient to prevent opioid use after discharge in more than 90% of cases (David S. Cohen, 2019).

Nonsteroidal anti-inflammatory drugs (NSAIDs) are also popularly used in pain management, and they have also been shown to reduce opioid use, nausea/vomiting, and ileus. In a prospective randomized control trial, Nguyen et al. concluded that ibuprofen provided equally effective pain control compared with hydrocodone/acetaminophen in outpatient otolaryngology procedures, including thyroidectomy and parathyroidectomy, with decreased opioid requirement. However, with the concern of bleeding, the perioperative use has not been momentous in head and neck surgeries. Postoperative bleeding after thyroidectomy has been associated with NSAID use postoperatively, although its clinical significance has been debated. NSAIDs are contraindicated in patients with renal insufficiency and gastric ulcers.

Tramadol is a different opioid with dual mechanisms of action. The reduced u-opioid receptor activation and the serotonin and norepinephrine reuptake inhibition may create a favorable profile for pain control. They may be used as a substitute for opioids, decreasing the opioid need in postoperative patients. The benefits of tramadol include lower abuse potential and less incidence of opioid side effects such as constipation.

Gamma-amino-butyric-acid analogs (gabapentin, pregabalin) and gabapentinoids have been postulated to desensitize patients to painful stimuli, reducing the need for other analgesic medication. When used as part of a multimodal preventative regimen, they are associated with lower postoperative pain scores and reduced opioid requirements. Hema et al. found that oral gabapentin was effective as preventative analgesia in reducing postoperative pain scores, total tramadol consumption, and prolonged time to rescue analgesia after thyroidectomy. Sanders and Dawes demonstrated that gabapentin seems to have a role in perioperative pain relief and decreased analgesic consumption in head and neck surgeries, including thyroidectomy. Lee et al. showed that preoperative oral gabapentin reduced the intensity and incidence of sore throat after thyroid surgery. Despite this, other studies have suggested that groups receiving a preoperative dose of gabapentin may have an increased opioid or APAP consumption. For this reason, additional studies specific to thyroid and parathyroid surgery are needed. Dizziness and sedation are common adverse effects, and dosing should be reduced for older patients or those with impaired renal function.

Multimodal Analgesia

Multiple studies encourage reducing opioid consumption and using multimodal analgesia for postoperative pain. Utilizing acetaminophen with a nonsteroidal anti-inflammatory drug and/or gabapentin has been described in the literature. Although there is a theoretical risk of bleeding with NSAIDs, they have not been substantiated in the literature. Some studies have reported that NSAIDs provide analgesia equivalent to that of opioids. The role of perioperative administration of corticosteroids in reducing postoperative pain and temporary recurrent laryngeal nerve palsy is controversial. Early studies demonstrated improvement in voice outcomes with perioperative steroid use. Additional studies have conflicting findings, with some studies demonstrating no change in pain or voice and others suggesting improvement in pain control with perioperative steroid use.

Managing Opioid Complications

While opioids are an effective choice of pain control, appropriate monitoring of sedation, hemodynamics, and respiratory status is recommended. Other side

effects such as nausea, vomiting, and opioid-induced constipation may be treated with anti-emetics and bowel regimens. Alternative analgesics may be used that have fewer side effects. Tramadol is effective after ambulatory surgery, but it is still associated with frequent side effects, including sedation, dizziness, and particularly postoperative nausea and vomiting. The mechanism of action of Tapentadol is dual-action and similar to that of tramadol, with comparable efficacy to oxycodone but with fewer GI adverse effects, such as nausea, vomiting, and constipation. Combining oral oxycodone with naloxone (Targinact) antagonizes the adverse GI effects, particularly preventing opioid-induced constipation.
Additionally, there is little effect on the analgesic effects because first-pass metabolism prevents much naloxone from reaching the central nervous system. Alvimopan is another peripherally acting μ-opioid (MOP) receptor antagonist used to reduce opioid-induced constipation. However, peripheral MOP receptors also may partially mediate opioid-associated postoperative nausea and vomiting, delayed gastric emptying, and urinary retention.

After head and neck surgeries, postoperative pain control encourages faster and more complete recovery, early mobilization, and increased patient comfort. Traditionally, after most head and neck procedures, pain management is done with intravenous or oral opiates. Amid the opioid epidemic and the risk of improper use that could lead to opioid addiction and overdose, there is a significant lack of guidance surrounding opioid prescription. The Center for Disease Control (CDC) issued recommendations for opioid prescriptions, but these guidelines are absent in otolaryngology. In a study done by Dang et al., patients with a higher score on the Charlson Comorbidity Index were associated with more extended opioid use, and prescription size was associated with increased opioid use. Other influencing factors in opioid use are cultural beliefs. Li et al. reported significantly less opioid use in Hong Kong patients (30). Other factors that were positive predictors of postoperative opioid use are male gender, tobacco use, and psychiatric medications.

Authors' Perspective

Educating the patients before any surgical procedure and setting reasonable expectations about their postoperative course would decrease their anxiety and help optimize pain management. We believe one of the keys is identifying the source of pain and using a multimodal analgesia approach with a synergistic combination of drugs that have been proved to be highly effective, allowing to decrease opioid consumption and their side effects. We strongly recommend using local anesthetic wound infiltration and routine NSAIDs and the use of opioids only for particular cases.

References

Ahmad, Raheel, Mehwish Changeez, Asim Tameez Ud Din, Anum Iftikhar, Hafiz Bilal Ahmad, Ahmed Mujtaba, Jahangir S Khan, and Mustafa N Malik. 2019. "Role of Prophylactic Dexamethasone Before Thyroidectomy in Reducing Postoperative Pain, Nausea and Vomiting." *Cureus*. https://doi.org/10.7759/cureus.4735.

Bhattacharyya, Neil. 2011. "The Increasing Workload in Head and Neck Surgery: An Epidemiologic Analysis." *Laryngoscope* 121 (1): 111–15. https://doi.org/10.1002/lary.21193.

Brookman, Jason C., Honorio T. Benzon, Asha Manohar, and Christopher L. Wu. 2013. "Postoperative Pain Management: Trends and Future Directions and Areas in Need of Investigation." *Practical Management of Pain: Fifth Edition*. https://doi.org/10.1016/B978-0-323-08340-9.00082-7.

Dang, Sophia, Alexander Duffy, Jonathan C. Li, Zachary Gandee, Tanvi Rana, Brittany Gunville, Tingting Zhan, et al., 2020. "Postoperative Opioid-Prescribing Practices in Otolaryngology: A Multiphasic Study." *Laryngoscope* 130 (3): 659–65. https://doi.org/10.1002/lary.28101.

Dhillon, Vaninder K., Babak Jahan-Parwar, and David S. Cohen. 2020. "Perioperative Analgesia for Thyroid and Parathyroid Surgery: A Review of Current Practices." *Otolaryngologic Clinics of North America* 53 (5): 779–87. https://doi.org/10.1016/j.otc.2020.05.007.

Dort, Joseph C., D. Gregory Farwell, Merran Findlay, Gerhard F. Huber, Paul Kerr, Melissa A. Shea-Budgell, Christian Simon, et al., 2017. "Optimal Perioperative Care in Major Head and Neck Cancer Surgery with Free Flap Reconstruction: A Consensus Review and Recommendations from the Enhanced Recovery after Surgery Society." *JAMA Otolaryngology - Head and Neck Surgery* 143 (3): 292–303. https://doi.org/10.1001/jamaoto.2016.2981.

Gemechu, Biruk Melkamu, Endale Gebreegziabher Gebremedhn, and Tadesse Belayneh Melkie. 2017. "Risk Factors for Postoperative Throat Pain after General Anaesthesia with Endotracheal Intubation at the University of Gondar Teaching Hospital, Northwest Ethiopia, 2014." *Pan African Medical Journal* 27 (127). https://doi.org/10.11604/pamj.2017.27.127.10566.

Genç, Aysun, Süleyman Utku Çelik, Volkan Genç, Derya Gökmen, and Birkan Sonel Tur. 2019. "The Effects of Cervical Kinesiotaping on Neck Pain, Range of Motion, and Disability in Patients Following Thyroidectomy: A Randomized, Double-Blind, Sham-Controlled Clinical Trial." *Turkish Journal of Medical Sciences* 49 (4): 1185–91. https://doi.org/10.3906/sag-1812-55.

Hadri, B., L. Emini, I. Arifaj, and I. Krasniqi. 2014. "Post Thyroidectomy Wound Infiltration for Postoperative Pain Relief." *European Journal of Anaesthesiology* 31: 229. https://doi.org/10.1097/00003643-201406001-00660.

Jaensson, M., L. L. Olowsson, and U. Nilsson. 2010. "Endotracheal Tube Size and Sore Throat Following Surgery: A Randomized-Controlled Study." *Acta Anaesthesiologica Scandinavica* 54 (2): 147–53. https://doi.org/10.1111/j.1399-6576.2009.02166.x.

Kelly, Dermot J., Mahmood Ahmad, and Sorin J. Brull. 2001. "Preemptive Analgesia I: Physiological Pathways and Pharmacological Modalities." *Canadian Journal of Anesthesia* 48 (10): 1000–1010. https://doi.org/10.1007/BF03016591.

Kim, Doyeon, Heejoon Jeong, Jihye Kwon, Sehee Kang, Bobae Han, Eun Kyung Lee, Sangmin M. Lee, and Ji Won Choi. 2019. "The Effect of Benzydamine Hydrochloride on Preventing Postoperative Sore Throat after Total Thyroidectomy: A Randomized-Controlled Trial." *Canadian Journal of Anesthesia* 66 (8): 934–42. https://doi.org/10.1007/s12630-019-01371-2.

Kim, Matthew, Ashutosh Kacker, David I. Kutler, Abtin Tabaee, Michael G. Stewart, Klaus Kjaer, and Anthony P. Sclafani. 2020. "Pain and Opioid Analgesic Use After Otorhinolaryngologic Surgery." Otolaryngology-Head *and Neck Surgery (United States)* 163 (6): 1178–85. https://doi.org/10.1177/0194599820933223.

Lee, Jae Ho, Hyun Kyu Lee, Na Hyung Chun, Yoon So, and Chi Young Lim. 2013. "The Prophylactic Effects of Gabapentin on Postoperative Sore Throat after Thyroid Surgery." *Korean Journal of Anesthesiology* 64 (2): 138–42. https://doi.org/10.4097/kjae.2013.64.2.138.

Lee, Minhyung, Jihye Rhee, Yoonjoong Kim, Young Ho Jung, Soon Hyun Ahn, and Woo Jin Jeong. 2019. "Perioperative Risk Factors for Post-Thyroidectomy Hematoma: Significance of Pain and Ketorolac Usage." *Head and Neck* 41 (10): 3656–60. https://doi.org/10.1002/hed.25895.

Li, Ryan J., Myriam Loyo Li, Enrique Leon, Cherrie W.K. Ng, Maisie Shindo, Katie Manzione, Peter Andersen, Daniel Clayburgh, Mark Wax, and Jason Y.K. Chan. 2018. "Comparison of Opioid Utilization Patterns after Major Head and Neck Procedures between Hong Kong and the United States." *JAMA Otolaryngology - Head and Neck Surgery* 144 (11): 1060–65. https://doi.org/10.1001/jamaoto.2018.1787.

Lou, Irene, Todd B. Chennell, Sarah C. Schaefer, Herbert Chen, Rebecca S. Sippel, Courtney Balentine, David F. Schneider, and Jacob Moalem. 2017. "Optimizing Outpatient Pain Management After Thyroid and Parathyroid Surgery: A Two-Institution Experience." *Annals of Surgical Oncology* 24 (7): 1951–57. https://doi.org/10.1245/s10434-017-5781-y.

Marshall, Sally M, and LeFever Joyce Kee. 2004. "Clinical Calculations: With Applications to General and Specialty Areas [2004]." *Elsevier Health Sciences*. http://uhn.summon.serialssolutions.com/2.0.0/link/0/eLvHCXMwY2AwNtIz0EUrE8wt05JTUlMNE4HVZZqxSWKapUGapWFSWoplkglo9yjoQL4Qo8gQ84AIYMQzwK5wRVrlDD5AFFx0F4I6k6CjI6AytqEefqpGBj6w7qUaeO0XMK8bgs4ZzLU1AvYqgGU0sKY2YGFgdQzz9YwA7_ACX7AMbP3ADn6C8o1AtUxGHg8Dk7EptJpxE2R.

Mayhew, D., N. Sahgal, R. Khirwadkar, J. M. Hunter, and A. Banerjee. 2018. "Analgesic Efficacy of Bilateral Superficial Cervical Plexus Block for Thyroid Surgery: Meta-

Analysis and Systematic Review." *British Journal of Anaesthesia* 120 (2): 241–51. https://doi.org/10.1016/j.bja.2017.11.083.

Nguyen, Khanh K., Yuan F. Liu, Crystal Chang, Jaimie J. Park, Cherine H. Kim, Brian Hondorp, Christopher Vuong, et al., 2019. "A Randomized Single-Blinded Trial of Ibuprofen- versus Opioid-Based Primary Analgesic Therapy in Outpatient Otolaryngology Surgery." *Otolaryngology - Head and Neck Surgery (United States)* 160 (5): 839–46. https://doi.org/10.1177/0194599819832528.

Noel, Julia E., Maxwell P. Kligerman, and Uchechukwu C. Megwalu. 2018. "Intraoperative Corticosteroids for Voice Outcomes among Patients Undergoing Thyroidectomy: A Systematic Review and Meta-Analysis." *Otolaryngology - Head and Neck Surgery (United States)* 159 (5): 811–16. https://doi.org/10.1177/0194599818793414.

Sada, Alaa, Daniel S. Ubl, Cornelius A. Thiels, Patricia A. Cronin, Benzon M. Dy, Melanie L. Lyden, Geoffrey B. Thompson, Travis J. McKenzie, and Elizabeth B. Habermann. 2020. "Optimizing Opioid-Prescribing Practices After Parathyroidectomy." *Journal of Surgical Research* 245: 107–14. https://doi.org/10.1016/j.jss.2019.07.039.

Sanders, James G., and Patrick J.D. Dawes. 2016. "Gabapentin for Perioperative Analgesia in Otorhinolaryngology-Head and Neck Surgery: Systematic Review." *Otolaryngology - Head and Neck Surgery (United States)* 155 (6): 893–903. https://doi.org/10.1177/0194599816659042.

Sanders, James G., Claire Cameron, and Patrick J.D. Dawes. 2017. "Gabapentin in the Management of Pain Following Tonsillectomy: A Randomized Double-Blind Placebo-Controlled Trial." *Otolaryngology - Head and Neck Surgery (United States)*. https://doi.org/10.1177/0194599817719883.

Schietroma, Mario, Emanuela Marina Cecilia, Francesco Carlei, Federico Sista, Giuseppe De Santis, Laura Lancione, and Gianfranco Amicucci. 2013. "Dexamethasone for the Prevention of Recurrent Laryngeal Nerve Palsy and Other Complications after Thyroid Surgery: A Randomized Double-Blind Placebo-Controlled Trial." *JAMA Otolaryngology - Head and Neck Surgery* 139 (5): 471–78. https://doi.org/10.1001/jamaoto.2013.2821.

Tharakan, Theresa, Sydney Jiang, Judd Fastenberg, Thomas J. Ow, Bradley Schiff, Richard V. Smith, and Vikas Mehta. 2019. "Postoperative Pain Control and Opioid Usage Patterns among Patients Undergoing Thyroidectomy and Parathyroidectomy." *Otolaryngology - Head and Neck Surgery (United States)* 160 (3): 394–401. https://doi.org/10.1177/0194599818797574.

Uhlmann, Rebecca A., Henry A. Reinhart, Eugene Postevka, Samuel K. Snyder, and Minerva Romero Arenas. 2019. "A Review of Postoperative Pain Management for Thyroid and Parathyroid Surgery." *Journal of Surgical Research* 241: 107–11. https://doi.org/10.1016/j.jss.2019.03.050.

Wilson, Caroline A., David Sommerfield, Thomas F.E. Drake-Brockman, Lita von Bieberstein, Anoop Ramgolam, and Britta S. von Ungern-Sternberg. 2016. "Pain after Discharge Following Head and Neck Surgery in Children." *Paediatric Anaesthesia* 26 (10): 992–1001. https://doi.org/10.1111/pan.12974.

Woolf, C. J., and M. S. Chong. 1993. "Preemptive Analgesia - Treating Postoperative Pain by Preventing the Establishment of Central Sensitization." *Anesthesia and Analgesia* 77 (2): 362–79. https://doi.org/10.1213/00000539-199377020-00026.

Zhang, Caiju, Mintao Zhou, and Man Li. 2018. "[Clinical Study of Electroacupuncture on Perioperative Analgesia in Patients with Thyroid Surgery under Cervical Plexus Block]." *Zhongguo Zhen Jiu = Chinese Acupuncture & Moxibustion*. https://doi.org/10.13703/j.0255-2930.2018.12.002.

Chapter 17

Postoperative Pain Management in Ophthalmic Plastic and Reconstructive Surgery

Gabriella Schmuter[1,*], MD
and Emery C. Jamerson[2], MD
[1]Department of Ophthalmology, Weill Cornell Medicine, New York, NY, USA
[2]Department of Oculoplastic & Orbital Surgery, Edward S. Harkness Eye Institute, Columbia University Irving Medical Center, New York, NY, USA

Postoperative pain has been associated with patient discomfort and a decrease in patient satisfaction. Ophthalmic plastic and reconstructive surgery has traditionally been viewed to cause little postoperative pain given its less invasive nature in comparison to other surgical procedures. Nevertheless, a variety of oculoplastic procedures, including enucleation and reconstructions, have been associated with severe postoperative pain. Orbital surgery is generally associated with greater pain than pure eyelid procedures. It is particularly essential to evaluate methods of mitigating postoperative pain as oculoplastic surgeries have been shifting to an ambulatory surgery in an outpatient setting from a traditional postoperative hospitalization.

Risk factors for postoperative pain in oculoplastic surgery include smoking history and prior surgery on the operative eye. A high level of preoperative anxiety has been found to potentially increase pain felt by the patient during and after eyelid surgery. Given this finding, oculoplastic surgeons are encouraged to implement psychological precautions in an attempt to mitigate the development of postoperative pain. Such precautions may include music therapy, anxiolytic medication, hypnosis, or virtual reality.

---

*Corresponding Author's Email: uxo9002@med.cornell.edu.

In: Postoperative Pain
Editors: Indraneil Mukherjee et al.
ISBN: 978-1-68507-971-0

This risk factor underscores the importance of providing comprehensive pre-operative information regarding each procedure.

The goal of medications used in post-operative surgery in this setting is to prevent the initial development of pain, rather than alleviating pain after its development. Nevertheless, it is increasingly essential to consider medications that minimize patients' risk of forming detrimentally addictive habits. As clinicians become increasingly aware of the risks associated with the use of opioid analgesics, many non-narcotic agents are increasingly used in the post-operative pain management after oculoplastic surgery. This shift in management is particularly notable given the rising epidemic of opioid abuse in the United States. Most patients require approximately 10-15 opioid tablets for adequate control of postoperative pain following facial plastic surgery. Major reconstructive head and neck procedures with free tissue transfer may be adequately managed with a limited amount of opioid medication. A variety of non-narcotic medications have been used in the context of oculoplastic surgery. For example, pregabalin has been documented to be efficacious in eyelid surgery and dacryocystorhinostomy; however, this medication is adversely associated with dizziness, ataxia, confusion, dysarthria, and blurred vision. Typical dosages for neuromodulators such as gabapentinoids include 300 mg daily of gabapentin or pregabalin.

It is advised to minimize use of non-steroidal anti-inflammatory drugs (NSAID) as much as possible after oculoplastic surgery to minimize risk of bleeding. Therefore, non-NSAID medications, such as acetaminophen, are generally preferred. Acetaminophen and ibuprofen are both widely used analgesics used post-operatively in eyelid surgery. Acetaminophen has additionally been studied in the context of orbital and Mohs surgeries. The typical recommendation is 500 mg of acetaminophen every 6 hours, 200 mg twice daily of celecoxib, or 30 mg once of intravenous ketorolac for adequate analgesia in this setting. Nevertheless, acetaminophen has its limitations in hepatic disease, while ibuprofen should be avoided in severe renal or gastrointestinal conditions. Memantine has reduced pain in dacryocystorhinostomy. Adverse effects of memantine include confusion, insomnia, and gastrointestinal side effects.

Local anesthesia is well-documented in its efficacy in enucleation, evisceration, secondary orbital implant placement, and dacryocystorhinostomy. Local anesthetics are strongly recommended and accepted as they have a rapid onset and are generally safe. Though, they may cause local irritation and toxicity if systematically absorbed. A minimal amount is needed to achieve analgesia. Lidocaine hydrochloride 1-2% without or with epinephrine (1:100,000 or 1:200,000) is the most commonly used injectable agent for local anesthesia. This vasoconstrictive dose of epinephrine for eyelid surgery provides hemostasis within one minute. About 2-3 mg/kg of bupivacaine or 5-7 mg/kg of lidocaine is sufficient in this setting. A regional supraorbital nerve block with 1 cc or less of lidocaine 2% with epinephrine has been recommended for upper blepharoplasty as it does not compromise the function of the levator. Nevertheless, this block may occasionally lead to formation of hematoma.

Alternative homeopathic agents, such as manuka honey or herbal medicines such as shosaikoto and goresian, have additionally been studied in the setting of upper eyelid blepharoplasties to reduce discomfort.

Future studies should consider focusing on the comparison of various analgesics after particular oculoplastic procedures. Studies would benefit from an increase in sample size to promote statistical power. Additionally, there is limited data on the use of neuropathic pain modulators after invasive oculoplastic surgery. Such investigations will allow clinicians to effectively guide patients toward the most suitable analgesic based on a specific surgery, consequently improving delivery and quality of care. Oculoplastic surgeons are encouraged to continue investigation of novel approaches for postoperative pain management in an effort to mitigate the impact of the opioid public health crisis.

References

"Understanding the Epidemic | Drug Overdose | CDC Injury Center. Centers for Disease Control and Prevention, National Center for Injury Prevention and Control." n.d. *Published*. https://www.cdc.gov/drugoverdose/epidemic/index.html.

Ing, Edsel B., Justine Philteos, Galina Sholohov, David Ta Kim, Navdeep Nijhawan, Patrick W. Mark, and Jaclyn Gilbert. 2019. "Local Anesthesia and Anxiolytic Techniques for Oculoplastic Surgery." *Clinical Ophthalmology* 13: 153–60. https://doi.org/10.2147/OPTH.S188790.

Ismail, Andre R., T. Anthony, D. J. Mordant, and H. MacLean. 2006. "Regional Nerve Block of the Upper Eyelid in Oculoplastic Surgery." *European Journal of Ophthalmology* 16 (4): 509–13. https://doi.org/10.1177/112067210601600401.

Korn, Bobby S., Don O. Kikkawa, Sunil N. Vasani, Mark J. Lucarelli, Geva E. Mannor, Robin R. Seaberg, and Marc Lewis. 2007. "Evaluation of Patient Comfort with Outpatient Orbital Surgery." *Orbit* 26 (1): 19–22. https://doi.org/10.1080/01676830600972708.

Lemaître, Stéphanie, and Miguel González-Candial. 2019. "Evaluation of Anxiety and Pain in Eyelid Surgery Patients: A Pilot Study." *Canadian Journal of Ophthalmology* 54 (6): 723–26. https://doi.org/10.1016/j.jcjo.2019.02.006.

Lesin, Mladen, Zeljka Duplancic Sundov, Marko Jukic, and Livia Puljak. 2014. "Postoperative Pain in Complex Ophthalmic Surgical Procedures: Comparing Practice with Guidelines." *Pain Medicine (United States)* 15 (6): 1036–42. https://doi.org/10.1111/pme.12433.

Meraj, Taha S., Amishav Bresler, and Giancarlo F. Zuliani. 2020. "Acute Pain Management Following Facial Plastic Surgery." *Otolaryngologic Clinics of North America* 53 (5): 811–17. https://doi.org/10.1016/j.otc.2020.05.010.

Myles, P. S., D. L. Williams, M. Hendrata, H. Anderson, and A. M. Weeks. 2000. "Patient Satisfaction after Anaesthesia and Surgery: Results of a Prospective Survey of 10,811 Patients." *British Journal of Anaesthesia* 84 (1): 6–10. https://doi.org/10.1093/oxfordjournals.bja.a013383.

Rahimzadeh, Poupak, Farnad Imani, Nasim Nikoubakht, Zahra Koleini, Seyed Hamid Reza Faiz, and Azadeh Sayarifard. 2017. "A Comparative Study on the Efficacy of Oral Memantine and Placebo for Acute Postoperative Pain in Patients Undergoing Dacryocystorhinostomy (DCR)." *Anesthesiology and Pain Medicine* 7 (3). https://doi.org/10.5812/aapm.45297.

Sheikh, Rafi, Ulf Dahlstrand, Khashayar Memarzadeh, Jonas Blohmé, Nina Reistad, and Malin Malmsjö. 2018. "Optimal Epinephrine Concentration and Time Delay to Minimize Perfusion in Eyelid Surgery: Measured by Laser-Based Methods and a Novel Form of Extended-Wavelength Diffuse Reflectance Spectroscopy." *Ophthalmic Plastic and Reconstructive Surgery* 34 (2): 123–29. https://doi.org/10.1097/IOP.0000000000000883.

Wei, Leslie A., Brett W. Davies, Eric M. Hink, and Vikram D. Durairaj. 2015. "Perioperative Pregabalin for Attenuation of Postoperative Pain after Eyelid Surgery." *Ophthalmic Plastic and Reconstructive Surgery* 31 (2): 132–35. https://doi.org/10.1097/IOP.0000000000000219.

Wladis, Edward J., Michael I. Rothschild, and Tal J. Rubinstein. 2020. "Management of Postoperative Pain in Ophthalmic Plastic Surgery: A Major Review." *Orbit (London)* 2020: 1–5. https://doi.org/10.1080/01676830.2020.1793373.

Chapter 18

Postoperative Pain Management for Colorectal Surgery

Jonathan Gardy Alabre*
City University of New York School of Medicine, New York, NY, USA

Protocols for the peri-operative management of colorectal surgery have their foundations based in Enhanced Recovery After Surgery (ERAS) procedures. ERAS guidelines have recommended that the standard of care to address post-operative pain (POP), is to begin with pre- and intra- operative interventions. These interventions include, but are not limited to, medical optimization and prophylactic treatment, implementation of patient education programs, and establishment of an efficient intra-operative plan. All of these pre-surgical interventions are necessary to help the patient anticipate their anticipated level of POP and minimize the incidence of post-operative complications which greatly contribute to patient discomfort. Once all other factors have been controlled for, the use of nonopioid analgesia is the main focus of reducing POP and maintaining patient comfort. Opioid use is often reserved for after surgery if the patient is not properly tolerating the initial form of pain management. However, the first step in eventually obtaining sufficient pain control must begin with a thorough evaluation of the patient's comorbidities and social risk factors for surgical complications.

Any patient undergoing colorectal surgery must be properly assessed for any potential medical or non-medical factors that may increase their risk of complication during or after surgery. These complications can range from myocardial infarction to pneumonia or infection. An unsuccessful post-

* Corresponding Author's Email: jalabre000@citymail.cuny.edu.

In: Postoperative Pain
Editors: Indraneil Mukherjee et al.
ISBN: 978-1-68507-971-0

operative course can often times delay discharge and increase the burden of pain a patient may experience. Thus, to establish proper post-operative pain management, clinicians must ensure that all risk factors are accounted for and optimized to the best degree possible. Initial evaluation typically includes a cardiac risk assessment that is comprehensive, including many factors that must be evaluated such as a patient's heart rate, blood pressure, and EKG readings. This is because patients with cardiovascular disease experience perioperative cardiac complications at a much higher incidence than those without. In a study of nearly 6,000 patients, a history of congestive heart failure, along with several other comorbid criteria, was identified as a strong predictive parameter for peri-operative death at 5.7% of surgical patients [8]. The cause for their increased morbidity and mortality is multifaceted. However, one identifiable reason is that major abdominal surgeries, such as colorectal surgeries, place a large amount of physiological stress on the patient's body. Stresses such as volume depletion, increased heart rate, and blood loss all contribute to temporary cardiac ischemia which can be catastrophic for patients with uncontrolled cardiovascular comorbidities. A separate study that evaluated approximately 70,000 patients who underwent colorectal surgery revealed that patients with cardiac complications were at increased risk for problems such as anastomotic leak and mortality [8]. It is possible that this association may be due to suboptimal perfusion and circulation secondary to the cardiac complication. Furthermore, another study observed an increased mortality rate following MI in patients who had colorectal surgery compared to other surgeries. Therefore, it is paramount that a patient's cardiac risk factors are accounted for and addressed prior to entering the operating room in order to optimize patient safety and increase the chance of an uncomplicated recovery course.

A pulmonary status and function assessment should also be conducted prior to colorectal surgery due to the risk of atelectasis, pneumonia, or respiratory failure post-operatively. The clinician may order Pulmonary Function Tests, chest radiographs, or oxygen saturation studies. Patients with chronic obstructive pulmonary disease, asthma, obstructive sleep apnea, or other underlying pulmonary disorders are at the greatest risk for complication. A study from the National Surgery Quality Improvement Program revealed that out of nearly 170,000 patients who completed major abdominal surgery, 6% experienced post-operative complications. A similar report stated that patients with pulmonary complications are at much greater risk for admission to the ICU and increased length of stay [6]. The general anatomic location of an abdominal surgery can influence the risk of pulmonary complication as well. The rate of significantly increases as the surgical site approaches the diaphragm, and subsequently decreases for lower abdominal surgeries. A systemic review published in 2006 evaluated the difference in complication rates for upper abdominal surgery versus lower abdominal surgery and found the rates differed by 12%, at 19.7% and 7.7% respectively. This comparison can be attributed to the proximity of these procedures to the diaphragm and respiratory muscles. The rates of complication can even be stratified for many abdominal surgeries depending on whether a patient is receiving an open or laparoscopic procedure. However, for colorectal cancer surgery specifically, a pooled analysis found that there was no significant difference in pulmonary complication rate for laparoscopic versus open surgery with an odds ratio of 0.65 but, a confidence interval of 0.28-1.49. Patients who remain in the hospital longer than the expected time to discharge often report inadequate pain control and require additional PRN opioid analgesics to manage their pain. Though cardiac and pulmonary examination are two major portions of the preoperative assessment, other medical disease and history must be taken into consideration as well. Social risk factors are equally as important to reduce or manage prior to surgery as well as they can greatly influence a patient's peri-operative course. If a patient has a history of smoking, they are advised to quit a minimum of 4 weeks prior to surgery. A 2014 study found that preoperative smoking was associated with an increased risk of post-op complications at a relative risk of 1.73. Moreover, the risk attributable to smoking is modified based on which procedure the patient is receiving. For cardiovascular and oncological procedures, including colorectal cancer resections, the incidence of complications in smokers was higher than in other surgeries. Once full medical clearance has been established by all necessary parties, the patient should be educated on the pre- and intra- operative basics of the procedure, as well as the expected pain level so that they can have a better understanding of their anticipated post-operative comfort level.

While it is already a standard that surgical teams must obtain informed consent from the patient prior to performing the surgery, there is now an emerging field of interest regarding patient education on multimodal analgesia and expected post-operative pain outcomes. Current literature regarding the efficacy of patient education on pain management is currently scarce, yet of the studies now available the results seem promising. One 2019 patient education study looked into the effect of implementing an educational "card" into the peri-operative management of total knee arthroplasty patients. This card was designed to inform patients about the various methods of non-opioid analgesia that they would be offered while also providing them a tool to precisely report their pain scale ratings. The study ultimately concluded that patient-morphine-usage actually decreased after one month of having the card. This decrease in opioid usage can be associated with a possible decrease in reported experienced POP. This report supports the idea that the psychological impact of a patient's expectations about their care can have great impact on their recovery course. A similar study evaluating the efficacy of a pre-operative education program for patients receiving laparoscopic cholecystectomy was conducted in 2015. Both patients in the intervention group and control group were to complete the American Pain Society Patient Outcome Questionnaire-Revised during their first post-operative visit 2 weeks after their procedure. The patients who received additional education about the procedure and expected pain outcomes reported experiencing less pain while also making more use of non-pharmacological pain control methods as compared to the control group. This suggests that enhanced methods of patient education can be beneficial for a patient's recovery after abdominal surgery if they anticipate their pain and normalize the experience. Thus, decreasing the need for post-operative opioid use. In addition to researching the efficacy of enhanced education patient programs, additional investigation has gone into understanding if certain methods of education such as verbal, video, or written instruction is optimal for patient understanding, and if the specific modality may impact their post-operative course. There is no set standard for medical literary among colorectal surgery patients, so depending on a patient's ability to read and education level, there can be variations in how receptive they are to the information provided. A study conducted in 2016 sought to evaluate whether patients undergoing colorectal surgery would have improved outcomes if they were educated on their surgeries via a literary pamphlet with additional video material, versus just with literature alone [7]. Interestingly, the study found that there was actually no statistical difference in surgical outcomes between patients who received a combined (video and literary) education versus solely literary. Further research into patient education on colorectal surgery must be conducted before conclusive statements about optimal education methods can be decided. In addition to educating the patient, the surgical team should consider the psychological impacts that a patient's surgical anxiety itself can have on their post-operative recovery and consider ways to mitigate that stress. While informing the patient about the risks and expected outcomes of the procedure can provide a sense of peace, sometimes education itself is not enough to manage a patient's anxiety. The physician should speak with the patient and extrapolate from them whether or not they are mentally and emotionally ready to undergo their colorectal procedure. In the event that a patient's concerns and stresses about the surgery haven't been properly addressed, their perception of their post-operative pain can be increased as their concern for common complaints may be greatly amplified. As patients' stress levels often rise as the day of the surgery approaches, it may be necessary to offer them a short acting anxiolytic pre-operatively. For example, some institutions have implemented policies in which patients can receive low dose short acting benzodiazepines prior to surgery if necessary. However, the side effects of benzodiazepines must be weighed against the benefits for each specific patient. Excess sedation and psychomotor impairment, sometimes seen with benzo use, can complicate the surgical procedure and increase a patient's risk of morbidity and mortality. According to the American Geriatrics Society Beers Criteria for Potentially Inappropriate Medication (PIM), use of benzos should be avoided in elderly patients due to this patient-populations extreme sensitivity to this class of drugs. Therefore, in geriatric patients it may be necessary to manage their stress with non-pharmacological methods such as repetition of the plan and reassurance, or even some form of alternative therapy. After all pre-surgical concerns and requirements have been completed, the next step in ensuring an uneventful recovery with optimal patient pain control is to enact pre-/intra-operative interventions that maximize patient comfort and decrease length of stay.

A common complication of colorectal surgery is post-operative nausea and vomiting (PONV), with nausea occurring in 30% and vomiting in 50% of all surgical patients. More than any other symptom, patients will complain of PONV, and if the degree is great enough, it can delay discharge and prolong the need for pain management. The leading causes of PONV are related to anesthetic use, opiate use, and the physiological stress of the procedure itself. Patients who receive volatile anesthesia are at increased risk as opposed to patients who are anesthetized with total intravenous anesthesia with propofol. Use of non-opiate multimodal analgesia can also mitigate the risk of developing PONV. However, the use of anti-emetic medication as prophylaxis is gaining popularity in many hospital settings. Patients may also be offered corticosteroids such as dexamethasone, or serotonin (5HT-3) antagonist like Ondansetron. A recently published study from the Dexamethasone Reduced Emesis After Major Gastrointestinal Surgery (DREAMS) trial, found that prophylactic administration of a single dose of Dexamethasone can reduce the need for rescue antiemetics for up to 72 hours in patients who've received open or laparoscopic bowel surgery for benign or malignant pathology. It should be stated that while individual use of these antiemetic drugs can establish a relative risk reduction of PONV by 25%, multi-modal antiemetic strategies has been found to be even more effective. Beyond prophylactic intervention, the choice of surgical approach also has major influence on the recovery course of the patient, which in turn influences the analgesic plan offered to the patient.

All patients who are eligible for open colorectal surgery should also be evaluated to see if they are candidates for laparoscopic surgery. Minimally invasive surgery causes less harm to the body and results in decreased inflammation and recovery time as opposed to open surgery. A study published in 2014 compared the reported levels of post-operative pain and fatigue in patients who underwent conventional (open) versus laparoscopic colorectal surgeries. The specific factors of comparison were post-operative use of patient-controlled analgesia (PCA), visual analog score at rest (VASR), and visual analog scale for fatigue (VASF). Visual analog scores are measures of assessment for patient pain but can be specified for other parameters as well. The study found that for the conventional group, the VASF and PCA dose administered until post-op day 4 was higher, yet there was no significant difference between the reported VASR of both groups. These results suggest that patients who undergo laparoscopic colorectal surgery, as opposed to open, experience less post-operative pain and therefore required a lesser number of opioids after their procedure. A similar prospective cohort study conducted in 2018 found that laparoscopic patients were more likely to experience "peak pain levels" (greater than or equal to 4 hours of pain) immediately after surgery as compared to open-surgery patients. However, conventional surgery patients experienced greater peak pain levels at mobilization at 72 hours. This too suggests that patients experience longer duration of pain after open-colorectal surgery as compared to laparoscopic patients. This increased level of patient discomfort has the potential to increase hospital length of stay (LOS) and delay discharge, as supported by a robust pool of research that compared the varying return of bowel function between both groups. A recent metanalysis of seven randomized controlled trials looked into how laparoscopic surgery with fast-track programs compared to traditional colorectal surgery with fast-track programs in terms of mortality rates, post-operative hospital stays, overall complication rate, and surgical complication rate. The results showed that while there was no significant difference in mortality or surgical complication rate between the two groups, overall complication rate, total hospital stay, and post-operative length of stay were significantly higher in the open colorectal group. This analysis further supports the idea that, if possible, a patient should be offered laparoscopic surgery to diminish their chances of prolonged postoperative pain from visceral discomfort, complications, or delayed recovery time. Consequently, the choice of surgical approach is of equal importance as the specific method of intra-operative analgesia administered when considering how to best manage a colorectal-surgery patient's pain.

The intra-operative period is critical in determining how the patient will recover after their surgery. It is paramount that the providers offer the most efficient form of analgesia to any colorectal surgery patient in order to assure a safe and comfortable post-operative course. There are wide variety of medications and strategies that can be employed when considering what is the best form of pain management. Though opiates are considered to be some of the strongest pain-killing agents available for use, they often cause unwanted side effects of constipation and ileus that can actually extend a patient's post-operative course and increase their discomfort and pain. A fairly recent shift in medicine has sought to discover alternative methods of pain management that are equally as effective, but do not carry the same side-effect profile or potential for abuse. By implementing a multimodal analgesic approach, there are many methods to which opioid sparing analgesia can be administered to patients undergoing colorectal surgery. While these methods may change depending on whether an open or laparoscopic approach is taken, they often include some variation of a combined regional and systemic anesthesia in order to achieve the desired effect. Establishment of regional anesthesia is a core component of ERAS protocols for colorectal surgery. The Transversus Abdominus Plane (TAP) block and the Quadratus Lumborum (QL) block are two of the major neuraxial routes through which analgesia is obtained. TAP blocks are typically performed under ultrasound guidance and are administered via a subcostal approach, lateral approach, or posterior approach. The anesthetic is released in the space between the internal oblique muscle and the transversus abdominus. Each approach causes pain relief from the superficial overlying skin to the deep parietal fascia and abdominal muscles. While the subcostal TAP block is often reserved for upper abdominal procedures, the lateral and posterior are more commonly used for lower abdominal surgery. Studies have shown that when compared to the lateral approach, the posterior TAP block actually results in longer duration of anesthesia and reduced use of morphine. Moreover, the use of TAP blocks for abdominal surgery has been found to decrease patients immediate 24-hour morphine require, while also delaying the time to first rescue analgesic dose. TAP blocks however have not been found to specifically effect post-operative nausea and vomiting. The QL block is a relatively new approach compared to the TAP, and it works by injection of local anesthetic that spreads through the thoracolumbar fascia and paravertebral space. Similarly, there are 3 techniques to the QL block including anterior approach, the anterolateral approach, and the posterior approach. The posterior approach is preferable because there is lower risk of intestinal injury with the needle tip kept separate from the peritoneum by the QL. However, compared to the TAP block the QL block is associated with an increased risk of post-operative lower extremity weakness as a complication. One study showed that the incidence of quadriceps muscle weakness in patients who received a QL block ranged from 1-65% depending on the approach. In addition to both of these techniques, thoracic epidural anesthesia has also proven to be an effective way to manage POP for open colorectal surgeries. Up until recently, epidural anesthesia was used for analgesia in patients undergoing either open or laparoscopic colorectal surgery. However, ERAS guidelines now no longer recommend thoracic epidural anesthesia for laparoscopic patients because studies have shown that it can increase hospital length of stay and time to ambulation without having a significant change in pain control. More often than not, these reginal therapies are used in conjunction with systemic analgesia to achieve an optimal effect.

The most used systemic therapies to achieve adequate post-operative pain control are Acetaminophen and non-steroidal anti-inflammatory drugs (NSAIDs). Acetaminophen has been proven to be a safe and effective drug for minimizing pain, while also reducing effective post-operative opioid consumption. According to a 2010 review of 12 trials in which post-operative acetaminophen was administered versus a placebo, patients in the experimental group had on average an 8.68 mg decrease in morphine consumption during the first 24 hours after surgery. Though greatly effective on its own, Acetaminophen is shown to have an even more robust effect when used synergistically with NSAIDS. When used in tandem, NSAIDS and Acetaminophen have shown to reduce post-operative opioid dosage by 38% and decrease post-operative VAS scores by 35%. This is not to say that use of NSAIDS does not pose its own risks. Some studies have brought to light a potential increase in anastomotic leakage that is associated with NSAID use for colorectal surgery. An increased duration of NSAID administration was positively correlated with increased risk of anastomosis leak. Alternative forms of systemic treatment include Lidocaine and Ketamine. Both Lidocaine and Ketamine have been shown to operative as effect agents in multimodal analgesia. Studies have shown that both drugs can effectively reduce post-operative pain within the first 24 hours after surgery. This effect was especially seen among patients who underwent laparoscopic abdominal surgery. In addition, use of Lidocaine is even associated with a reduced risk of developing post-operative ileus. Ketamine, while strongly evident in its ability to decrease POP, raises some concern among health care officials due to its potential to cause neuropsychiatric side effects. A 2011 metanalysis that evaluated the influence of Ketamine on procedure related pain found that it decreased VASC scores, PONV, and post-operative opioid requirements. However, when the results were stratified to exclude studies in which Ketamine was not found to be efficacious, the incidence of neuropsychiatric side effects rose significantly by approximately 4%. In addition to Lidocaine and Ketamine, Gabapentinoids served as an alternative form of systemic analgesia. As of fall 2020 however, they have been recently rejected as an effective form of treatment. A metanalysis of 24,000 surgical patients revealed that use of gabapentinoids perioperatively did not cause a clinically significant difference in pain control yet, they increased the patients' risk for developing adverse events such as dizziness and visual disturbances. Moreover, gabapentinoids are associated with decreased respiratory drive and delirium in geriatric patients and therefore are no longer recommended as routine treatment for surgical patients unless otherwise indicated.

Management of a colorectal surgery patient's post-operative pain is an intricate task that requires intervention at multiple stages throughout the peri-operative process. With the establishment of ERAS protocols for colorectal surgery, a degree of convention has been developed for how to properly control these patients' pain levels and optimize them for a success recovery. These protocols describe evidence-based guidelines for sufficient care during the pre intra and post-operative stages that are all necessary to achieve sufficient post-operative pain control.

References

[1] Deng, W., Xiaofei Long, Manjun Li, Chang Li, Liwei Guo, Guohai Xu, and Shuchun Yu. 2019. "Quadratus Lumborum Block versus Transversus Abdominis Plane Block for Postoperative Pain Management after Laparoscopic Colorectal Surgery: A Randomized Controlled Trial." *Medicine (United States)* 98 (52): 18448. https://doi.org/10.1097/MD.0000000000018448.

[2] Grønkjær, M., Marie Eliasen, Lise Skrubbeltrang Skov-Ettrup, Janne Schurmann Tolstrup, Anne Hjøllund Christiansen, Stine Schou Mikkelsen, Ulrik Becker, and Trine Flensborg-Madsen. 2014. "Preoperative Smoking Status and Postoperative Complications: A Systematic Review and Meta-Analysis." *Annals of Surgery* 259 (1): 52-71. https://doi.org/10.1097/SLA.0b013e3182911913.

[3] Ihedioha, U., S. Vaughan, J. Mastermann, B. Singh, and S. Chaudhri. 2013. "Patient Education Videos for Elective Colorectal Surgery: Results of a Randomized Controlled Trial." *Colorectal Disease* 15 (11): 1436-41. https://doi.org/10.1111/codi.12348.

[4] Stampfer, M. J., F. Grodstein, and S. Bechtel. 1994. "Postmenopausal Estrogen and Cardiovascular Disease." *Contemporary Internal Medicine* 6 (9): 342-343. https://doi.org/10.1056/nejm198702053160613.

[5] "Dexamethasone versus Standard Treatment for Postoperative Nausea and Vomiting in Gastrointestinal Surgery: Randomised Controlled Trial (DREAMS Trial)." 2017. *BMJ (Clinical Research Ed.)*. https://doi.org/10.1136/bmj.j1455.

[6] Simpson, J. Creswell, Xiaodong Bao, and Aalok Agarwala. 2019. "Pain Management in Enhanced Recovery after Surgery (ERAS) Protocols." *Clinics in Colon and Rectal Surgery* 32 (2): 121-28. https://doi.org/10.1055/s-0038-1676477.

[7] Schwenk, W., B. Böhm, and J. M. Müller. 1998. "Postoperative Pain and Fatigue after Laparoscopic or Conventional Colorectal Resections: A Prospective Randomized Trial." *Surgical Endoscopy* 12 (9): 1131-36. https://doi.org/10.1007/s004649900799.

[8] Smetana, G. W., Valerie A. Lawrence, and John E. Cornell. 2006. "Preoperative Pulmonary Risk Stratification for Noncardiothoracic Surgery: Systematic Review for the American College of Physicians." *Annals of Internal Medicine* 144 (8): 581-95. https://doi.org/10.7326/0003-4819-144-8-200604180-00009.

[9] Schmid, M., Akshay Sood, Logan Campbell, Victor Kapoor, Deepansh Dalela, Dane E. Klett, Felix K. H. Chun, et al., 2015. "Impact of Smoking on Perioperative Outcomes after Major Surgery." *American Journal of Surgery* 210 (2): 221-229.e6. https://doi.org/10.1016/j.amjsurg.2014.12.045.

[10] Yang, C. K., Annabelle Teng, David Y. Lee, and Keith Rose. 2015. "Pulmonary Complications after Major Abdominal Surgery: National Surgical Quality Improvement Program Analysis." *Journal of Surgical Research* 198 (2): 441-49. https://doi.org/10.1016/j.jss.2015.03.028.

[11] Yajnik, M., Jonay N. Hill, Oluwatobi O. Hunter, Steven K. Howard, T. Edward Kim, T. Kyle Harrison, and Edward R. Mariano. 2019. "Patient Education and Engagement in Postoperative Pain Management Decreases Opioid Use Following Knee Replacement Surgery." *Patient Education and Counseling* 102 (2): 383-87. https://doi.org/10.1016/j.pec.2018.09.001.

[12] Lei, Q. C., Xin-Ying Wang, Hua-Zhen Zheng, Xian-Feng Xia, Jing-Cheng Bi, Xue-Jin Gao, and Ning Li. 2015. "Laparoscopic Versus Open Colorectal Resection Within Fast Track Programs: An Update Meta-Analysis Based on Randomized Controlled Trials." *Journal of Clinical Medicine Research* 7 (8): 594-601. https://doi.org/10.14740/jocmr2177w.

[13] Park, J. S., Gyu Seog Choi, Seon Hahn Kim, Hyeong Rok Kim, Nam Kyu Kim, Kang Young Lee, Sung Bum Kang, et al., 2013. "Multicenter Analysis of Risk Factors for Anastomotic Leakage after Laparoscopic Rectal Cancer Excision: The Korean Laparoscopic Colorectal Surgery Study Group." *Annals of Surgery* 257 (4): 665-71. https://doi.org/10.1097/SLA.0b013e31827b8ed9.

[14] Møller, A. M., R. Maaløe, and T. Pedersen. 2001. "Postoperative Intensive Care Admittance: The Role of Tobacco Smoking." *Acta Anaesthesiologica Scandinavica* 45 (3): 345-48. https://doi.org/10.1034/j.1399-6576.2001.045003345.x.

[15] Itawi, E. A., Lisa M. Savoie, Amy J. Hanna, and George Y. Apostolides. 2011. "Alvimopan Addition to a Standard Perioperative Recovery Pathway." *Journal of the Society of Laparoendoscopic Surgeons* 15 (4): 492-98. https://doi.org/10.4293/108680811X13176785204076.

[16] N. A. 2014. "Consensus Guidelines for the Management of Postoperative Nausea and Vomiting (Anesthesia and Analgesia (2014) 118(85-113))." *Anesthesia and Analgesia* 118 (3): 689. https://doi.org/10.1213/ANE.0000000000000140.

[17] Fernandez-Bustamante, A., Gyorgy Frendl, Juraj Sprung, Daryl J. Kor, Bala Subramaniam, Ricardo Martinez Ruiz, Jae Woo Lee, et al., 2017. "Postoperative Pulmonary Complications, Early Mortality, and Hospital Stay Following Noncardiothoracic Surgery: A Multicenter Study by the Perioperative Research Network Investigators." *JAMA Surgery* 152 (2): 157-66. https://doi.org/10.1001/jamasurg.2016.4065.

[18] Lyden, J., and Ingrid A. Binswanger. 2019. "The United States Opioid Epidemic." *Seminars in Perinatology* 43 (3): 123-31. https://doi.org/10.1053/j.semperi.2019.01.001.

[19] "Erratum: Perioperative Use of Gabapentinoids for the Management of Postoperative Acute Pain ((Anesthesiology (2020) 133 (265-279) doi: 10.1097/ALN.0000000000003428)." 2020. *Anesthesiology* 133 (5): 1159. https://doi.org/10.1097/ALN.0000000000003549.

[20] Kirchhoff, P., Pierre Alain Clavien, and Dieter Hahnloser. 2010. "Complications in Colorectal Surgery: Risk Factors and Preventive Strategies." *Patient Safety in Surgery* 4 (1): 5. https://doi.org/10.1186/1754-9493-4-5.

[21] Duncan, C., Jiasian Teh, and Nathan Lawrentschuk. 2019. "Alvimopan for Post-Radical Cystectomy Ileus: What Should We Know?" *Translational Andrology and Urology* 8 (S1): S96-98. https://doi.org/10.21037/tau.2019.02.01.

[22] Keller, D. S., Juan Ramon Flores-Gonzalez, Sergio Ibarra, Ali Mahmood, and Eric M. Haas. 2016. "Is There Value in Alvimopan in Minimally Invasive Colorectal Surgery?" *American Journal of Surgery* 212 (5): 851-56. https://doi.org/10.1016/j.amjsurg.2016.02.016.

[23] Sultan, S., Bernadette Coles, and Philipp Dahm. 2017. "Alvimopan for Recovery of Bowel Function after Radical Cystectomy." *Cochrane Database of Systematic Reviews* 2017 (5). https://doi.org/10.1002/14651858.CD012111.pub2.

[24] Marderstein, E. L., and Conor P. Delaney. 2008. "Management of Postoperative Ileus: Focus on Alvimopan." *Therapeutics and Clinical Risk Management* 4 (5): 965-73. https://doi.org/10.2147/tcrm.s3147.

[25] Dunn, L. K., Robert H. Thiele, Michelle C. Lin, Edward C. Nemergut, Marcel E. Durieux, Siny Tsang, Mark E. Shaffrey, Justin S. Smith, Christopher I. Shaffrey, and Bhiken I. Naik. 2019. "The Impact of Alvimopan on Return of Bowel Function after Major Spine Surgery - A Prospective, Randomized, Double-Blind Study." *Neurosurgery* 85 (2): E233-39. https://doi.org/10.1093/neuros/nyz005.

[26] Mark, J., Deanna M. Argentieri, Camille A. Gutierrez, Kayla Morrell, Kevin Eng, Alan D. Hutson, Paul Mayor, et al., 2018. "Ultrarestrictive Opioid Prescription Protocol for Pain Management After Gynecologic and Abdominal Surgery." *JAMA Network Open* 1 (8): e185452. https://doi.org/10.1001/jamanetworkopen.2018.5452.

[27] Coussens, N. P., G. Sitta Sittampalam, Samantha G. Jonson, Matthew D. Hall, Heather E. Gorby, Amir P. Tamiz, Owen B. McManus, Christian C. Felder, and Kurt Rasmussen. 2019. "The Opioid Crisis and the Future of Addiction and Pain Therapeutics." *Journal of Pharmacology and Experimental Therapeutics* 371 (2): 396-408. https://doi.org/10.1124/jpet.119.259408.

[28] Samuel, M. J. 2015. "American Geriatrics Society 2015 Updated Beers Criteria for Potentially Inappropriate Medication Use in Older Adults." *Journal of the American Geriatrics Society* 63 (11): 2227-46. https://doi.org/10.1111/jgs.13702.

[29] Hensley, P., Margaret Higgins, Alison Rasper, Ali Ziada, Stephen Strup, Clyde Coleman, Kathryn Ruf, and Shubham Gupta. 2021. "Efficacy and Safety of Alvimopan Use in Benign Urinary Tract Reconstruction." *International Urology and Nephrology* 53 (1): 77-82. https://doi.org/10.1007/s11255-020-02621-9.

[30] Apfel, C. C., Beverly K. Philip, Ozlem S. Cakmakkaya, Ashley Shilling, Yun-Ying Shi, John B. Leslie, Martin Allard, et al., 2013. "Who Is at Risk for Postdischarge Nausea and Vomiting After Ambulatory Surgery?" *Survey of Anesthesiology* 57 (1): 1. https://doi.org/10.1097/sa.0b013e31827f2d6b.

Chapter 19

Postoperative Pain Management in Urological Surgery

Mark El-Miniawi[1,*] and Miguel Pineda[2], MD
[1]City University of New York School of Medicine, New York, NY, USA
[2]Staten Island University Hospital - Northwell Health, New York, NY, USA

Introduction

Urology is a surgical field in which focuses on the genitourinary system. With advances in anesthesia, surgical techniques, and equipment, more procedures are able to be done in an ambulatory setting as opposed to an inpatient setting. When implementing the use of endoscopic, percutaneous, and open surgery, urologists require comprehensive pain management recommendations in order to reduce pain. Untreated pain is not only unacceptable for the patient, but it also increases the risk of complications. Untreated pain increases physiological stress during the recovery period. When considering post-operative pain management, one must consider the setting of the procedure, the access site for the procedure, the long-term outcomes, and the patients' comorbidities. At this time, there are no universally accepted guidelines for pain management in urology. A study looking at opioid prescribing patterns in the management of kidney stones in 22,609 patients, it found a very wide variation in prescribing patterns and showcases a need for standard pain management protocols (Salami 2021). In this chapter, a comprehensive review on current practices in post-operative pain management in the field of urology for common procedures will be reviewed.

---

* Corresponding Author's Email: mark.elminiawi@gmail.com.

In: Postoperative Pain
Editors: Indraneil Mukherjee et al.
ISBN: 978-1-68507-971-0

In Patient versus Outpatient Treatment

When discussing pain management options for patients undergoing procedures in the inpatient or outpatient setting, it is important to understand the individual needs and concerns for the patient. A general understanding of when inpatient services should be utilized over the outpatient setting is important as well. In a German study that utilized quality assurance documentation to assess quality management of pain therapy in the outpatient and inpatient setting, it found that patients in an inpatient setting were much older, female, and were more likely to have multiple localizations of pain. Inpatient setting demographics also had a significantly poorer physical and mental health-related quality of life. They also had higher rates of depression, anxiety, and stress levels (Hüppe et al. 2017). This may indicate that patients in the inpatient setting may potentially require more chronic and advanced pain management options in order to manage higher pain chronicity and stress. On the other hand, in the outpatient setting, advanced pain managements such as narcotic medications may be unnecessary. Although narcotics are effective analgesics for all types of pain, it was found to be no more effective than NSAIDS for pain relief in a study of patients undergoing ureteroscopy or transurethral resection of bladder tumor in the ambulatory setting (Tabib, Cwach, and Schwartz 2019). Comparing post vasectomy patients prescribed opioids to patients not prescribed, there was found to be no statistically significant difference in scrotal pain between the two groups. In fact, 7.8% of patients who were prescribed opiates continued to use it at 3-6 months after their procedure. The lack of universally accepted guidance for pain management care in outpatient procedures may be a possible contribution to the over prescription of opioids (Barham et al. 2019).

Scope Procedures

In comparison to open surgery, laparoscopic surgery results in a decrease in post-operative pain and shorter recovery. During laparoscopic procedures, one may be concerned how the location and size of port incisions may impact post-operative pain. A study of 41 men undergoing laparoscopic radical prostatectomy, found no correlation between size of the port incision and pain. It did, however, find location to be an attributing factor to pain. Port site pain was found to be lowest in the left lateral port location and highest in the umbilical port location. It is thought that the incision in the fascia, rather than the port incision itself, and size of the extracted specimen (causing increased stretching of the rectus muscle) may account for the higher pain in the umbilical location. Therefore, there is no apparent need to modify the port location based on the likelihood of exacerbating post-operative pain (LaGrange and Strup 2007). Alternative means of pain management can also be utilized to remedy post-operative pain. In a study at Virginia Mason Medical Center, a rectal suppository was evaluated for post-operative analgesic effects. The suppository consisted of belladonna, a naturally occurring muscarinic antagonist, along with atropine, scopolamine, and opium and was placed after induction of anesthesia. The group of patients that took suppository had improved post-operative pain and had lower 24 hour morphine requirement (Babayan 2011). Intercostal nerve block may also be an option to utilize in laparoscopic procedures. Particularly, in laparoscopic surgeries that utilize the upper abdomen since nerves T7-T11 supply the skin, muscles, and parietal peritoneum in that region. If a bilateral intercostal block is utilized to extend the area of analgesia from a transversus abdominis plane block, intercostal nerves nine, ten, and eleven can be covered and blocked as well (Batley et al. 2015).

As discussed in the chapter on NSAIDs, IV ketorolac shows excellent efficacy in laparoscopic procedures for pain management. The use of IV ketorolac is associated with improved pain scores and reduced post-operative ileus. NSAIDs can be tolerated well, but critical attention and care should be taken in patients with known renal insufficiency, a history of esophageal reflux, or peptic ulcer disease. For procedures such as ureteroscopy for kidney stone management, pain management can be achieved without the need for narcotic pain pills. In a retrospective analysis of patients undergoing ureteroscopy, only 17% of patients who underwent ureteroscopy without prescribed narcotics sought additional pain management with narcotics and only 10% of patients who were prescribed narcotics sought additional pain management for pain control (Salami 2021).

Open Surgery

When other measures are not ideal, open surgery may be the only feasible method of care which could lead to higher post-operative medication prescriptions. Unsurprisingly, in a study of 820 patients that required narcotic refill following discharge, the open surgery procedures with the highest rates of post-operative medication refills were male reconstruction or traumas. The next highest was neurourologic or female reconstruction procedures. Statistically significant patient demographics that correlate with narcotic refill after discharge include diabetes, a history of tobacco use, and use of illicit drugs. It should be noted that of all refill prescriptions ordered in the post-operative period, only 20.4% were placed by the operating urologist (Ellis et al. 2021). Further investigation may be warranted to see why other providers besides the surgeon are prescribing narcotics.

There are several other ways to address pain control in the perioperative period. For patients undergoing procedures that require extensive retroperitoneal or transperitoneal surgery, continuous epidural techniques can be used because of their excellent analgesia and facilitation with enhanced recovery in the post-operative period (Ellis et al. 2021). In a study that utilized the National Surgical Quality Inpatient program database (NSQIP) (a nationally validated program that improves quality of surgical care), it was found that in comparison to general anesthesia alone, epidural anesthesia was reported to have an increased risk of perioperative complications, longer hospitalization, and readmission (Mishra et al. 2020). The risk to benefit should be addressed, but may be beneficial if there is a high probability that a procedure may need to be converted to an open procedure (Batley et al. 2015). An alternative that can be potentially used is liposomal bupivacaine, a slow-release depofoam formulation that can be injected into the subfascia at the incision site to provide 72-hour analgesia for after surgery. Patients in a prospective cohort found it to be tolerable, reported better pain scores (compared to historical controls), and had shorter length of stay (Chu et al. 2019). It is thought that preemptive anesthesia reduces post-operative pain by preventing central sensitization and hyperexcitability.

It is without question that robotic surgery reduces post-operative pain. There are several reasons for this, such as reduction in incision size and handling of tissue. However, pain could potentially worsen up to three days after surgery. A reason for pain that is seen in robotic/laparoscopic surgery, but not in open surgery is peritoneal pain due to distension from carbon dioxide filling the abdominal cavity. This is due to rapid insufflation tearing the blood vessels and causing traction to nerves. Insufflation can cause visceral pain and shoulder tip pain. To manage this, it is better to utilize lower pressure pneumoperitoneum and aspirating any residual gas at the end of the procedure. Studies that have examined analgesia in the setting of robot assisted urologic procedures are limited and make it difficult to make any strong recommendations. A 2015 literature review attempted to remedy this situation by expanding their search to include colorectal and gynecologic studies. As a result, paracetamol, intravenous lidocaine, magnesium, intrathecal clonidine, and steroids were all shown to be promising forms of analgesia in their prospectively reviewed studies, however more data is needed to make firm recommendations and guidance to be universally used. Multimodal analgesia, using different classes of analgesics and different sites of administration, were shown to have improved recovery without symptoms of opiate side effects (Batley et al. 2015).

Pediatric Population

In the pediatric urologic setting, there is no clear guideline or standardization of care for post-operative analgesia. In fact, many pediatric urologists have reported frequently prescribing opioids after routine ambulatory procedures despite believing that patients (infant, children, and adolescents) do not take the most of their prescribed medications. This leaves a significant amount of unused medication in the family home. In addition, due to little education in the pre-operative setting, many patients and their parents improperly handle and dispose of excess narcotics (Garren et al. 2019). Measures are in place, to provide analgesia that can last well into the post-operative period.

In a survey assessing pain management to members of the Society for Pediatric Urology, local or regional block was the most commonly used for intraoperative anesthesia followed by epidural anesthesia. Pediatric urologists have either one of two methods to prescribing post-operative pain medications. Either they prescribe without any age restriction, or they wait until the patient is at least 6 months old. 63% responded that ketorolac was prescribed for pain management if the patient had normal renal function. 20% responded that ketorolac is acceptable so long as there was confirmation of adequate urine output if a bilateral renal procedure was performed (Morrison et al. 2014).

Protocols

Despite the shortcomings of a universal plan that is well utilized for pain management in the urologic setting, several studies have found that existing protocols can be effective in managing post-operative pain for patients.

Enhanced recovery after surgery (ERAS) protocols are multimodal perioperative care standards that aid in achieving better outcomes for patients. A retrospective study on radical cystectomy for bladder cancer that utilized ERAS protocol, found that patients under the protocol used significantly fewer opioid analgesics. In turn, those patients had fewer opioid related symptoms such as ileus and shorter hospital stays (Xu et al. 2015). In detail, ERAS protocol encompasses standards in counseling in the pre-operative setting, nutrition optimization, and regiments for anesthesia and analgesia. This is done to moderate physiological and psychological responses to the surgery in the way that optimizes better outcomes for patients after surgery. One component of ERAS protocol that is recommended for radical cystectomy is to abandon the conservative use of manual bowel prep. Not only does mechanical bowel prep cause abdominal pain and bloating post-operation, but it also leads to higher incidence of post-operative ileus, a slower initiation of diet, a longer hospital stay, and a greater risk of wound dehiscence. Another component for radical cystectomy, as stated, includes proper nutrition. ERAS also acknowledges the autonomic, endocrine response to surgery that induces a hyperglycemic and insulin resistant state in patients. This can lead to poor wound healing, infection, and an increased length of stay. Therefore, management to reduce this state includes pain relief, carbohydrate loading, and reducing the time between preoperative fasting and surgery. Other components covered include nutrition in the post-operative period as well as preventing prolonged post-operative ileus (Melnyk et al. 2011). 70-90% of urological cancer patients can be treated following the World Health Organization's Recommendations for cancer pain control which encompasses the use of cancer pain relief, therapeutic radiotherapy to treat metastases and pain, and psychosocial and spiritual interventions (Zimmer, Greul, and Meißner 2013).

Inflatable penile implants (IPP) are considered the gold standard for men with erectile dysfunction. Patients may be apprehensive to elect this procedure due to concerns of pain management although it is considered an equal line option in comparison to conservative measures such as phosphodiesterase-5-inhibitors, vacuum assisted devices, intracavernosal injections, and intraurethral suppositories. Patients are justifiably apprehensive as the penile tissue has an increased number of free nerve endings and corpuscular receptors. Pain outcomes in the post-operative period vary between patients. NSAIDs and gabapentin/pregabalin have been proven to be effective measures to control pain when initiated preoperatively. So far, no studies have shown a difference between different NSAIDs in effectiveness in pain management, but surgeons may opt to utilize COX-2 inhibitors for its more selective properties. Gabapentin and pregabalin can also be utilized and have the advantage of being neuropathic and antiepileptic. In a 2020 study that examined these medications in different surgical specialties (as there are few studies in urology alone), it found supporting evidence that these medications used either alone or in combination can help to reduce the requirement of opiates to manage pain. Nerve blockade may be utilized in the intraoperative period as well. Since the free nerve endings and corpuscular receptors converge into the dorsal penile nerve, have afferent signaling into the pudendal nerve, and communicate with the S2-S4 level of the spinal cord, they are excellent targets for nerve blockade. This can be performed using local anesthetic such as short acting lidocaine or long-acting bupivacaine. It is still unclear if nerve block should be performed prior to incision or at the conclusion of the procedure, but it may be more of a risk at the end of the procedure as an implant component may be inadvertently damaged by needlestick. A combination of a penile ring and ropivacaine dorsal penile nerve block has some potential efficacy according to a study of 131 men undergoing IPP. As of 2020, no studies compared pain reduction strategies between different approaches to IPP placement. The Einstein Healthcare Network has investigated the aforementioned pain management options and proposed their own multimodal analgesia protocol:

In the preoperative period, 975 mg of acetaminophen, 300 mg of gabapentin, and 7.5 or 15 mg of meloxicam can be given. Intraoperatively, 40 cc of 1% lidocaine and 0.5% bupivacaine injected as a dorsal penile nerve and pudendal nerve block. Post operatively, 975 mg of acetaminophen can be given every 6 hours with 300 mg of gabapentin every 8 hours. 7.5 or 15 mg of meloxicam around the clock. Oxycodone can be given 5 mg every 4 hours for breakthrough pain. On discharge, 975 mg of acetaminophen every 6 hours, 300 mg of gabapentin every 8 hours, 7.5 or 15 mg meloxicam daily around the clock. And 5 mg every 4 hours as needed for breakthrough pain. Overall, studies identifying strong post operative pain management strategies for IPP are limited and more will need to be done.

Alternative Pain Management Therapies

Besides medication and analgesia in the peri-operative and post-operative setting such as narcotics, NSAIDS, and epidurals, alternative therapies can be utilized to manage post-operative pain. In the setting of percutaneous nephrolithotomy, a gold standard for treating large renal calculi, electro-acupuncture was examined against no acupuncture and "sham" acupuncture. Acupuncture has been used as an adjunctive treatment outside of the field of urology in abdominal, spinal, and orthopedic surgeries. It can be easily performed and is noninvasive. Electro-acupuncture has the added benefit of providing electrical stimulation which is thought to release central endorphins. This study found that electro-acupuncture significantly reduced not only narcotic use, but also post-operative pain after surgery (Parkhomenko et al. 2017).

It may also be viable to provide care options that are less invasive. For example, rather than utilizing transurethral resection of the prostate (TURP) to treat benign prostatic hyperplasia, one may opt to consider embolization of the prostate artery. This procedure is not mainstream, but is an advanced technique performed by an interventional radiologist. In comparison to TURP which is sometimes performed in the inpatient setting, embolization is performed in the ambulatory setting. This may be beneficial to a subset of patients who are hesitant to proceed with surgery at first. It is important to note, however, that although it is effective at reducing prostate symptoms, it is not as effective as TURP. Despite its lower effectiveness, it does have a higher safety profile and allows for a quicker return to normal activities. It also has a lower rate of hospital readmission. Patients who underwent embolization had statistically significant improvement in their maximum flow rate and had significant reduction in prostate volume. The reoperation rate for this procedure is only 5% before 12 months and 15% after. The complication rate of embolization is quite low. Of the 215 individuals studied, the most common complications were due to hematomas (4 patients) or arterial dissections (4 patients) (Ray et al. 2018).

Pain Syndromes

It is common after procedures for patients to experience pain. After all diagnoses are excluded, one must begin to consider psychosomatic causes for pain, even in the post-operative period. Examples can include post prostatectomy incontinence of psychosomatic cause, somatoform overactive bladders, chronic pelvic pain syndrome, and enuresis. Considering the 12-month prevalence of psychological disorders in the general adult population is 28%, one should be cautious to recommend treatment attempts for pain that may not be otherwise indicated. Unnecessary treatment may lead to further worsening of pain and other complications. Hence why multimodal treatment regimens are utilized. A program that utilizes progressive muscle relaxing, trains the perception of the body, and provides psychotherapy to reduce psychosocial stressors the patient may be facing may be an effective approach. By providing training, patients can regain control of physiological voiding by having more focus on regulating the external urethral sphincter (Hohenfellner 2019). One helpful form of psychotherapy is cognitive behavioral therapy. This may be utilized by any urologist, or at the very least, introduced to the patient prior to referral to a therapist. It can even be used in conjunction with relaxation exercising, coping skills training, stress management, and more. It is important to help the patient identify and correct any distorted beliefs that are maladaptive in nature through self-awareness. By bringing these thoughts to awareness that can be contributing to pain, one can utilize a behavioral response to correct the situation. Practicing this technique can be done through various exercises or scenarios (Lebow 2021).

Urology is an ever-evolving field. With advances come newer procedures that may be less invasive and cause less pain in the post-operative period. Creating new means is important, however without comprehensive data it is difficult for the everyday urologist to know what the standard recommendations to patient care are. Although pain management practices have proven to be effective, more studies are needed in order to improve patient care further. Additionally, creating a multimodal analgesia program or following a protocol from the WHO or ERAS have also shown to be promising. Care should be taken in knowing the age, contraindications, and chronicity of illness prior to going to the operating room. This allows for a modification of treatment strategies to decrease risk and improve outcomes for patients.

References

Babayan, Richard K. 2011. "Does a Perioperative Belladonna and Opium Suppository Improve Postoperative Pain Following Robotic Assisted Laparoscopic Radical Prostatectomy? Results of a Single Institution Randomized Study: Editorial Comments." *Journal of Urology* 186 (1): 110. https://doi.org/10.1016/j.juro.2011.03.077.

Barham, David W., Leah P. McMann, John E. Musser, John Q. Schisler, Ryan W. Speir, Seth P. Olcese, Joseph R. Sterbis, Timiyin M. E-Nunu, and George B. Stackhouse. 2019. "Routine Prescription of Opioids for Post-Vasectomy Pain Control Associated with Persistent Use." *Journal of Urology* 202 (4): 806-10. https://doi.org/10.1097/JU.0000000000000304.

Batley, Sian E., Venkat Prasad, Nikhil Vasdev, and Gowrie Mohan-S. 2015. "Post-Operative Pain Management in Patients Undergoing Robotic Urological Surgery." *Current Urology*. https://doi.org/10.1159/000442843.

Chu, Carissa, Lauren Law, Lee-Lynn Chen, Candy Tsourounis, Kirsten Greene, Maxwell Meng, and Sima Porten. 2019. "Mp38-12 Liposomal Bupivacaine (Exparel®) Administration in Open Radical Cystectomy Is Associated With Decreased Post-Operative Pain, Length of Stay, and Opioid Use." *Journal of Urology* 201 (Supplement 4). https://doi.org/10.1097/01.ju.0000556082.70020.89.

Ellis, Jeffrey L., Eric M. Ghiraldi, Joshua A. Cohn, Matthew Nitti, Justin I. Friedlander, Serge Ginzburg, Steven N. Sterious, et al. 2021. "Prescribing Trends in Post-Operative Pain Management After Urologic Surgery: A Quality Care Investigation for Healthcare Providers." *Urology* 153 (Supplement 4): 156-63. https://doi.org/10.1016/j.urology.2020.11.070.

Garren, B. R., M. B. Lawrence, P. P. McNaull, R. Sutherland, T. P. Bukowski, M. E. Nielsen, N. Woody, et al. 2019. "Opioid-Prescribing Patterns, Storage, Handling, and Disposal in Postoperative Pediatric Urology Patients." *Journal of Pediatric Urology* 15 (3): 260.e1-260.e7. https://doi.org/10.1016/j.jpurol.2019.02.009.

Hohenfellner, Ulrike. 2019. "Psychosomatic Urology: How to Treat Chronic Urological Diseases." *Aktuelle Urologie* 50 (2): 184-89. https://doi.org/10.1055/a-0834-5989.

Hüppe, M., S. Kükenshöner, F. Bosse, H. R. Casser, T. Kohlmann, G. Lindena, M. Pfingsten, F. Petzke, and B. Nagel. 2017. "Schmerztherapeutische Versorgung in Deutschland - Was Unterscheidet Ambulante Und Stationäre Patienten Zu Behandlungsbeginn?: Eine Auswertung Auf Basis Des KEDOQ-Schmerz-Datensatzes." *Schmerz* 31 (6): 559-67. https://doi.org/10.1007/s00482-017-0240-z.

LaGrange, Chad A., and Stephen E. Strup. 2007. "811: Effect of Laparoscopic Port Incision Size and Location on Post-Operative Pain Following Laparoscopic Radical Prostatectomy." *Journal of Urology* 177 (4S): 271-271. https://doi.org/10.1016/s0022-5347(18)31051-6.

Lebow, Jay. 2021. "Overview of Psychotherapies." 2021.

Melnyk, Megan, Rowan G. Casey, Peter Black, and Anthony J. Koupparis. 2011. "Enhanced Recovery after Surgery (Eras) Protocols: Time to Change Practice?" *Journal of the Canadian Urological Association*. https://doi.org/10.5489/cuaj.11002.

Mishra, Kirtishri, Austin Fernstrum, Amr Mahran, Vasu Sidagam, Brittany Adamic, Anjali Shekar, Adam Calaway, Carvell Nguyen, Lee Ponsky, and Laura Bukavina. 2020. "Epidural Anesthesia Is Associated With Increased Complications in Cystectomy Patients: A NSQIP Analysis." *Urology* 138 (April): 77-83. https://doi.org/10.1016/j.urology.2020.01.002.

Morrison, Kasey, Katherine Herbst, Sean Corbett, and C. D. Anthony Herndon. 2014. "Pain Management Practice Patterns for Common Pediatric Urology Procedures." *Urology* 83 (1): 206-10. https://doi.org/10.1016/j.urology.2013.08.041.

Parkhomenko, Egor, Rohit Chugh, Jillian Capodice, Timothy Tran, Julie Thai, Kyle Blum, and Mantu Gupta. 2017. "Pd35-01 a Randomized Double-Blind Controlled Study Assessing Electro-Acupuncture for the Management of Post-Operative Pain After

Percutaneous Nephrolithotomy." *Journal of Urology* 197 (4S). https://doi.org/10.1016/j.juro.2017.02.1537.

Ray, Alistair F., John Powell, Mark J. Speakman, Nicholas T. Longford, Ranan DasGupta, Timothy Bryant, Sachin Modi, et al. 2018. "Efficacy and Safety of Prostate Artery Embolization for Benign Prostatic Hyperplasia: An Observational Study and Propensity-Matched Comparison with Transurethral Resection of the Prostate (the UK-ROPE Study)." *BJU International* 122 (2): 270-82. https://doi.org/10.1111/bju.14249.

Salami, Simpa. 2021. "Principles of Urologic Surgery: Perioperative Care." In: *Campbell-Walsh-Wein Urology*, Twelfth, 119-34. Elsevier Inc.

Tabib, Christian, Kevin Cwach, and Michael Schwartz. 2019. "Mp15-20 Effectiveness of Narcotics After Ambulatory Endoscopic Procedures: Patient Reported Outcomes." *Journal of Urology* 201 (Supplement 4). https://doi.org/10.1097/01.ju.0000555336.04396.3f.

Xu, Weichen, Hamed Ahmadi, Jie Cai, Gus Miranda, Anne Shuckman, Siamak Daneshmand, and Hooman Djaladat. 2015. "Mp27-10 Post-Operative Pain Management After Radical Cystectomy: Comparing Traditional and Enhanced Recovery After Surgery Protocol At Usc." *Journal of Urology* 193 (4S). https://doi.org/10.1016/j.juro.2015.02.1172.

Zimmer, A., F. Greul, and W. Meißner. 2013. "Schmerztherapie in Der Urologie." *Urologe - Ausgabe A* 52 (4): 585-97. https://doi.org/10.1007/s00120-013-3164-y.

Chapter 20

Postoperative Pain Management in the Vascular Patient

Thomas Kania*, MD and Kiara Singer, DO
Staten Island University Hospital – Northwell Health, New York, NY, USA

Introduction

There are a wide variety of pain management interventions available to vascular surgery patients. One must first consider the specific comorbidities that complicate the care of the vascular surgery patient. Therefore, preoperative evaluation and risk assessment is of utmost importance when choosing a particular pain management intervention. Second, the astute provider should appreciate the wide gambit of vascular surgeries from open abdominal surgery to minimally invasive endovascular procedures, as the pain management for these operations varies widely. The goal of pain management should be to ultimately provide improvement in the care and outcomes of vascular surgery patients. In this chapter, we will discuss pain management for the vascular patient categorized by the various etiologies of pain, including nociceptive, inflammatory, and neuropathic pain. To close, we will review hemodynamic, renal, and other considerations when treating the vascular patient with pain.

* Corresponding Author's Email: tkania@northwell.edu.

In: Postoperative Pain
Editors: Indraneil Mukherjee et al.
ISBN: 978-1-68507-971-0

Preoperative Evaluation, Risk Stratification, and Expectation Management

Before an operation, it is advised that surgeons discuss postoperative pain management with their patients. Preoperative evaluation allows for the estimation of procedural risks and benefits and provides the team the opportunity to optimize any other comorbidities or preexisting conditions. This can be as simple as blood pressure control for a hypertensive patient or as complicated as a multidisciplinary approach to a patient with cardiac disease requiring cardiac catheterization. In some cases, medical optimization can lead to decreased postoperative pain and lessen the need for analgesics. For example, it has been shown that quitting smoking prior to surgery may lead to decreased postoperative pain compared to tobacco-dependent counterparts (Zhao et al., n.d.).

In addition to educating patients about the surgery itself, education regarding the anticipated postoperative course and the postoperative pain management plan can lead to improved understanding and provide reassurance to patients. Having these conversations helps patients regain a sense of control in regards to their care. Patients are better prepared for the postoperative pain they may experience and better informed on possible postoperative complications. Patients who receive preoperative pain management education report less severe pain postoperatively than those who do not receive this education.(O'Donnell, n.d.) It is thought that anxiety, the need for analgesics, and the length of hospital stay can be reduced with quality preoperative education (Kitching and O'Neill, n.d.).

The enhanced recovery after surgery program or "ERAS" involves pre-, peri-, and post-operative guidelines, stressing the importance of education in the preoperative period and multimodal pain management in the postoperative period. It is already standard for colorectal surgery and is currently being implemented and studied in vascular surgery. Though there is not enough evidence yet to form a program unique to vascular surgery, it further demonstrates the importance of education and pain control in all subspecialties of surgery to help lessen pain and therefore ultimately decrease hospital stays and improve outcomes as well as patient satisfaction (Ljungqvist, Francis, and Urman, n.d.).

Nociceptive Pain

Nociceptive pain is the most common form of pain overall as well as the most common form of pain experienced after surgery. Physical or mechanical trauma such as incisions, and chemical/thermal damage such as electrocautery cause nociceptive pain. Nociceptive pain is commonly described as aching, sharp, or throbbing. Concerning vascular disease, nociceptive pain can be the result of surgery itself, pain from PAD, intermittent claudication, aortic aneurysms, and varicose veins to name a few (Seretny and Colvin, n.d.).

Visceral and somatic pain receptor stimulation can both lead to nociceptive pain; fortunately, most analgesics are effective at treating this kind of pain. On a cellular level, treating nociceptive pain involves targeting specific receptors, such as nociceptors on unmyelinated C fibers or small, myelinated Aδ fibers involved in local tissue injury (Seretny and Colvin, n.d.).

First-line therapy for nociceptive pain is NSAIDs, followed by acetaminophen, COX-2 inhibitors, and aspirin. For opioids, codeine, oxycodone, fentanyl, morphine, hydromorphone, and meperidine are the most used. In addition to systemic oral and intravenous medications, there are other anti-analgesic modalities for nociceptive pain such as topical, local/injectable anesthetic agents, and local or regional blocks.

Inflammatory Pain

With every surgery it should be expected that there will be some degree of local inflammation post-operatively as a result of tissue disruption. Inflammation is the body's response to a harmful stimulus. Classically, inflammation is characterized by erythema, swelling, heat, pain, and sometimes loss of function. It results from local immune, vascular and inflammatory cell responses. Important micro events occur during the inflammatory process which include vascular permeability changes, leukocyte recruitment and accumulation, and inflammatory mediator release (L. Chen, Deng, and Cui, n.d.). In order to treat pain due to inflammatory processes, inflammation mediators must be targeted.

Prostaglandin E2 (PGE2) is a cyclooxygenase (COX) product. It is one of the best-known lipid mediators that contributes to inflammatory pain. Nonsteroidal anti-inflammatory drugs (NSAIDs), inhibitors of COX-1 and/or

COX-2, can suppress inflammatory pain by reducing prostanoid production (Kawabata, n.d.).

Acetaminophen and opioids have no anti-inflammatory properties and therefore should not be used with the intention of treating inflammation. Using hot or cold compress can help with inflammation.

Neuropathic Pain and Phantom Limb Pain

Neuropathic pain is most associated with painful diabetic neuropathy, trigeminal neuralgia, and spinal cord injury. In relation to vascular surgery, the most common association is phantom limb pain after amputation. There is no specific protocol for treating neuropathic pain, and each patient is different. In this section we will focus on postamputation pain and phantom limb pain, as it is thought that phantom limb pain develops in 45–85% of patients who undergo major amputations (Kuffler, n.d.). This is no small portion of society. There are approximately 2 million people living with limb loss in the United States and among those with limb loss, the main causes are vascular disease (54%). This includes diabetes and peripheral arterial disease; the second leading cause istrauma representing 45% of cases (Ziegler-Graham et al., n.d.). Approximately 185,000 amputations occur in the United States each year and it is important to know how to take care of these patient postoperatively to try and avoid chronic pain (Kozak and Owings, n.d.).

Neuropathic pain can stem from multiple levels of the peripheral or central nervous system. Unlike nociceptive pain, which is brought on by pain receptors being stimulated, neuropathic pain is a result of damage or dysfunction of parts of the nervous system.

Pain in the amputated limb can occur for many different reasons and must not be taken lightly. If a patient is having postamputation pain it is imperative to rule out infection and ischemia first. Once those have been ruled out, one can then begin neuropathic pain management. Neuropathic pain is often described as a shooting or burning pain without associated skin changes. There are two predominant periods when phantom pain may develop, the first is approximately one week postoperatively and the other is approximately one year postoperatively (Kuffler, n.d.). Neuropathic pain is usually a chronic condition, but can present intermittently as well.

Treatment of neuropathic pain is multimodal. Treatment modalities include injection therapy, pharmacotherapy, complementary and alternative therapy, surgical therapy, and interventions aimed at prevention. Neuropathic pain will respond to opioids, but they are not a favorable long-term solution. In fact, there is strongly recommended that one use tricyclic antidepressants, serotonin-noradrenaline reuptake inhibitors, pregabalin, and/or gabapentin over strong opioids and botulinum toxin A.

Aspirin and NSAIDs

Aspirin (or Acetylsalicylic acid) is a non-selective inhibitor and irreversibly inhibits cyclooxygenase-1 (COX-1) and cyclooxygenase-2 (COX-2) thereby disrupting the production of prostaglandins throughout the body. Prostaglandins are hormone-like substances that contribute to pain and inflammation, amongst their other functions. Aspirin has been used for over 100 years and the usual adult dose can provide 4-6 hours of pain relief. In the vascular setting, the prescription of aspirin postoperatively is often not for pain but rather for its anti-platelet properties and consideration must be given regarding bleeding risks when NSAIDs are used. Aspirin is commonly given to patients after carotid endarterectomy, as well as infrainguinal vein and prosthetic bypasses. It is often used as an adjunct with other analgesics.

The most used NSAIDs include diclofenac, ketorolac, ibuprofen, indomethacin, naproxen, celecoxib, mefenamic acid, and aspirin. All NSAIDs can be taken by mouth, but diclofenac and ketorolac can be given by injection. Diclofenac also comes in a topical form. NSAIDs, as previously discussed with aspirin, decrease the production of prostaglandins and therefore reduce the sensation of pain. At higher doses, NSAIDs can exhibit anti-inflammatory properties as well. In the postoperative setting, inflammation is often synonymous with pain. While most NSAIDs block COX-1 and COX-2, celecoxib is a selective COX-2 inhibitor and is associated with thrombotic complications.

Acetaminophen

Acetaminophen's exact mechanism of action is not completely understood, but its pain-relieving qualities are comparable to aspirin, without the anti-inflammatory or antithrombotic effects, which makes it a good choice for vascular patients, especially those already receiving anticoagulation or antithrombotic therapy (Kitching et al., n.d.). Acetaminophen can be taken in multiple routes including oral, intravenous, and per rectum. Acetaminophen is also a relatively inexpensive, well-known, well-studied drug and is thought to be generally safe. In high doses it can affect the liver and therefore should be avoided in patients with hepatic pathology, such as cirrhosis, hepatitis, or liver cancer.

Opioids

Opioid medications, or narcotics, are well known for their powerful pain relief as well as their addictive qualities. They are availablein oral, intravenous, and topical formulations. Opioids are not commonly used for mild pain, yet are often the mainstay for moderate and severe nociceptive pain. Opioids are often used in the peri- and postoperative settings. Opioids bind mu-opioid receptors in the peripheral nervous system and inhibitory pain circuits. (Nicholson, n.d.) Tolerance to opioids can build quickly and it is important for providers to attempt multimodal pain management and not use opioids alone. This is particularly important in the vascular surgery patient as side effects with higher doses such as bradycardia and vasodilation can occur leading to hypotension along with other detrimental consequences (A. Chen and Ashburn, n.d.).

Local Injections and More

While oral medications are the mainstay for postoperative pain management, regional anesthesia is another excellent option. For open abdominal aortic aneurysm repair (AAA) combined general and epidural anesthesia is associated with superior analgesia, lower pulmonary complications, and shorter intensive care stay when compared with general anesthesia and systemic analgesia. Transversus abdominis plane and other truncal blocks are examples of regional blocks which represent excellent alternative analgesic options (MacFarlane, Vlassakov, and Elkassabany, n.d.).

For carotid endarterectomy, cervical plexus block is gaining favor as an alternative to direct local injection and is associated with benefits such as decreased expense, postoperative resource utilization, and length of hospital stay (Stoneham, Stamou, and Mason, n.d.). Epidural, combined spinal epidural, and spinal anesthesia are all acceptable regional anesthetic techniques for infrainguinal revascularization procedures. Axillary, infraclavicular, or supraclavicular brachial plexus blocks may all be used for arteriovenous fistulas (AVF).

Application of lidocaine to the dorsal root ganglion (DRG) or intrathecally has been show to give rapid relief to phantom limb pain (PLP). Epidural analgesia can decrease the severity of residual limb pain and the prevalence of PLP after lower extremity amputation (Kuffler, n.d.).

Antidepressants are commonly used in the treatment of neuropathic pain. Their mechanism of action is antagonism of the NMDA receptor and sodium channel blockade. Although tricyclic antidepressants are commonly used, they do not work for all patients and are often used as an adjunct for PLP. Acetaminophen and NSAIDs as previously described are among the most prevalent medications used for PLP. The data on gabapentin and pregabalin is mixed, however, these anti-convulsant medications remain to be among the most used medications for PLP and neuropathic pain in general (Kuffler, n.d.).

The use of regional anesthesia offers an alternative and/or adjunct to systemic pharmacotherapy. A potential benefit of regional anesthesia is prevention and management of postamputation pain (PAP). PAP can be categorized into neuropathic phantom limb pain and phantom sensations, as well as nociceptive residual limb pain or "stump pain." Regional anesthesia appears to be more effective in the treatment of stump pain compared with PLP although the duration of pain relief is highly variable. Superior early pain control and a reduction in opioid requirements up to 1 week after surgery has been reported with peripheral nerve blocks and/or epidural analgesia when compared with general or spinal anesthesia (MacFarlane, Vlassakov, and Elkassabany, n.d.).

Inadequately treated PAP puts patients at risk for developing chronic persistent pain. Observational data suggest the use of peripheral nerve block (PNB) for prolonged periods (median 30 days) may decrease PLP in addition to decreasing acute stump pain for up to 12 months (MacFarlane, Vlassakov, and Elkassabany, n.d.).

Ketamine

As providers continue to search for non-opioid alternatives, a promising option is ketamine. Ketamine can be administered byintravenous (IV) route and provides analgesia via antagonism of N-Methyl-D-Asparate (NMDA) receptors. IV ketamine has been shown to provide postoperative analgesia in many clinical trials. However, IV administration of ketamine has limitations as it can only be given in a monitored setting. Therefore, the use of oral ketamine for management of acute pain after trauma or postoperative surgery is highly desirable and is being examined in clinical trials. Oral administration would broaden its utility and permit the drug to be used in a rehabilitation facility or at home after hospital discharge (Buvanendran et al., n.d.).

Hemodynamic and Renal Considerations

Many opiate medications can cause significant hemodynamic changes, which can further exacerbate a patient's tenuous perfusion status. Hypotension is a complication of neuraxial blockade and can be a complication of both opioid and spinal analgesia. Diabetes is another common comorbidity which potentially adds to the risk of regional anesthesia associated nerve injury (MacFarlane, Vlassakov, and Elkassabany, n.d.).

Many vascular patients have concomitant renal disease, in such settings, non-steroidal anti-inflammatory drugs should be used with caution. NSAIDs are not recommended in the immediate postoperative period due to the associated risk of platelet dysfunction and bleeding. Due to these associations, the lowest effective dose should be used for the shortest amount of time for these particular patients, and the use of other analgesics is preferred. It is very common to use IV contrast loads during endovascular procedures thus furthering the risk of potential renal injury. Providers can consider acetaminophen as an alternative if there is moderate pain and/or opioids if there is moderate to severe pain. IV hydration may help and one must monitor renal function via Creatinine, BUN, and GFR.

Summary

It is clear that quality postoperative analgesia and pain management is important for patient outcomes. It also helps minimize the stress response to vascular surgery, which can cause anxiety, tachycardia, hypertension, and vasoconstriction, all of which are detrimental to both the patient overall as well as the results of their particular vascular procedure.

References

Buvanendran A, Kroin J S, Rajagopal A, Robison S J, Moric M, Tuman K J. Oral Ketamine for acute pain management after amputation surgery. *Pain Medicine (United States).* 2018;19(6):1265-1270. doi:10.1093/pm/pnx229.

Buvanendran, A, J S Kroin, A Rajagopal, S J Robison, M Moric, and K J Tuman. n.d. "Oral Ketamine for Acute Pain Management after Amputation Surgery." *Pain Medicine (United States* 19 (6): 1265–1270. https://doi.org/10.1093/pm/pnx229.

Chen A, Ashburn M A. Cardiac Effects of Opioid Therapy. *Pain Medicine*. 2015;16(suppl 1). doi:10.1111/pme.12915.

Chen L, Deng H and Cui. H, n.d. *Inflammatory Responses and Inflammation-Associated Diseases in Organs*.

Chen L, Deng H, Cui H, et al. *Inflammatory Responses and Inflammation-Associated Diseases in Organs*. Vol 9.; 2018.

Chen, A, and M A Ashburn. n.d. "Cardiac Effects of Opioid Therapy." *Pain Medicine* 16 (suppl 1). https://doi.org/10.1111/pme.12915.

Kawabata A. Prostaglandin E2 and Pain-An Update. *Biological and Pharmaceutical Bulletin*. 2011;34(8). doi:10.1248/bpb.34.1170.

Kawabata, A. n.d. "Prostaglandin E2 and Pain-An Update." *Biological and Pharmaceutical Bulletin* 34 (8). https://doi.org/10.1248/bpb.34.1170.

Kitching, A J, and S S O'Neill. n.d. "Fast-Track Surgery and Anaesthesia." *Continuing Education in Anaesthesia, Critical Care and Pain* 9 (2): 39–43. https://doi.org/10.1093/bjaceaccp/mkp006.

Kitching, A J, S S O'Neill, L J Kozak, M F Owings, S Zhao, F Chen, D Wang, et al. n.d. "Treatment of Pain." Edited by R K Albert, D Birnbaumer, and G Braunstein. *British Journal of Anaesthesia* 9 (3): 1265–1270. https://doi.org/10.1093/pm/pnx229.

Kozak L J, Owings M F. Ambulatory and inpatient procedures in the United States, 1995. *Vital Health Stat*. 1995;13:1-116.

Kozak, L J, and M F Owings. n.d. "Ambulatory and Inpatient Procedures in the United States, 1995." *Vital Health Stat* 13: 1–116.

Kuffler D P. Coping with phantom limb pain. *Molecular Neurobiology*. 2018;55(1):70-84. doi:10.1007/s12035-017-0718-9.

Kuffler, D P. n.d. "Coping with Phantom Limb Pain." *Molecular Neurobiology* 55 (1): 70–84. https://doi.org/10.1007/s12035-017-0718-9.

Ljungqvist, O, N K Francis, and R D Urman. n.d. *Enhanced Recovery After Surgery*. Springer International Publishing. https://doi.org/10.1007/978-3-030-33443-7.

MacFarlane A J R, Vlassakov K, Elkassabany N. Regional anesthesia for vascular surgery: Does the anesthetic choice influence outcome? *Current Opinion in Anaesthesiology*. 2019;32(5):690-696. doi:10.1097/ACO.0000000000000781.

MacFarlane, A J R, K Vlassakov, and N Elkassabany. n.d. "Regional Anesthesia for Vascular Surgery: Does the Anesthetic Choice Influence Outcome?" *Current Opinion in Anaesthesiology* 32 (5): 690–696. https://doi.org/10.1097/ACO.0000000000000781.

Nicholson, B. n.d. "Responsible Prescribing of Opioids for the Management of Chronic Pain." *Drugs* 63 (1). https://doi.org/10.2165/00003495-200363010-00002.

O'Donnell, K F. n.d. "Preoperative Pain Management Education: A Quality Improvement Project." *Journal of Perianesthesia Nursing* 30 (3): 221–227. https://doi.org/10.1016/j.jopan.2015.01.013.

Seretny, M, and L A Colvin. n.d. "Pain Management in Patients with Vascular Disease." *British Journal of Anaesthesia* 117:ii95-i. https://doi.org/10.1093/bja/aew212.

Stoneham MD, Stamou D, Mason J. Regional anaesthesia for carotid endarterectomy. *British Journal of Anaesthesia*. 2015;114(3). doi:10.1093/bja/aeu304.

Stoneham, M D, D Stamou, and J Mason. n.d. "Regional Anaesthesia for Carotid Endarterectomy." *British Journal of Anaesthesia* 114 (3). https://doi.org/10.1093/bja/aeu304.

Zhao, S, F Chen, D Wang, H Wang, W Han, and Y Zhang. n.d. "Effect of Preoperative Smoking Cessation on Postoperative Pain Outcomes in Elderly Patients with High Nicotine Dependence." *Medicine (United States* 98 (3). https://doi.org/10.1097/MD.0000000000014209.

Ziegler-Graham K, MacKenzie EJ, Ephraim PL, Travison TG, Brookmeyer R. Estimating the Prevalence of Limb Loss in the United States: 2005 to 2050. *Archives of Physical Medicine and Rehabilitation*. 2008;89(3). doi:10.1016/j.apmr.2 007.11.005.

Ziegler-Graham, K, E J MacKenzie, P L Ephraim, T G Travison, and R Brookmeyer. n.d. "Estimating the Prevalence of Limb Loss in the United States: 2005 to 2050." *Archives of Physical Medicine and Rehabilitation* 89 (3). https://doi.org/10.1016/j.apmr.2007.11.005.

Chapter 21

Obstetric Postoperative Pain

Alexandra Over* and Ana Christina Reyes

Touro School of Osteopathic Medicine, New York, NY, USA

Abstract

Obstetric operations are unique in that they are preceded by a patient's experience of pregnancy and sometimes labor. This context is crucial to understanding obstetric postoperative recovery because it can affect not only the degree of preoperative trauma, but also the patient's expectations and perception of pain. (Lowe 2002, J. Pan et al. 2020, Lim et al. 2020) Childbirth pain is a deeply rooted part of human culture, predating the first analgesia by thousands of years. Even with modern medications available for direct injection into the central nervous system (neuraxial anesthesia), labor and delivery is frequently an intensely painful event. (Andrews et al. 2008, East et al. 2012, Butwick et al. 2018) The rapid and extreme anatomic changes that occur during labor and delivery result in spontaneous perineal tears in up to 46% of vaginal deliveries. (Fynes et al. 1999, East et al. 2012) Women who deliver by cesarean section might avoid labor, but will likely have more pain in the first week postpartum and face a longer recovery. (Burrows, Meyn, and Weber 2004; Buhimschi and Buhimschi 2006) Persistent pain is reported at 24 hours in up to 92% of women after vaginal delivery and 85% of women after cesarean delivery, resolving after an average of 14 or 21 days, respectively. (Komatsu, Carvalho, and Flood 2017, Cappell and Pukall 2017, Andrews et al. 2008, Chin, Vincent, and Wilkie 2014) Although pain is a natural part of the birth process, excessive pain can cause long-term harm to mothers and their babies. Severe postpartum pain has been shown to delay mother-baby bonding, interfere with breastfeeding, and increase the risk of postpartum depression. (Karaçam

* Corresponding Author's E-mail: aover@student.touro.edu.

In: Postoperative Pain
Editors: Indraneil Mukherjee et al.
ISBN: 978-1-68507-971-0

and Eroğlu 2003, Karlström et al. 2007, East et al. 2012, Cappell and Pukall 2017, Lim et al. 2020) For all these reasons, obstetric postoperative pain is a topic of universal interest with many conflicting opinions. This chapter aims to outline a few of the important variables to consider in the pathogenesis and treatment of obstetric postoperative pain.

Mechanisms of Injury and Pain During Childbirth

Birth-related trauma depends primarily on mode of delivery. Vaginal deliveries can be broadly categorized into spontaneous, induced, and assisted. Cesarean deliveries can be differentiated in three main ways—planned vs. emergency, primary vs. repeat, and with vs. without a preceding trial of labor. Although researchers disagree about the optimal mode of delivery, it is well established that operative interventions, especially when unplanned, increase the risk of trauma and complications. Here we will discuss in greater detail the types of pain and potential injury associated with each mode of delivery.

Most women begin delivery with labor—uterine contractions resulting in cervical dilation. Labor pain is complex and multimodal, involving both nociceptive and neuropathic components. Nociception, or the sensation of tissue damage from stretching, tearing and inflammation, is transmitted through two different neurological pathways during vaginal delivery—visceral and somatic.

During the first stage of labor, dilation of the endocervix and lower uterine segment trigger visceral nociceptors with every contraction. Unmyelinated C fibers running parallel to sympathetic efferents carry this impulse back to the sympathetic chain ganglia, and then disperse the signal along projections to multiple spinal cord levels. This produces the diffuse sensation of visceral pain described as "cramping", "heavy", or "pulling", and can also cause constant, referred pain to the T10-L1 dermatomes that is sometimes referred to as "back labor". (Lowe 2002)

During the second stage of labor, fetal descent through the birth canal is primarily felt via myelinated, somatosensory A-delta fibers, including the cutaneous branches of the ilioinguinal or genitofemoral nerve, and the pudendal nerves that travel with parasympathetic efferents. The pain during the final stretch of the perineum when the baby is crowning has been called the "ring of fire" by both Aristotle and modern-day obstetricians. (Dahlen et al. 2009) This "burning" "cracking" or "breaking" sensation at the end of the second stage can be attributed to a combination of sharply localized perineal nociception and neuropathic pain from direct nerve damage. (Dahlen et al. 2009) Computer models of the pelvic floor at maximal descent indicate the inferior rectal nerve and perineal nerve to the anal sphincter are at greatest risk of injury. (Lien et al. 2005) Compression or stretching of the sacral plexus can additionally cause neuropathic pain referral to the lower lumbar or sacral dermatomes. (Hutton et al. 2009)

If labor does not begin spontaneously, labor can be induced with uterotonic medications or procedures such as an amniotomy. Over 22% of pregnant women in the United States undergo artificial labor induction in order to limit the duration of high-risk pregnancies or to prevent full-term babies from growing too large and causing further trauma during delivery. ("ACOG Practice Bulletin No. 107: Induction of Labor" 2009) The main danger of this intervention is that hyperstimulation of the uterus before the cervix is sufficiently ripened can cause fetal hypoxia and require conversion to an emergency cesarean section. Cervical ripening can be hastened with synthetic prostaglandins or mechanical dilation of the cervix using a foley catheter. The ARRIVE trial published in 2018 found that labor induction at 39 weeks actually reduced the rate of C-sections, as well as the reported pain during delivery. (Grobman et al. 2018) Of note, pharmaceutical induction has been found to be less successful in overweight women— requiring longer labor, larger dosages of oxytocin, and more frequently resulting in cesarean delivery. (Ellis et al. 2019) Considering that fetal macrosomia is a frequent indication for early labor induction, maternal diabetes and obesity are important comorbidities to keep in mind.

For laboring patients who are unable to progress through the second stage, obstetricians can assist in delivery of the neonate with tools like obstetric forceps or a vacuum. In 2017, operative vaginal deliveries comprised 3.1% of all deliveries in the United States. (Martin et al. 2017) The decision to use these instruments can be high-risk, high-reward. Success might save a patient from emergency cesarean section but failed attempts can cause more pain and significant perineal or anorectal damage. One recent study found that successful instrumental deliveries were associated with a 45% reduction in severe maternal morbidity, but failed attempts led to a 214% increase in severe maternal morbidity and a 78% increase in severe unexpected neonatal morbidity. (Panelli et al. 2021) Vacuums are used in cases of relatively easy extraction, whereas forceps are both more difficult to use and more effective at grasping the fetal head. (Mohamed-Ahmed, Hinshaw, and Knight 2019) Use of forceps often requires additional anesthesia such as an epidural top-off or a regional nerve block because it causes additional stretching to the birth canal. Mothers recovering from an operative vaginal delivery are therefore more likely to have severe perineal tears, anorectal trauma, and long-term dyspareunia. (N. O. Rosen and Pukall 2016; Karaçam and Eroğlu 2003; Andrews et al. 2008)

Historically, obstetricians routinely facilitated vaginal deliveries with episiotomy, which is an incision made to widen the birth canal. Although episiotomies are intended to reduce maternal and fetal trauma, routinely performed episiotomies have been found to cause higher overall rates of obstetric anal sphincter injuries (OASIS) and severe perineal laceration in both concurrent and future deliveries. In 1996, the World Health Organization began advocating for a reduction in episiotomy rate to only 10% of deliveries. ("Care in Normal Birth: A Practical Guide. Technical Group, World Health Organization" 1997) Since then, episiotomies have declined in the United States—down to 11.6% in 2012. However, many developing countries around the world continue to have an episiotomy rate of over 70%. (Clesse et al. 2018)

New guidelines state that episiotomies are only indicated in select cases when there are signs of fetal distress, high risk for 3rd or 4th degree laceration, anatomical narrowing of the introitus (such as scarring from genital cutting), or for better positioning of instruments for an operative vaginal delivery. (Smith, n.d.) There are multiple options for episiotomy technique but the most supportive evidence exists for mediolateral incision, as it does not increase the risk of anal sphincter laceration. (Karbanova et al. 2014) Similar to forceps delivery, analgesia for episiotomy may be added to an existing epidural or provided via separate pudendal nerve block.

For non-vertex fetal presentations, or for women who have recently had uterine surgery, a planned cesarean delivery without a trial of labor might be a safer option. Some low-risk mothers may also request this option to avoid the daunting pain of labor. In the past, even obstetricians reported a personal preference for c-section when they or their partner delivered, citing fear of perineal or anorectal trauma as the primary reason. (Fynes et al. 1999, Arikan et al. 2011) Rates of cesarean deliveries have been rising globally since the 1970s, reaching 31.7% in United States during 2019, but the cause and effects of this trend are still not fully understood. (Martin et al. 2019, Buhimschi and Buhimschi 2006) The relative convenience and controlled atmosphere of a scheduled surgery by comparison to a vaginal birth raises the concern that our shift towards C-sections is being driven by motives other than patient health. Although this remains a highly debated topic, it is well established that cesarean sections result in prolonged, more painful postpartum rehabilitation during a sensitive period when mother-infant interaction is vital. This is partly due to a higher rate of infections, particularly endometritis. A longer, more painful recovery period has been used to connect C-sections with difficulty breastfeeding, postpartum depression, and lower overall satisfaction with birth experience. As one example, a 2020 meta-analysis of 1.8 million deliveries found that risk of mild postpartum depression was 33% higher after elective cesarean delivery compared to a spontaneous vaginal delivery. (Sun, Wang, and Li 2020) Other authors have contrastingly shown that postpartum depression is not correlated with mode of delivery, but rather with severe, acute pain in the first 36 hours after delivery. (Lavand'Homme 2018, Eisenach et al. 2008) More evidence is still needed to evaluate these arguments but researchers and physicians nonetheless agree that maternal pain after cesarean section is a key issue in obstetric practice. (Eshkevari, Trout, and Damore 2013; Leung 2004; Hardy-Fairbanks et al. 2013; Lavand'Homme 2018; Karlström et al. 2007)

Emergency cesarian section is the last resort for mothers or babies who are in distress and cannot complete a vaginal delivery. Once the decision is made to perform an emergency C-section, delivery should occur within thirty minutes. (Wilson et al. 2018, Knigin, Avidan, and Weiniger 2020) Emergency C-sections have the highest risk of intraoperative hemorrhage, bladder injury, and failed neuraxial anesthesia, which in turn can result in a horrifically painful surgery or necessary conversion to general anesthesia. (Allen, O'Connell, and Baskett 2006; Yang and Sun 2017; Erdem, Ege, and Bagli 2020; Buhimschi and Buhimschi 2006; Burrows, Meyn, and Weber 2004) After delivery, emergency C-sections confer the highest risk of surgical site infection, endometritis, puerperal fever, DIC, and wound dehiscence. (Yang and Sun 2017) These complications exact a psychological toll as well, leading to even higher rates of postpartum depression and difficulty breastfeeding than elective cesarean. (Trowell 1982, Hobbs et al. 2016) The best way to combat the morbidity and mortality of emergency cesarians is by planning ahead and preparing for who might need it.

Treatment of Intrapartum Pain

Addressing acute pain during delivery is the first step to preventing chronic postpartum pain. As described above, that involves treating visceral nociception, somatic nociception, and neuropathic pain. Visceral pain, transmitted in a diffuse pattern by unmyelinated C fibers, has been shown to respond best to opioids in both human and animal studies. (Dallel, Dualé, and Molat 1998, Ma et al. 1998, Robertson 1996) These drugs mirror the powerful effects of endogenous opioids, which modulate C fiber signals at their many synaptic interfaces across the spinal cord. Somatic pain, by contrast, is more effectively treated with local anesthetics. A-delta fibers, having less unmyelinated axonal surface area to cover, can be quickly suppressed by small concentrations of ion channel blockers. (Liu, Kopacz, and Carpenter 1995)

Neuraxial anesthesia allows both lipid soluble opioids and local anesthetics to be injected into the spinal cord where visceral and somatic pain pathways converge. It is therefore, predictably, the most effective treatment for pain during childbirth and is reportedly used in 73% of deliveries in the United Sates. (Butwick et al. 2018) The two most common neuraxial techniques for labor are epidural and combined spinal-epidural (CSE). Both involve placing an epidural catheter at L2-L3 where drugs can be administered continuously, at programmed intermittent intervals, and/or by the patient herself. Optimal analgesia during labor using these techniques should be carefully titrated to achieve a selective sensory blockade of T10-L1 in stage one, extending down to S2-S4 in stage two. With only a continuous epidural infusion, it may take several hours before the anesthesia spreads down to cover the sacral levels involved during the second stage of labor. Spinal injections provide onset in 3-5 minutes but increase the risk for pruritis, nausea, post-dural puncture headache, fetal bradycardia, and maternal hypotension, which can decrease placental perfusion (Grangier et al. 2020, Knigin, Avidan, and Weiniger 2020) Other potential complications of both types of neuraxial anesthesia include epidural hematoma, pneumocephalus, and Local Anesthetic Systemic Toxicity (LAST), which can cause rapid respiratory or cardiac arrest. (Hawkins et al. 2007; Russell 1995) Neuraxial analgesia is contraindicated in patients with coagulopathy, significant hypotension, increased intracranial pressure, or an intracranial mass. Further specific information about neuraxial techniques and complications can be found in the chapter regarding epidural anesthesia.

Although neuraxial anesthesia is the gold standard for pain control, it may not provide a pain-free delivery for several possible reasons. First, labor analgesia is necessarily limited to avoid a motor blockade that could hinder a mother's ability to push. (Hawkins et al. 2007) High concentrations of neuraxial anesthesia have previously been linked to a prolonged second stage of labor and increased rates of instrumental delivery. (Hawkins et al. 2007, Butwick et al. 2020) In the past, this led to a common practice of reducing or discontinuing analgesia during the second stage of labor to help preserve maternal effort with contractions. Current neuraxial techniques, dosing regimens, and drug formulations are designed to minimize motor blockade and have since been proven safe for use in the second stage without increased risk of cesarean section. (Zheng et al. 2020) However, maintaining adequate anesthesia while a mother is rapidly transitioning from first to second stage labor is not always feasible using the spaced boluses and minimal concentrations that prevent overdosing. (Arnolds and Scavone 2021; P. H. Pan, Bogard, and Owen 2004) This is particularly true for multiparous women who are more likely to transition rapidly. (P. H. Pan, Bogard, and Owen 2004)

Second, procedural errors in needle or catheter placement can lead to incorrect injection location. Even epidural catheters that are initially effective may kink or migrate with manipulation, especially in patients with more soft tissue overlying their spinal cord. The overall failure rate of neuraxial anesthesia for labor has been reported at 12-17%, with a higher rate of failure for epidural only at 14% and a lower rate of failure for CSE at 10%. (P. H. Pan, Bogard, and Owen 2004) The difference in failure rate between techniques may be because CSE technique enables confirmation of the correct anatomical space by obtaining CSF before placement of the catheter. (Arnolds and Scavone 2021) Factors that increase the likelihood of failure include patient obesity, poor patient positioning, practitioner inexperience, and unanticipated instrumentation or operation. (Arnolds and Scavone 2021; P. H. Pan, Bogard, and Owen 2004) It is therefore crucial to consider placing an epidural early during a high-risk delivery that might require surgery. (Wilson et al. 2018)

Third, there are alternate "back roads" for pain communication to the brain that circumvent the area of anesthetized spinal cord. Abdominal visceral pain fibers running together with sympathetic nerves through various intra-abdominal plexuses may enter the spinal cord as high as T5, far above what would be covered for a vaginal delivery. (Russell 1995) Pressure on abdominal organs and stretching of the peritoneum can transmit pain at higher levels or through the vagus nerve. More evidence of these alternate pain pathways can be seen in the fact that anesthesia during cesarean delivery requires dermatomal block up to the level of T4, despite the incision occurring at the dermatomal level around T10-T12. (Liu, Kopacz, and Carpenter 1995; Russell 1995)

If a patient experiences breakthrough pain despite standard doses of neuraxial anesthesia, or if operative delivery becomes unexpectedly necessary, additional boluses can be added via an existing epidural or separate spinal injection. However, if a patient requires more than two unscheduled boluses through an epidural, there is a much higher risk of neuraxial failure during the progression of labor or surgery and the catheter should be replaced. (Hawkins et al. 2007; Wilson et al. 2018) A dangerous consequence of inadequate obstetric analgesia is the necessity for general anesthesia, which uses lipophilic induction agents that can rapidly traverse the placenta, depress fetal vital signs and cause lower one minute Apgar scores. (Obi and J. Umeora 2018) In addition, the volatile inhaled anesthetics used for maintenance of general anesthesia cause dose dependent uterine relaxation and atony, leading to increased blood loss. To avoid fetal exposure to the lipophilic anesthetics, cesarean section under general anesthesia must be completed as quickly as possible. Induction-to-delivery intervals of over eight minutes, or uterine incision-to-delivery intervals of greater than 3 minutes, have been shown to cause neonatal acidosis. (Andersen et al. 1987) This priority on speed may lead to an increased risk of accidental injury. General anesthesia can also cause amnesia of the birth experience that may be extremely distressing to mothers. (Trowell 1982) For all of these reasons, access to alternative or supplementary analgesics is vital.

Systemic opioids, like fentanyl or remifentanil, are the second-choice pharmaceutical option for pain control during the first stage of labor, as they have been shown to reduce pain scores more than any other systemic analgesic. (Hale et al. 2020, Grangier et al. 2020) Unfortunately, systemic opioids can also cross the placenta and cause respiratory depression in both mother and baby, so they must be used sparingly. (Grangier et al. 2020) Another option is nitrous oxide, a tasteless, odorless gas that is one of the oldest anesthetics still in use. It has the benefits of easy administration, fast elimination, and no known fetal toxicity, but it can also cause nausea and transient drowsiness, which may reduce maternal effort during the second stage. (Collins et al. 2012) Anxiolytic adjuncts like benzodiazepines and barbiturates can also be added during the first stage to reduce sympathetic tone and help provide rest that is especially important after many hours of labor.

Regional nerve blocks have proven effective at addressing somatic pain during delivery. The pudendal nerve block is most commonly used to relieve pain from perineal tears, instrumentation, or episiotomy, and can be ultrasound-guided for increased precision. (Patel and Zakowski 2021, Wong 2019, Minzter and Devarajan 2018) Fascial plane blocks are most frequently administered for postpartum analgesia immediately after cesarean section, but can also be used prior to cesarean section in cases of neuraxial failure. (P. H. Pan, Bogard, and Owen 2004) Paracervical blocks were historically used to inhibit visceral pain during the first stage of labor but are no longer recommended because they do not inhibit perineal pain and can cause fetal bradycardia. (M. A. Rosen 2002) Similar to neuraxial anesthesia, regional nerve blocks interrupt the process of central sensitization that transforms acute pain into chronic pain. (Patel and Zakowski 2021)

Non-pharmacologic childbirth analgesics are countless, ranging from psychological techniques like the Lamaze method to aromatherapy and music. Almost every cultural background describes a unique remedy for this universal experience. Some physical techniques like the application of hot or cold packs to the perineum have been adapted for frequent modern-day use. (Eshkevari, Trout, and Damore 2013) Others are have recently gathered increasing evidence-based support. (Abedian et al. 2020, Dahlen et al. 2009, Robertson 1996; Eshkevari, Trout, and Damore 2013, Carolina et al. 2012, Abedian et al. 2020) For example, sterile subcutaneous injections of water and transcutaneous electrical nerve stimulation (TENS) therapy have both been used successfully to treat back pain during the first stage of labor. (Hutton et al. 2009, Carolina et al. 2012) The proposed mechanism is similar to that of acupuncture and relies on the "gate-control" theory of pain perception, where hyper-stimulation of one type of nerve fiber can drown-out the signal from another. (Hutton et al. 2009, Carolina et al. 2012) Acupressure, reflexology, music, and aromatherapy are other examples of low-cost, non-invasive options that may improve maternal satisfaction. (Abedian et al. 2020, Simavli et al. 2014, Nik Yusof Fuad et al. 2020)

Treatment of Postpartum Pain

After an uncomplicated vaginal delivery, most women report resolution of daily pain within 2-3 weeks. Dyspareunia and discomfort with certain activities may continue for weeks or months afterwards but chronic pain after vaginal delivery is generally rare. (Cardaillac et al. 2020) Women recovering from an operative vaginal delivery, an episiotomy, or a cesarean section are much more likely to experience persistent postpartum pain and morbidity. (Lebraud et al. 2021; Mohamed-Ahmed, Hinshaw, and Knight 2019; Panelli et al. 2021; East et al. 2012; Andrews et al. 2008) Pre-partum factors that can influence the persistence of pain include parity, age, cephalopelvic disproportion, and presence of pre-existing chronic pain syndromes. (Hunter et al. 2013; Kalsi and Zambare 2020; Cardaillac et al. 2020) Intra-partum factors, as discussed above, are primarily the mode of delivery and extent of tissue trauma. Although the pathophysiology of chronic pain is complex and incompletely understood, research suggests that acute pain transforms into chronic pain because repetitive peripheral stimulation, especially of C-fibers, changes and intensifies central perception. (You, Lei, and Arendt-Nielsen 2009; Minzter and Devarajan 2018; Cardaillac et al. 2020) Rational treatment of chronic pain involves preventing or breaking the progressive cycle of central sensitization.

In the past, pharmaceutical treatment for postpartum pain meant sending new mothers home with a two-week prescription for oral opioids. Given their documented ability to suppress C-fiber nociception, opioids are understandably powerful tools for relieving postoperative pain. However, opioids can transfer through breastmilk to affect newborns, or cause mothers to feel drowsy or become addicted. (Zipursky and Juurlink 2020, Juurlink et al. 2012; Leung 2004) This issue was brought to light in 2006 by a highly publicized case study of an infant in Toronto who died from opioid toxicity. (Zipursky and Juurlink 2020) The FDA and other regulatory agencies subsequently published warnings against prescribing codeine to breastfeeding mothers. (Zipursky and Juurlink 2020) Further research has shown that other opioids besides codeine are similarly unsafe in the postpartum period and can have unpredictable effects because they are metabolized at different rates depending on genetic enzyme differences. (Juurlink et al. 2012) In response to this growing body of evidence and the ongoing opioid crisis in the United States, new protocols like the "Enhanced Recovery After Cesarean delivery" (ERAC) guidelines have emphasized alternative analgesia strategies that limit oral opioid prescriptions. (Patel and Zakowski 2021)

All current protocols for pain management begin with harm-limiting preoperative and intraoperative practices, as described in the previous section. These include careful consideration of delivery mode, anticipating difficult labor with early epidural placement, evidence-based choices of instrument and incisional technique, and preemptive treatment with analgesia. (Patel and Zakowski 2021; Wilson et al. 2018) Another crucial intraoperative intervention is infection prevention via sterile technique and antibiotics. Prophylactic antibiotics alone can reduce the rate of infections by 60%. (Mohamed-Ahmed, Hinshaw, and Knight 2019) Although some factors of operative outcome are not easily controlled, such as hospital resources or surgical skill, any delivery team can improve patient experience by planning to avoid pain.

Neuraxial opioids given just after delivery can continue to treat acute post-cesarean pain for 24 hours. (Goodman et al. 2005) Low concentrations of intrathecal morphine have been found to provide better post-cesarean analgesia than higher concentrations of systemic opioids. (Grangier et al. 2020) This treatment takes advantage of pregnancy-induced sensitivity to neuraxial anesthesia. Although doses have not been tested extensively in pregnancy for ethical reasons, pregnant women have an estimated 25% lower dose requirement for spinal or epidural anesthesia. (Wong 2019, Bromage 1962) Proposed neurohormonal mechanisms for this observation include increased meningeal vascularity and permeability, increased plasma endorphins, decreased plasma Substance P, and increased CSF progesterone and oxytocin. (Datta et al. 1986, Condés-Lara et al. 2009) Neuraxial adjuvants can also be added to prolong the effect of postoperative analgesia, including clonidine, neostigmine, and dexmedetomidine. (Arroyo-Fernández, Calderón Seoane, and Torres Morera 2020) There is insufficient evidence about these drugs to recommend their use but they have been reported to decrease postpartum pain and opioid use at the cost of causing hypotension and nausea. (Ohnesorge et al. 2020, Bhatia et al. 2017) Neuraxial opioids (and possibly adjuvants) should be considered for women with chronic pain conditions who require more analgesia and have an increased tolerance to opioids. (Patel and Zakowski 2021, Arroyo-Fernández, Calderón Seoane, and Torres Morera 2020) Such cases can also occasionally benefit from an extended hospital stay for neuraxial treatment. (Arroyo-Fernández, Calderón Seoane, and Torres Morera 2020) Otherwise, neuraxial treatment is not applicable beyond the first 24 hours and must be combined with other medications.

The synergistic combination of non-steroidal anti-inflammatory drugs and acetaminophen are a well-established pillar of postoperative analgesia, especially in an opioid-sparing context. (See chapter on NSAIDs and acetaminophen) Acetaminophen and NSAIDs should be used cautiously in patients with cirrhosis, coagulopathy, or kidney disease, but are otherwise considered safe in healthy patients. (Fu, Wang, and Lin 2020; Eshkevari, Trout, and Damore 2013; Arroyo-Fernández, Calderón Seoane, and Torres Morera 2020, Wuytack, Smith, and Cleary 2016) Although both types of drugs may transfer small amounts into breastmilk at high maternal doses, there are no reports of significant effects in neonates. (Fu, Wang, and Lin 2020) A valuable update in the postpartum application of acetaminophen/ NSAIDs is a shift from PRN to scheduled dosing. Scheduled drug administration to prevent pain has been shown to reduce the need for opioids and improve pain scores without changing the amount of medication given. (Patel and Zakowski 2021, J. Pan et al. 2020)

The drug metamizole, or dipyrone, is an analgesic that is sometimes misclassified as an NSAID, but does not have the same mechanism of action or benign profile. Metamizole is banned in the United States, Canada, the United Kingdom, Sweden, and India because it can rarely cause agranulocytosis. It is still widely used in other parts of the world where the risk of myelotoxicity is weighed to be less than its benefits. Metamizole and its metabolites have been found in breastmilk at relatively high concentrations and thus is not recommended for analgesia in lactating mothers. ("Dipyrone - Drugs and Lactation Database (LactMed) - NCBI Bookshelf," n.d.)

Limited evidence exists to support other pharmaceutical adjuncts for postpartum pain. Ketamine has been proposed as a treatment for both postpartum pain and postpartum depression, with mixed clinical results. (Arroyo-Fernández, Calderón Seoane, and Torres Morera 2020) Animal models show that NMDA receptor antagonists prevent central sensitization and ketamine's side effect profile is relatively favorable. (Eshkevari, Trout, and Damore 2013) However, the benefits of ketamine are unclear and its potential effect on neonates via breastmilk are unknown. Pregabalin and gabapentin treat neuropathic pain and do not seem to accumulate significantly in breast milk, but have so far demonstrated only small, if any, changes to postpartum pain. (Arroyo-Fernández, Calderón Seoane, and Torres Morera 2020, You, Lei, and Arendt-Nielsen 2009) One of the more promising adjuvants is the glucocorticoid dexamethasone, either injected locally into a cesarean incision or given intravenously. (Maged et al. 2018) Systemically, dexamethasone has been shown to decrease postoperative nausea and vomiting, and some evidence suggests it can decrease postoperative pain as well. (Maged et al. 2018, Leung 2004) However, researchers disagree about whether there is a clinically significant improvement in postpartum pain. (Ohnesorge et al. 2020) The accumulation of dexamethasone in breastmilk is unknown but similar glucocorticoids transfer negligibly. Further research into ketamine, gabapentinoids, and glucocorticoids may identify niche applications for these drugs with clearer benefits. (Arroyo-Fernández, Calderón Seoane, and Torres Morera 2020; Ohnesorge et al. 2020)

Non-pharmacologic adjuncts for post-operative pain are similar to those described previously for labor, but will likely be performed at home, without medical supervision. The longer time frame for treatment means gradual healing methods like physical therapy, pelvic floor exercises, and herbal remedies to play a larger role. Although some herbal remedies are supported by randomized control trials, the effect of herbal ingestion on neonates is unpredictable and may be linked with increased risk of jaundice. (Abedian et al. 2020; Nik Yusof Fuad et al. 2020) Culturally competent discussion of these options is crucial to creating an effective postpartum discharge plan.

The last component of postpartum pain treatment is frequent and empathetic reevaluation of patient progress, both in the hospital and at early follow up appointments. Although that may seem obvious, multiple recent studies have demonstrated that racial and ethnic bias is interfering with this step and preventing many women from receiving the attention and analgesia they need. Black and Hispanic women are being reevaluated less often and receiving less pain medication despite higher pain scores. (Johnson et al. 2019, Minehart et al. 2021, Herb et al. 2021) Opioids in particular, are least likely to be prescribed for black women. (Mullen et al. 2020) Standardized universal protocols that use scheduled, preemptive analgesia have been effective at combatting some of these disparities but this problem is far from resolved. (Patel and Zakowski 2021; Herb et al. 2021) Black women are still 3 to 4 times more likely to die from pregnancy and birth-related causes, regardless of socioeconomic background. (Minehart et al. 2021) The systemic discrimination belied by that statistic suggests that black women are suffering more at every level of quality control. Other types of bias that can also hinder maternal care and should be kept in mind include bias against same-sex partners, physical disabilities, neurocognitive differences, and obesity.

Conclusion

The pain that mothers endure before, during, and after childbirth is both an ancient monument to their strength and a measurement of modern medicine's weaknesses. Labor itself is a complex painful experience but women who undergo instrumentation, episiotomies, or cesarean sections will predictably face an even more difficult recovery. Physicians cannot afford to dismiss postpartum pain as an expected eventuality because it can have permanent, and widely-felt consequences for women, their children, and society. (Hannah et al. 2002; Leung 2004; Lim et al. 2020; Cappell and Pukall 2017) Recent procedural updates have shifted away from using escalating opioid prescriptions to overpower worsening pain. (Patel and Zakowski 2021) Instead, new protocols emphasize a multidisciplinary and prophylactic approach, including preoperative preparation, intraoperative harm-reduction, and early postoperative analgesia with scheduled dosing. (Patel and Zakowski 2021, Wilson et al. 2018) These methods interrupt the process of central sensitization to peripheral nociception that leads to chronic pain. Women with a history of opiate dependence or with unreliable access to outpatient follow up are particularly vulnerable to inadequate pain management and may benefit from multimodal therapy. Pharmacologic options for analgesia are limited by their potential to transfer through the placenta or into breastmilk and new drugs need further research before safe use. Although much debate continues regarding the optimal techniques and tools for delivery, researchers and clinicians agree that improved planning beforehand, and frequent, standardized evaluations afterwards, are essential to ensure quality care. The dense cultural and traditional context around childbirth can also present unique challenges to achieving adequate pain control and must be individually considered in designing each patient's treatment plan.

References

Abedian, Sara, Parvin Abedi, Shayesteh Jahanfar, Mina Iravani, and Maryam Zahedian. 2020. "The Effect of Lavender on Pain and Healing of Episiotomy: A Systematic Review." *Complementary Therapies in Medicine*. Churchill Livingstone. https://doi.org/10.1016/j.ctim.2020.102510.

"ACOG Practice Bulletin No. 107: Induction of Labor." 2009. *Obstetrics and Gynecology*. https://doi.org/10.1097/AOG.0b013e3181b48ef5.

Allen, Victoria M., Colleen M. O'Connell, and Thomas F. Baskett. 2006. "Maternal Morbidity Associated With Cesarean Delivery Without Labor Compared With Induction of Labor at Term." *Obstetrics & Gynecology* 108 (2): 286–94. https://doi.org/10.1097/01.aog.0000215988.23224.e4.

Andersen, H. Frank, Gail H. Auster, Gertie F. Marx, and Irwin R. Merkatz. 1987. "Neonatal Status in Relation to Incision Intervals, Obstetric Factors, and Anesthesia at Cesarean Delivery." *American Journal of Perinatology* 4 (4): 279–83. https://doi.org/10.1055/s-2007-999791.

Andrews, Vasanth, Ranee Thakar, Abdul H. Sultan, and Peter W. Jones. 2008. "Evaluation of Postpartum Perineal Pain and Dyspareunia-A Prospective Study." *European Journal of Obstetrics and Gynecology and Reproductive Biology* 137 (2): 152–56. https://doi.org/10.1016/j.ejogrb.2007.06.005.

Arikan, Deniz Cemgil, Ali Özer, Ilker Arikan, Ayhan Coskun, and Hakan Kiran. 2011. "Turkish Obstetricians' Personal Preference for Mode of Delivery and Attitude toward Cesarean Delivery on Maternal Request." *Archives of Gynecology and Obstetrics* 284 (3): 543–49. https://doi.org/10.1007/s00404-010-1682-z.

Arnolds, D., and B. Scavone. 2021. "Neuraxial Labor Analgesia Failure Rates in Women with a Body Mass Index ≥ 50 Kg/M2: A Single-Center Retrospective Study." *International Journal of Obstetric Anesthesia*, May, 103176. https://doi.org/10.1016/j.ijoa.2021.103176.

Arroyo-Fernández, F. J., J. E. Calderón Seoane, and L. M. Torres Morera. 2020. "Strategies of Analgesic Treatment after Cesarean Delivery. Current State and New Alternatives." *Revista Española de Anestesiología y Reanimación (English Edition)* 67 (3): 167–75. https://doi.org/10.1016/j.redare.2019.11.002.

Bhatia, Upasna, Premal Soni, Udit Khilji, and YaminiN Trivedi. 2017. "Clonidine as an Adjuvant to Lignocaine Infiltration for Prolongation of Analgesia after Episiotomy." *Anesthesia: Essays and Researches* 11 (3): 651. https://doi.org/10.4103/0259-1162.204204.

Bromage, P. R. 1962. "Spread of Analgesic Solutions in the Epidural Space and Their Site of Action: A Statistical Study." *British Journal of Anaesthesia* 34 (3): 161–78. https://doi.org/10.1093/bja/34.3.161.

Buhimschi, Catalin S., and Irina A. Buhimschi. 2006. "Advantages of Vaginal Delivery." In *Clinical Obstetrics and Gynecology*, 49:167–83. Clin Obstet Gynecol. https://doi.org/10.1097/01.grf.0000198186.71542.03.

Burrows, Lara J., Leslie A. Meyn, and Anne M. Weber. 2004. "Maternal Morbidity Associated with Vaginal versus Cesarean Delivery." *Obstetrics and Gynecology*. https://doi.org/10.1097/01.AOG.0000124568.71597.ce.

Butwick, Alexander J., Jason Bentley, Cynthia A. Wong, Jonathan M. Snowden, Eric Sun, and Nan Guo. 2018. "United States State-Level Variation in the Use of Neuraxial Analgesia During Labor for Pregnant Women." *JAMA Network Open* 1 (8): e186567. https://doi.org/10.1001/jamanetworkopen.2018.6567.

Butwick, Alexander J., Cynthia A. Wong, Henry C. Lee, Yair J. Blumenfeld, and Nan Guo. 2020. "Association between Neuraxial Labor Analgesia and Neonatal Morbidity after Operative Vaginal Delivery: A Retrospective Cross-Sectional Study." *Anesthesiology* 134 (1): 52–60. https://doi.org/10.1097/ALN.0000000000003589.

Cappell, Jaclyn, and Caroline F. Pukall. 2017. "Clinical Profile of Persistent Genito-Pelvic Postpartum Pain." *Midwifery* 50 (July): 125–32. https://doi.org/10.1016/j.midw.2017.04.002.

Cardaillac, Claire, Bérénice Delga, Thibault Thubert, Jean Jacques Labat, Amélie Levesque, Norbert Winer, Thibault Riant, and Stéphane Ploteau. 2020. "Description and Classification of Postpartum Chronic Pain: A Multicentric Prospective Study." *Journal of Gynecology Obstetrics and Human Reproduction* 49 (9). https://doi.org/10.1016/j.jogoh.2020.101769.

"Care in Normal Birth: A Practical Guide. Technical Group, World Health Organization." 1997. *Birth* 24 (2): 121–23. https://doi.org/10.1111/j.1523-536x.1997.00121.pp.x.

Carolina, Ana, Rodarti Pitangui, Ligia De Sousa, Flávia Azevedo Gomes, Cristine Homsi, Jorge Ferreira, Ana Márcia, and Spanó Nakano. 2012. "High-Frequency TENS in Post-Episiotomy Pain Relief in Primiparous Puerpere: A Randomized, Controlled Trialj Og_1824 980..987." https://doi.org/10.1111/j.1447-0756.2011.01824.x.

Chin, Emily G., Catherine Vincent, and Diana Wilkie. 2014. "A Comprehensive Description of Postpartum Pain after Cesarean Delivery." *JOGNN - Journal of Obstetric, Gynecologic, and Neonatal Nursing* 43 (6): 729–41. https://doi.org/10.1111/1552-6909.12483.

Clesse, Christophe, Joëlle Lighezzolo-Alnot, Sylvie De Lavergne, Sandrine Hamlin, and Michèle Scheffler. 2018. "Health Care for Women International Statistical Trends of Episiotomy around the World: Comparative Systematic Review of Changing Practices." https://doi.org/10.1080/07399332.2018.1445253.

Collins, Michelle R, Sarah A Starr, Judith T Bishop, and Curtis L Baysinger. 2012. "Nitrous Oxide for Labor Analgesia: Expanding Analgesic Options for Women in the United States." *Reviews in Obstetrics & Gynecology* 5 (3–4): e126-31.

Condés-Lara, Miguel, Gerardo Rojas-Piloni, Guadalupe Martínez-Lorenzana, Mónica López-Hidalgo, and Javier Rodríguez-Jiménez. 2009. "Hypothalamospinal Oxytocinergic Antinociception Is Mediated by GABAergic and Opiate Neurons That Reduce A-Delta and C Fiber Primary Afferent Excitation of Spinal Cord Cells." *Brain Research* 1247 (January): 38–49. https://doi.org/10.1016/j.brainres.2008.10.030.

Dahlen, Hannah G., Caroline S. E. Homer, Margaret Cooke, Alexis M. Upton, Rosalie A. Nunn, and Belinda S. Brodrick. 2009. "'Soothing the Ring of Fire': Australian Women's and Midwives' Experiences of Using Perineal Warm Packs in the Second Stage of Labour." *Midwifery* 25 (2): e39–48. https://doi.org/10.1016/j.midw.2007.08.002.

Dallel, Radhouane, Christian Dualé, and Jean Louis Molat. 1998. "Morphine Administered in the Substantia Gelatinosa of the Spinal Trigeminal Nucleus Caudalis Inhibits Nociceptive Activities in the Spinal Trigeminal Nucleus Oralis." *Journal of Neuroscience* 18 (10): 3529–36. https://doi.org/10.1523/jneurosci.18-10-03529.1998.

Datta, S., R. J. Hurley, J. S. Naulty, P. Stern, D. H. Lambert, M. Concepcion, D. Tulchinsky, J. B. Weiss, and G. W. Ostheimer. 1986. "Plasma and Cerebrospinal Fluid Progesterone Concentrations in Pregnant and Nonpregnant Women." *Anesthesia and Analgesia* 65 (9): 950–54. https://doi.org/10.1213/00000539-198609000-00007.

"Dipyrone - Drugs and Lactation Database (LactMed) - NCBI Bookshelf." n.d.

East, Christine E., Margaret Sherburn, Catherine Nagle, Joanne Said, and Della Forster. 2012. "Perineal Pain Following Childbirth: Prevalence, Effects on Postnatal Recovery and Analgesia Usage." *Midwifery* 28 (1): 93–97. https://doi.org/10.1016/j.midw.2010.11.009.

Eisenach, James C., Peter H. Pan, Richard Smiley, Patricia Lavand'homme, Ruth Landau, and Timothy T. Houle. 2008. "Severity of Acute Pain after Childbirth, but Not Type of Delivery, Predicts Persistent Pain and Postpartum Depression." *Pain* 140 (1): 87–94. https://doi.org/10.1016/j.pain.2008.07.011.

Ellis, Jessica A., Carolyn M. Brown, Brian Barger, and Nicole S. Carlson. 2019. "Influence of Maternal Obesity on Labor Induction: A Systematic Review and Meta-Analysis." *Journal of Midwifery and Women's Health*. John Wiley and Sons Inc. https://doi.org/10.1111/jmwh.12935.

Erdem, Selami, Serhat Ege, and İhsan Bagli. 2020. "Comparison of Maternal Morbidity in Emergency and Elective Cesarean Section." *Aegean Journal of Obstetrics and Gynecology* 2 (3): 10–13. https://doi.org/10.46328/aejog.v2i3.56.

Eshkevari, Ladan, Kimberly K. Trout, and Jennifer Damore. 2013. "Management of Postpartum Pain." *Journal of Midwifery and Women's Health*. John Wiley and Sons Inc. https://doi.org/10.1111/jmwh.12129.

Fu, Shao Chi, Chen Yu Wang, and Chi Kang Lin. 2020. "Do Postpartum Nonsteroidal Antiinflammatory Drugs (NSAIDs) Affect Neonatal Hyperbilirubinaemia?" *Taiwanese Journal of Obstetrics and Gynecology* 59 (6): 891–94. https://doi.org/10.1016/j.tjog.2020.09.015.

Fynes, Michelle, Valerie Donnelly, Michael Behan, P. Ronan O'Connell, and Colm O'Herlihy. 1999. "Effect of Second Vaginal Delivery on Anorectal Physiology and Faecal Continence: A Prospective Study." *Lancet* 354 (9183): 983–86. https://doi.org/10.1016/S0140-6736(98)11205-9.

Goodman, Stephanie R., Ana M. Drachenberg, Sally A. Johnson, Maria A. Negron, Susan H. Kim-Lo, and Richard M. Smiley. 2005. "Decreased Postpartum Use of Oral Pain Medication after a Single Dose of Epidural Morphine." *Regional Anesthesia and Pain Medicine* 30 (2): 134–39. https://doi.org/10.1016/j.rapm.2004.11.010.

Grangier, L., B. Martinez de Tejada, G. L. Savoldelli, O. Irion, and G. Haller. 2020. "Adverse Side Effects and Route of Administration of Opioids in Combined Spinal-Epidural Analgesia for Labour: A Meta-Analysis of Randomised Trials." *International Journal of Obstetric Anesthesia*. Churchill Livingstone. https://doi.org/10.1016/j.ijoa.2019.09.004.

Grobman, William A., Madeline M. Rice, Uma M. Reddy, Alan T. N. Tita, Robert M. Silver, Gail Mallett, Kim Hill, et al. 2018. "Labor Induction versus Expectant Management in Low-Risk Nulliparous Women." *New England Journal of Medicine* 379 (6): 513–23. https://doi.org/10.1056/nejmoa1800566.

Hale, Susan, Catherine M. Hill, Melanie Hermann, Angel Kinzig, Carol Lawrence, Nicole McCaughin, Cheryl Parker, et al. 2020. "Analgesia and Anesthesia in the Intrapartum Period." *JOGNN - Journal of Obstetric, Gynecologic, and Neonatal Nursing* 49 (2): e1–60. https://doi.org/10.1016/j.jogn.2020.01.004.

Hannah, Mary E., Walter J. Hannah, Ellen D. Hodnett, Beverley Chalmers, Rose Kung, Andrew Willan, Kofi Amankwah, et al. 2002. "Outcomes at 3 Months after Planned Cesarean vs Planned Vaginal Delivery for Breech Presentation at Term: The International Randomized Term Breech Trial." *Journal of the American Medical Association* 287 (14): 1822–31. https://doi.org/10.1001/jama.287.14.1822.

Hardy-Fairbanks, Abbey J., Michele R. Lauria, Todd Mackenzie, and Martin Mccarthy. 2013. "Intensity and Unpleasantness of Pain Following Vaginal and Cesarean Delivery: A Prospective Evaluation." *Birth* 40 (2): 125–33. https://doi.org/10.1111/birt.12039.

Hawkins, Joy L., James F. Arens, Brenda A. Bucklin, Richard T. Connis, Patricia A. Dailey, David R. Gambling, David G. Nickinovich, et al. 2007. "Practice Guidelines for Obstetric Anesthesia: An Updated Report by the American Society of Anesthesiologists Task Force on Obstetric Anesthesia." *Anesthesiology*. Lippincott Williams and Wilkins. https://doi.org/10.1097/01.anes.0000264744.63275.10.

Herb, Joshua N., Brittney M. Williams, Kevin A. Chen, Jessica C. Young, Brooke A. Chidgey, Peggy P. McNaull, and Karyn B. Stitzenberg. 2021. "The Impact of Standard Postoperative Opioid Prescribing Guidelines on Racial Differences in Opioid Prescribing: A Retrospective Review." In *Surgery (United States)*. Mosby Inc. https://doi.org/10.1016/j.surg.2020.12.034.

Hobbs, Amy J., Cynthia A. Mannion, Sheila W. McDonald, Meredith Brockway, and Suzanne C. Tough. 2016. "The Impact of Caesarean Section on Breastfeeding Initiation, Duration and Difficulties in the First Four Months Postpartum." *BMC Pregnancy and Childbirth* 16 (1): 1–9. https://doi.org/10.1186/s12884-016-0876-1.

Hunter, Corey, Nimish Davé, Sudhir Diwan, and Timothy Deer. 2013. "Neuromodulation of Pelvic Visceral Pain: Review of the Literature and Case Series of Potential Novel Targets for Treatment." *Pain Practice* 13 (1): 3–17. https://doi.org/10.1111/j.1533-2500.2012.00558.x.

Hutton, E. K., M. Kasperink, M. Rutten, A. Reitsma, and B. Wainman. 2009. "Sterile Water Injection for Labour Pain: A Systematic Review and Meta-Analysis of Randomised Controlled Trials." *BJOG: An International Journal of Obstetrics and Gynaecology* 116 (9): 1158–66. https://doi.org/10.1111/j.1471-0528.2009.02221.x.

Johnson, Jasmine D., Ifeyinwa V. Asiodu, Christine P. McKenzie, Christine Tucker, Kristin P. Tully, Katherine Bryant, Sarah Verbiest, and Alison M. Stuebe. 2019. "Racial and Ethnic Inequities in Postpartum Pain Evaluation and Management." *Obstetrics and Gynecology* 134 (6): 1155–62. https://doi.org/10.1097/AOG.0000000000003505.

Juurlink, David N, Tara Gomes, Astrid Guttmann, Chelsea Hellings, Marco L A Sivilotti, Marie-Andrée Harvey, Muhammad M Mamdani, and Marie-andr E É Harvey. 2012. "Clinical Toxicology Postpartum Maternal Codeine Therapy and the Risk of Adverse Neonatal Outcomes: A Retrospective Cohort Study Postpartum Maternal Codeine Therapy and the Risk of Adverse Neonatal Outcomes: A Retrospective Cohort Study." https://doi.org/10.3109/15563650.2012.681052.

Kalsi, Jasmine, and Sonal Zambare. 2020. "Chronic Pain After Cesarean Delivery." *Topics in Pain Management* 36 (1): 1–8. https://doi.org/10.1097/01.tpm.0000694228.69712.2e.

Karaçam, Zekiye, and Kafiye Eroğlu. 2003. "Effects of Episiotomy on Bonding and Mothers' Health." *Journal of Advanced Nursing* 43 (4): 384–94. https://doi.org/10.1046/j.1365-2648.2003.02727.x.

Karbanova, Jaroslava, Zdenek Rusavy, Lucie Betincova, Magdalena Jansova, Pavlina Necesalova, and Vladimir Kalis. 2014. "Clinical Evaluation of Early Postpartum Pain and Healing Outcomes after Mediolateral versus Lateral Episiotomy." *International Journal of Gynecology and Obstetrics* 127 (2): 152–56. https://doi.org/10.1016/j.ijgo.2014.05.025.

Karlström, Annika, Regina Engström-Olofsson, Karl Gustaf Norbergh, Mats Sjöling, and Ingegerd Hildingsson. 2007. "Postoperative Pain after Cesarean Birth Affects Breastfeeding and Infant Care." *JOGNN - Journal of Obstetric, Gynecologic, and Neonatal Nursing* 36 (5): 430–40. https://doi.org/10.1111/j.1552-6909.2007.00160.x.

Knigin, David, Alexander Avidan, and Carolyn F. Weiniger. 2020. "The Effect of Spinal Hypotension and Anesthesia-to-Delivery Time Interval on Neonatal Outcomes in Planned Cesarean Delivery." *American Journal of Obstetrics and Gynecology* 223 (5): 747.e1-747.e13. https://doi.org/10.1016/j.ajog.2020.08.005.

Komatsu, Ryu, Brendan Carvalho, and Pamela D. Flood. 2017. "Recovery after Nulliparous Birth: A Detailed Analysis of Pain Analgesia and Recovery of Function." *Anesthesiology* 127 (4): 684–94. https://doi.org/10.1097/ALN.0000000 000001789.

Lavand'Homme, Patricia. 2018. "Postoperative Cesarean Pain: Real but Is It Preventable?" *Current Opinion in Anaesthesiology*. Lippincott Williams and Wilkins. https://doi.org/10.1097/ACO.0000000000000585.

Lebraud, Margaux, Romain Griffier, Salwa Hmila, Yves Aubard, Tristan Gauthier, Olivier Parant, and Paul Guerby. 2021. "Comparison of Maternal and Neonatal Outcomes after Forceps or Spatulas-Assisted Delivery." *European Journal of Obstetrics and Gynecology and Reproductive Biology* 258 (March): 126–31. https://doi.org/10.1016/j.ejogrb.2020.12.057.

Leung, Albert Y. 2004. "Postoperative Pain Management in Obstetric Anesthesia-New Challenges and Solutions." *Journal of Clinical Anesthesia.* Elsevier Inc. https://doi.org/10.1016/j.jclinane.2003.02.012.

Lien, Kuo Cheng, Daniel M. Morgan, John O. L. Delancey, and James A. Ashton-Miller. 2005. "Pudendal Nerve Stretch during Vaginal Birth: A 3D Computer Simulation." *American Journal of Obstetrics and Gynecology* 192 (5 SPEC. ISS.): 1669–76. https://doi.org/10.1016/j.ajog.2005.01.032.

Lim, Grace, Kelsea R. Lasorda, Lia M. Farrell, Ann M. McCarthy, Francesca Facco, and Ajay D. Wasan. 2020. "Obstetric Pain Correlates with Postpartum Depression Symptoms: A Pilot Prospective Observational Study." *BMC Pregnancy and Childbirth* 20 (1): 1–14. https://doi.org/10.1186/s12884-020-02943-7.

Liu, S., D. J. Kopacz, and R. L. Carpenter. 1995. "Quantitative Assessment of Differential Sensory Nerve Block after Lidocaine Spinal Anesthesia." *Anesthesiology* 82 (1): 60–63. https://doi.org/10.1097/00000542-199501000-00009.

Lowe, Nancy K. 2002. "The Nature of Labor Pain." *American Journal of Obstetrics and Gynecology* 186 (5): S16–24. https://doi.org/10.1016/s0002-9378(02)70179-8.

Ma, D., S. M. Sapsed-Byrne, M. K. Chakrabarti, and J. G. Whitwam. 1998. "Synergistic Antinociceptive Interaction between Sevoflurane and Intrathecal Fentanyl in Dogs." *British Journal of Anaesthesia* 80 (6): 800–806. https://doi.org/10.1093/bja/80.6.800.

Maged, Ahmed M., Wesam Sayed Deeb, Sahar Elbaradie, Ahmed R. Elzayat, Ahmed A. Metwally, Mohamed Hamed, and Ahmed Shaker. 2018. "Comparison of Local and Intra Venous Dexamethasone on Post Operative Pain and Recovery after Caesersam Section. A Randomized Controlled Trial." *Taiwanese Journal of Obstetrics and Gynecology* 57 (3): 346–50. https://doi.org/10.1016/j.tjog.2018.04.004.

Martin, Joyce A, Brady E Hamilton, Michelle J K Osterman, and Anne K Driscoll. 2019. "National Vital Statistics Reports Volume 70, Number 2, March 23 Births: Final Data for 2019."

Martin, Joyce A, Brady E Hamilton, Michelle J K Osterman, Anne K Driscoll, and Patrick Drake. 2017. "National Vital Statistics Reports Volume 67, Number 8, November 7, 2018." *National Vital Statistics Reports.* Vol. 67.

Minehart, Rebecca D., Allison S. Bryant, Jaleesa Jackson, and Jaime L. Daly. 2021. "Racial/Ethnic Inequities in Pregnancy-Related Morbidity and Mortality." *Obstetrics and Gynecology Clinics of North America.* W. B. Saunders. https://doi.org/10.1016/j.ogc.2020.11.005.

Minzter, Beth H., and Jagan Devarajan. 2018. "Mechanisms of Labor Analgesia." In *Fundamentals of Pain Medicine*, 127–40. Springer International Publishing. https://doi.org/10.1007/978-3-319-64922-1_15.

Mohamed-Ahmed, Olaa, Kim Hinshaw, and Marian Knight. 2019. "Operative Vaginal Delivery and Post-Partum Infection." *Best Practice and Research: Clinical Obstetrics and Gynaecology.* Bailliere Tindall Ltd. https://doi.org/10.1016/j.bpobgyn.2018.09.005.

Mullen, Courtney Olivia, Jonathan Shepherd, Bonnie Campbell, and Richard Feinn. 2020. "Opioid Prescription Practices in the Postpartum Period." *Journal of the American College of Surgeons* 231 (4): S182–83. https://doi.org/10.1016/j.jamcollsurg.2020.07.297.

Nik Yusof Fuad, Nik Farah, Siew Mooi Ching, Dayangku Hayaty Awg Dzulkarnain, Ai Theng Cheong, and Zainul Amiruddin Zakaria. 2020. "Complementary Alternative Medicine Use among Postpartum Mothers in a Primary Care Setting: A Cross-Sectional Study in Malaysia." *BMC Complementary Medicine and Therapies* 20 (1): 197. https://doi.org/10.1186/s12906-020-02984-7.

Obi, VitusOkwuchukwu, and OdidikaUgochukwu J. Umeora. 2018. "Anesthesia for Emergency Cesarean Section: A Comparison of Spinal versus General Anesthesia on Maternal and Neonatal Outcomes." *African Journal of Medical and Health Sciences* 17 (1): 31. https://doi.org/10.4103/ajmhs.ajmhs_33_18.

Ohnesorge, Henning, Veronika Günther, Matthias Grünewald, Nicolai Maass, and İbrahim Alkatout. 2020. "Postoperative Pain Management in Obstetrics and Gynecology." *Journal of the Turkish German Gynecology Association* 21 (4): 287–97. https://doi.org/10.4274/jtgga.galenos.2020.2020.0024.

Pan, Jingru, Ziqing Hei, Liping Li, Dan Zhu, Hongying Hou, Huizhen Wu, Chulian Gong, and Shaoli Zhou. 2020. "The Advantage of Implementation of Enhanced Recovery After Surgery (ERAS) in Acute Pain Management During Elective Cesarean Delivery: A Prospective Randomized Controlled Trial." https://doi.org/10.2147/TCRM.S244039.

Pan, P. H., T. D. Bogard, and M. D. Owen. 2004. "Incidence and Characteristics of Failures in Obstetric Neuraxial Analgesia and Anesthesia: A Retrospective Analysis of 19,259 Deliveries." *International Journal of Obstetric Anesthesia* 13 (4): 227–33. https://doi.org/10.1016/j.ijoa.2004.04.008.

Panelli, Danielle M., Stephanie A. Leonard, Noor Joudi, Anna I. Girsen, Amy E. Judy, Yasser Y. El-Sayed, William M. Gilbert, and Deirdre J. Lyell. 2021. "Severe Maternal and Neonatal Morbidity after Attempted Operative Vaginal Delivery." *American Journal of Obstetrics & Gynecology MFM* 3 (3): 100339. https://doi.org/10.1016/j.ajogmf.2021.100339.

Patel, Kishan, and Mark Zakowski. 2021. "Enhanced Recovery After Cesarean: Current and Emerging Trends." *Current Anesthesiology Reports*. Springer. https://doi.org/10.1007/s40140-021-00442-9.

Robertson, A. 1996. "The Pain of Labour." *Midwifery Today and Childbirth Education* 2 (37): 15–19. https://doi.org/10.1177/204946370800200205.

Rosen, Mark A. 2002. "Paracervical Block for Labor Analgesia: A Brief Historic Review." *American Journal of Obstetrics and Gynecology* 186 (5): S127–30. https://doi.org/10.1016/s0002-9378(02)70187-7.

Rosen, Natalie O., and Caroline Pukall. 2016. "Comparing the Prevalence, Risk Factors, and Repercussions of Postpartum Genito-Pelvic Pain and Dyspareunia." *Sexual Medicine Reviews*. Elsevier B. V. https://doi.org/10.1016/j.sxmr.2015.12.003.

Russll, I. F. 1995. "Levels of Anaesthesia and Intraoperative Pain at Caesarean Section under Regional Block." *International Journal of Obstetric Anesthesia* 4 (2): 71–77. https://doi.org/10.1016/0959-289X(95)82995-M.

Simavli, Serap, Ikbal Kaygusuz, Ilknur Gumus, Betul Usluogullari, Melahat Yildirim, and Hasan Kafali. 2014. "Effect of Music Therapy during Vaginal Delivery on Postpartum Pain Relief and Mental Health." *Journal of Affective Disorders* 156: 194–99. https://doi.org/10.1016/j.jad.2013.12.027.

Smith, Elizabeth. n.d. "ICEA Position Paper Episiotomy Position." Raleigh, NC.

Sun, Lei, Su Wang, and Xi Qian Li. 2020. "Association between Mode of Delivery and Postpartum Depression: A Systematic Review and Network Meta-Analysis." *Australian and New Zealand Journal of Psychiatry*, September. https://doi.org/10.1177/0004867420954284.

Trowell, Judith. 1982. "Possible Effects of Emergency Caesarian Section on the Mother-Child Relationship." *Early Human Development* 7 (1): 41–51. https://doi.org/10.1016/0378-3782(82)90006-8.

Wilson, R. Douglas, Aaron B. Caughey, Stephen L. Wood, George A. Macones, Ian J. Wrench, Jeffrey Huang, Mikael Norman, et al. 2018. "Guidelines for Antenatal and Preoperative Care in Cesarean Delivery: Enhanced Recovery After Surgery Society Recommendations (Part 1)." *American Journal of Obstetrics and Gynecology* 219 (6): 523.e1-523.e15. https://doi.org/10.1016/j.ajog.2018.09.015.

Wong, Cynthia. 2019. "Obstetric Pain." In *Bonica's Management of Pain Fifth Edition*, edited by Jane C. Ballantyne, Scott M. Fishman, and James P. Rathmell, 5th ed., 940–54. Philadelphia: Wolters Kluwer.

Wuytack, Francesca, Valerie Smith, and Brian J. Cleary. 2016. "Oral Non-Steroidal Anti-Inflammatory Drugs (Single Dose) for Perineal Pain in the Early Postpartum Period." *Cochrane Database of Systematic Reviews*. John Wiley and Sons Ltd. https://doi.org/10.1002/14651858.CD011352.pub2.

Yang, Xiao Jing, and Shan Shan Sun. 2017. "Comparison of Maternal and Fetal Complications in Elective and Emergency Cesarean Section: A Systematic Review and Meta-Analysis." *Archives of Gynecology and Obstetrics* 296 (3): 503–12. https://doi.org/10.1007/s00404-017-4445-2.

You, H. J., J. Lei, and L. Arendt-Nielsen. 2009. "Selective Inhibitory Effects of Pregabalin on Peripheral C but Not A-Delta Fibers Metadiated Nociception in Intact and Spinalized Rats." *Neuroscience* 164 (4): 1845–53. https://doi.org/10.1016/j.neuroscience.2009.09.047.

Zheng, Sheng Xing, Wenwen Zheng, Tianqi Zhu, Haiyan Lan, Qian Wang, Xiao Sun, and Ming Pin Hu. 2020. "Continuing Epidural Analgesia during the Second Stage and ACOG Definition of Arrest of Labor on Maternal-Fetal Outcomes." *Acta Anaesthesiologica Scandinavica* 64 (8): 1187–93. https://doi.org/10.1111/aas.13611.

Zipursky, Jonathan, and David N. Juurlink. 2020. "The Implausibility of Neonatal Opioid Toxicity from Breastfeeding." *Clinical Pharmacology and Therapeutics*. Nature Publishing Group. https://doi.org/10.1002/cpt.1882.

Chapter 22

Analgesia for Office and Ambulatory Procedures

Nikhilesh Chitibomma[1,*], Juan Garces[1] and Gregory Haskin[2]
[1]Staten Island University Hospital – Northwell Health, New York, NY, USA
[2]Touro College of Osteopathic Medicine, New York, NY, USA

Ambulatory surgery has evolved over the latter half of the last century due to an increased demand for non-urgent procedures. In the late 1950s and early 1960s, outpatient surgery facilities were introduced to relieve waitlists for elective surgery in hospitals (Reed and Ford 1976). From 1981 to 2011 outpatient procedures grew nearly 10-fold, accounting for 19% to more than 60% of all surgeries performed in the United States in 2011 (Adair et al., 2019). Ambulatory procedures have become a standard practice and provide high-quality care and convenience while decreasing the expenses encountered by patients, their families, surgical providers, and medical institutions.

The application of technological advances and adaptive surgical techniques have improved patient outcomes and expanded the range of procedures possible in the outpatient setting, while minimizing the risks and costs associated with general anesthesia for otherwise minor procedures.

The intent of this chapter is to identify the unique aspects of modern outpatient analgesia with an emphasis on optimizing outcomes and patient experience while reducing costs.

* Corresponding Author's Email: nchitibomma@northwell.edu.

In: Postoperative Pain
Editors: Indraneil Mukherjee et al.
ISBN: 978-1-68507-971-0

Preoperative Assessment and Preparation

Ambulatory procedures are not just surgical procedures followed by a patient being discharged home. More specifically, ambulatory surgery refers to minimally invasive surgical techniques and short-acting anesthetics with an emphasis on patient safety, comfort, and recovery; this allows for the prevention of even the most insignificant postoperative conditions. To optimize patient satisfaction, it is essential to understand their expectations for the procedure, including: a safe procedure with minimal pain, slight nausea or abdominal discomfort, and a rapid return to their daily activities with minimal burden to their caretakers.

Preoperative assessment is an essential step in determining whether a patient is a good candidate for an ambulatory procedure. The focus of this assessment should include a complete knowledge of the patient's comorbid conditions as well as the factors that shape a patient's access to healthcare resources. A complete understanding of the patient's medical needs allows for an accurate anticipation of surgical preparation, anesthetic requirements, procedure duration, and postoperative recovery. A thorough preoperative assessment can also decrease the likelihood of unexpected events during and after the procedure (Painter and Ludbrook 2013).

As with any surgical procedure, ambulatory procedures require the patient to be provided with a complete and detailed description of the procedure, including what to expect before and after the procedure. Adequately prepared patients are more likely to be relaxed and comply with pre and post-operative surgical protocols (Afonso et al., 2019). All information must be communicated directly to the patient along with written instructions in their preferred language, this is particularly important in the management of medications during the preoperative period. In example, there are several common medications that patients need to discontinue prior to any surgical procedure and patients also need to be educated on when and how to resume taking their medications after the procedure. Patients must be counseled on their use of over-the-counter products, herbal products, and even certain habits or activities that can interfere with recovery (Afonso et al., 2019).

Preoperative Analgesia

Traditionally, the intent of preoperative drug administration is to reduce anxiety prior to the procedure. However, analgesic premedication also plays an essential role in the management of pain in the early postoperative period and is important in improving outcomes. Nearly two thirds of ambulatory surgical patients exhibit some manifestation of anxiety related symptoms, as a result different anxiolytic regimens have been developed to alleviate these symptoms and enhance patient experience during and after the procedure (Bailey 2010).

A typical regimen might include the administration of acetaminophen, gabapentin or pregabalin, and a nonsteroidal anti-inflammatory drug (NSAIDs) during the preoperative period. The goal is to initiate preventive analgesia so that serum concentrations are at therapeutic levels prior to aversive surgical stimuli, this reduces the potential for secondary hyperalgesia, postoperative opioid dependence, and other opioid-related side effects (Verla and Iqbal 2021).

While some ambulatory centers give oral acetaminophen in the preoperative holding area, IV administration just prior to surgical incision is associated with faster onset and a more predictable rate of absorption. IV administration is typically followed by a transition to an oral medication as soon as the patient can tolerate it, this is typical of Enhanced recovery after surgery (ERAS) protocols (Luo and Min 2017). Beginning in the early 1990s, ERAS protocols were developed for colorectal surgery and more recently have been integrated into many clinical subspecialties. ERAS protocols are centered around educating patients and promoting self-health before and after the operation, subsequently promoting a quick return to regular activities. Enhanced Recovery Programs (ERPs/ ERAS) often use NSAIDs and COX-2 agents preoperatively which work to reduce inflammation, decreasing postoperative pain. Ketorolac is an NSAID commonly used in ambulatory surgical centers; however, renal dosage adjustments should be kept in mind in certain patient populations (Cheung et al., 2022). A double-blind placebo-controlled study found improvements in recovery and pain management in patients pretreated with ibuprofen (1200 mg/d) and celecoxib (400 mg/d), which was associated with decreased need for rescue analgesia in early postoperative patients following an ambulatory procedure. The timing of COX-2 inhibitor dosing is important; most clinicians recommend preoperative rather than postoperative administration. Celecoxib (400 mg orally) administered on the day of surgery and continued 3 days following the procedure has been found to improve pain management as well as speed of recovery following plastic surgery, better than postoperative dosing alone (Afonso et al., 2019). A study on orthopedic surgery patients, found comparable analgesia with a single dose of celecoxib and a combination of hydrocodone/acetaminophen in a sample of over 400 patients (Afonso et al., 2019).

Both gabapentin and pregabalin are γ-aminobutyric acid (GABA) analogues that have historically been used as antiepileptics, they have also been found to exhibit anticonvulsant, analgesic, and anxiolytic effects. The addition of preemptive pregabalin at both 150 mg and 300 mg doses has demonstrated decreased pain scores and postoperative fentanyl usage in patients following a laparoscopic procedure in a dose-dependent manner without any differences in side effects (Balaban et al., 2012). While GABA analogues are an effective tool for postoperative pain treatment, care must be taken when managing ambulatory patients. Although these analogues are generally well-tolerated, side effects such as sedation and dizziness can be hazardous for certain patient populations, such as the elderly (Schmidt et al., 2013).

Several studies have demonstrated benefit in acute pain management when 1200 mg gabapentin was administered orally prior to the procedure. One study also incorporated a limited postoperative dosing course (10 days after breast surgery) and reported lower opioid requirements and pain scores with ambulation (Hanna, Ouanes, and Tomas 2014). A study on abdominal hysterectomies, found that the use of gabapentin (400 mg four times a day for 1 day preoperatively and 5 days postoperatively) led to lower pain scores 1 month following surgery, but not during the immediate postoperative period (Hanna, Ouanes, and Tomas 2014).

Intraoperative Analgesia

Opioid-sparing multimodal analgesia should be a major focus of ERPs given the concern surrounding opioid dependence. Local anesthesia–based techniques, including wound infiltration, regional nerve blocks, and neuraxial anesthesia, have increasingly become a key component of opioid-sparing pain management strategies for ambulatory surgery. These techniques are recommended by the American Society of Anesthesiologists Task Force on Acute Pain Management. Ultrasound guidance has advanced the clinical practice of regional anesthesia and more anesthesiologists are becoming comfortable using this as standard practice. A review of the utility of regional anesthetic techniques for common outpatient procedures with a focus on transversus abdominis plane (TAP) block for laparoscopic surgery and chest wall blocks for breast surgery will follow (Charipova et al., 2020).

Transversus Abdominis Plane Blocks

The TAP block is a fascial plane block in which local anesthesia is injected between the transversus abdominis and internal oblique muscles to provide analgesia to the anterior abdominal wall. TAP blocks have been described for postoperative pain management in a variety of procedures. A number of hospitals utilized liposomal bupivacaine for procedures involving abdominal incisions, as it has been associated with reduced time to ambulation and shorter hospital stays when compared with other regimens among patients undergoing cesarean birth (Villadiego and Baker 2021). A small study of patients undergoing laparoscopic colorectal surgery, found that TAP blocks reduced mean hospital stays and overall opioid consumption compared to historic controls (Ris et al., 2014). A meta-analysis of randomized controlled trials by De Oliveira and colleagues, in 2014 investigated pain outcomes after laparoscopic surgery with TAP blocks. This study found that patients who received preoperative TAP blocks had less pain at rest during both early and late stages of recovery but no improvement in pain with movement throughout recovery (De Oliveira et al., 2014). Furthermore, improved quality of recovery was observed in patients who received preoperative TAP blocks for laparoscopic gynecologic procedures, but no improvement in recovery or pain scores was observed in patients undergoing laparoscopic hysterectomies with postoperative TAP blocks (Zhou et al., 2018). More evidence is needed to support the routine use of TAP blocks for outpatient laparoscopic procedures, but current research indicates that there is minimal risk to the patient and they may be a useful tool in multimodal analgesic plan (Tran et al., 2019).

Chest Wall Blocks

Complex breast surgeries are being performed in the outpatient setting more frequently. Both acute and chronic pain are a significant complication of breast surgery (Chang, Mehta, and Langford 2009). The paravertebral block (PVB) is considered the gold standard of regional anesthetic techniques for breast surgery. The use of PVBs in combination with total intravenous anesthesia or general anesthesia is associated with decreased pain scores, postoperative analgesic consumption, PONV, LOS, and the incidence of chronic pain. This PVB combination also demonstrated higher patient satisfaction and superior quality of recovery when compared with general anesthesia alone (Abdallah et al., 2014). Although the classic approach was a landmark-based technique, an ultrasound-guided approach has also been described. The risk of pneumothorax with PVB using ultrasound guidance is decreased greatly. More recently, fascial plane blocks have emerged as alternative regional anesthetic options for breast surgery (Abdallah et al., 2014).

Post-operative Analgesia: Multimodal Analgesia and Systematic Pain Management

Pain is a highly individualized, unpleasant sensory and an emotional experience. For this reason, the assessment of pain should be multidimensional. Surgical pain should be distinguished from chronic pain, as well as anxiety or emotionally somatic pain. A systematic approach to pain care seeks to adequately manage pain, minimize side effects, and prevent postoperative and post-discharge discomfort through risk stratification and treatment planning. Some practitioners argue that the three most important aspects include: identification, implementation, and intervention. The ASA practice guidelines on acute pain management recommend individualized care that prioritizes efficacy with minimal adverse events. Counseling patients prior to surgery on the potential for pain following the procedure and the methods that will be used ease it may also influence patient satisfaction (Charipova et al., 2020).

Implementing an opioid-sparing, multimodal pain plan that incorporates regional anesthesia enables effective analgesia and minimizes side effects. Intradermal local anesthesia reduces opioid exposure during preoperative regional anesthesia techniques. Avoiding the administration of opioids prior to the postoperative period may lessen PONV. Increased postoperative sedation and opioid requirements are associated with preoperative and intraoperative opioid use (Afonso et al., 2019). Multiple studies support preoperative administration of pregabalin and gabapentin, COX-2 inhibitors, intraoperative β-adrenergic blockers, ketorolac, sub-anesthetic dose ketamine, magnesium, dexamethasone, methylprednisolone, dexmedetomidine, and intravenous lidocaine infusions to diminish the need for postoperative opioids, alleviate acute postoperative pain, and reduce PONV and time to discharge. With countless non-opioid analgesics available, it is a disservice to the patient to not explore other drugs that may be suitable for outpatient procedures requiring pain management (Verla and Iqbal 2021).

When multimodal analgesia falls short, the ambulatory anesthesia provider must intervene in a timely and potent manner. After a multidimensional assessment of pain, additional non-opioids are administered during the assessment for a potential neural blockade. Opioids may be warranted for severe uncontrolled postoperative pain, but the potential for delayed discharge because of PONV and other opioid-related adverse events must be taken into consideration. Non-pharmacologic techniques for pain management should also be incorporated (Afonso et al., 2019).

Office-Based Anesthesia and analgesia

Historically, ASCs were thought to be a safer location to perform surgery than in an office. The arguments in favor of this theory include: a higher level of attention per case and in selecting appropriate patients, as well as the on-site preparations practiced by freestanding ASCs. However, studies have found that office-based anesthesia can be as safe as hospital and ASC-based procedures (Shapiro et al., 2014). Office accreditation, provider credentialing, proper procedures and patient selection, patient safety checklists, and the implementation of professional society guidelines can improve safety in office-based procedures (Urman, Punwani, and Shapiro 2012).

Dental surgery, plastic surgery, and an ever-growing variety of surgical procedures are now being performed in offices rather than ambulatory surgical facilities or hospitals. The office setting is convenient, private, and cost-effective. Facility requirements, case selection, and anesthesia techniques for approved surgical office establishments have been well defined (Urman, Punwani, and Shapiro 2012). A comparison of the risks for anesthesia and surgery in the office, ASCs, or hospitals is difficult because reporting mechanisms insufficient. The Institute for Safety in Office-Based Surgery has developed a safety checklist to improve preparedness for office-based procedures. Most remote-site injuries related to anesthesia occur due to inadequate monitoring, not errors in patient selection. Factors that were associated with increased risk in the office setting include the use of unqualified surgical or anesthesia staff, a lack of proper equipment and training for resuscitation and other emergencies, and a lack of access to hospitals for the occasional life-threatening emergency. If these factors are eliminated, office-based anesthesia administered by qualified providers in an accredited facility appears to be equally safe (Shapiro et al., 2014).

Summary

Given the growth of the ambulatory surgical field alongside chronic issues related opioid misuse it is essential for modern outpatient analgesia providers to continuously evaluate and improve upon protocols to optimize patient outcomes and reduce healthcare costs. Current research suggests that appropriate preoperative analgesia or preventative analgesia may have a significant effect on postoperative pain and opioid requirements. Typical regimens include acetaminophen, gabapentin or pregabalin, and a nonsteroidal anti-inflammatory drug (NSAIDs) during the preoperative period. Preoperative administration of these medications has demonstrated significantly reduced opioid consumption in the post-anesthesia care unit (PACU) and initial and maximum pain scores following ambulatory procedures (Barker et al., 2018). Furthermore, the application of local anesthetics such as TAP blocks, have also demonstrated decreased PACU narcotic requirements and decreased pain scores (Villadiego and Baker 2021) (Barker et al., 2018). Therefore, the use of oral preoperative multimodal analgesia regimens in combination with intraoperative local anesthetic for ambulatory should be considered when evaluating methods for improving patient outcomes.

Implementing multimodal pain plans that incorporate non-opioid preoperative preventive analgesia as well as intraoperative regional anesthesia enables effective analgesia and minimizes side effects. It is imperative that analgesia protocols are designed to limit risks to society while maintaining patient satisfaction. Analgesia providers should also emphasize counseling patients prior to surgery on the potential for pain following the procedure and the methods that will be used to modulate pain while also ensuring patient safety.

References

Abdallah, Faraj W, Pamela J Morgan, Tulin Cil, Andrew McNaught, Jaime M Escallon, John L Semple, Wei Wu, and Vincent W Chan. 2014. "Ultrasound-Guided Multilevel Paravertebral Blocks and Total Intravenous Anesthesia Improve the Quality of Recovery after Ambulatory Breast Tumor Resection." *Anesthesiology* 120 (3): 703–13. https://doi.org/10.1097/ALN.0000436117.52143.bc.

Adair, Marcus, Stephen Markowiak, Hollis Merrick, James Macho, Kara Richardson, Moriah Muscaro, Munier Nazzal, and F Charles Brunicardi. 2019. "Ambulatory Surgery." In *Schwartz's Principles of Surgery, 11e*, edited by F Charles Brunicardi,

Dana K Andersen, Timothy R Billiar, David L Dunn, Lillian S Kao, John G Hunter, Jeffrey B Matthews, and Raphael E Pollock. New York, NY: McGraw-Hill Education.

Afonso, Anoushka M, Hanae K Tokita, Patrick J McCormick, and Rebecca S Twersky. 2019. "Enhanced Recovery Programs in Outpatient Surgery." *Anesthesiology Clinics* 37 (2): 225–38. https://doi.org/10.1016/j.anclin.2019.01.007.

Bailey, Laila. 2010. "Strategies for Decreasing Patient Anxiety in the Perioperative Setting." *AORN Journal* 92 (4): 445–60. https://doi.org/10.1016/j.aorn.2010.04.017.

Balaban, Fatih, Seyhan Yağar, Ayşegül Özgök, Mihrican Koç, and Hayriye Güllapoğlu. 2012. "A Randomized, Placebo-Controlled Study of Pregabalin for Postoperative Pain Intensity after Laparoscopic Cholecystectomy." *Journal of Clinical Anesthesia* 24 (3): 175–78. https://doi.org/10.1016/j.jclinane.2011.06.027.

Barker, Jenny C, Kaitlin DiBartola, Corinne Wee, Nicole Andonian, Mahmoud Abdel-Rasoul, Deborah Lowery, and Jeffrey E Janis. 2018. "Preoperative Multimodal Analgesia Decreases Postanesthesia Care Unit Narcotic Use and Pain Scores in Outpatient Breast Surgery." *Plastic and Reconstructive Surgery* 142 (4): 443e–50. https://doi.org/10.1097/PRS.0000000000004804.

Chang, Serene H., Vivek Mehta, and Richard M. Langford. 2009. "Acute and Chronic Pain Following Breast Surgery." *Acute Pain* 11 (1): 1–14. https://doi.org/10.1016/j.acpain.2009.01.001.

Charipova, Karina, Kyle L Gress, Ivan Urits, Omar Viswanath, and Alan D Kaye. 2020. "Maximization of Non-Opioid Multimodal Analgesia in Ambulatory Surgery Centers." *Cureus* 12 (9): e10407–e10407. https://doi.org/10.7759/cureus.10407.

Cheung, Christopher K, Janet O Adeola, Sascha S Beutler, and Richard D Urman. 2022. "Postoperative Pain Management in Enhanced Recovery Pathways." *Journal of Pain Research* 15 (January): 123–35. https://doi.org/10.2147/JPR.S231774.

Hanna, Marie N, Jean-Pierre P Ouanes, and Vicente Garcia Tomas. 2014. *"18 - Postoperative Pain and Other Acute Pain Syndromes."* In, edited by Honorio T Benzon, James P Rathmell, Christopher L Wu, Dennis C Turk, Charles E Argoff, and Robert W B T - *Practical Management of Pain* (Fifth Edition) Hurley, 271-297.e11. Philadelphia: Mosby. https://doi.org/10.1016/B978-0-323-08340-9.00018-9.

Luo, Jie, and Su Min. 2017. "Postoperative Pain Management in the Postanesthesia Care Unit: An Update." *Journal of Pain Research* 10 (November): 2687–98. https://doi.org/10.2147/JPR.S142889.

Oliveira, Gildasio S Jr De, Lucas Jorge Castro-Alves, Autoun Nader, Mark C Kendall, and Robert J McCarthy. 2014. "Transversus Abdominis Plane Block to Ameliorate Postoperative Pain Outcomes after Laparoscopic Surgery: A Meta-Analysis of Randomized Controlled Trials." *Anesthesia and Analgesia* 118 (2): 454–63. https://doi.org/10.1213/ANE.0000000000000066.

Painter, T, and G L Ludbrook. 2013. "Reducing System Errors in the Preoperative Assessment Process." *BJA: British Journal of Anaesthesia* 110 (6): 1060–61. https://doi.org/10.1093/bja/aet148.

Reed, W A, and J L Ford. 1976. "Development of an Independent Outpatient Surgical Center." *International Anesthesiology Clinics* 14 (2): 113–30. https://doi.org/10.1097/00004311-197614020-00007.

Ris, F, J M Findlay, R Hompes, A Rashid, J Warwick, C Cunningham, O Jones, N Crabtree, and I Lindsey. 2014. "Addition of Transversus Abdominis Plane Block to Patient Controlled Analgesia for Laparoscopic High Anterior Resection Improves Analgesia, Reduces Opioid Requirement and Expedites Recovery of Bowel Function." *Annals of the Royal College of Surgeons of England* 96 (8): 579–85. https://doi.org/10.1308/003588414X13946184900921.

Schmidt, Peter C, Gabriela Ruchelli, Sean C Mackey, and Ian R Carroll. 2013. "Perioperative Gabapentinoids: Choice of Agent, Dose, Timing, and Effects on Chronic Postsurgical Pain." *Anesthesiology* 119 (5): 1215–21. https://doi.org/10.1097/ALN.0b013e3182a9a896.

Shapiro, Fred E, Nathan Punwani, Noah M Rosenberg, Arnaldo Valedon, Rebecca Twersky, and Richard D Urman. 2014. "Office-Based Anesthesia: Safety and Outcomes." *Anesthesia and Analgesia* 119 (2): 276–85. https://doi.org/10.1213/ANE.0000000000000313.

Tran, De Q, Daniela Bravo, Prangmalee Leurcharusmee, and Joseph M Neal. 2019. "Transversus Abdominis Plane Block: A Narrative Review." *Anesthesiology* 131 (5): 1166–90. https://doi.org/10.1097/ALN.0000000000002842.

Urman, Richard D, Nathan Punwani, and Fred E Shapiro. 2012. "Patient Safety and Office-Based Anesthesia." *Current Opinion in Anaesthesiology* 25 (6): 648–53. https://doi.org/10.1097/ACO.0b013e3283593094.

Verla, Mariatu A, and Atif Iqbal. 2021. "Multimodal Analgesia: Opioid-Sparing Strategies for Pain Management." *Seminars in Colon and Rectal Surgery* 32 (3): 100830. https://doi.org/10.1016/j.scrs.2021.100830.

Villadiego, Lea, and B Wycke Baker. 2021. "Improving Pain Management After Cesarean Birth Using Transversus Abdominis Plane Block With Liposomal Bupivacaine as Part of a Multimodal Regimen." *Nursing for Women's Health* 25 (5): 357–65. https://doi.org/10.1016/j.nwh.2021.07.009.

Zhou, Hong, Xuefeng Ma, Jinghua Pan, Hanlin Shuai, Shanshan Liu, Xin Luo, and Ruiman Li. 2018. "Effects of Transversus Abdominis Plane Blocks after Hysterectomy: A Meta-Analysis of Randomized Controlled Trials." *Journal of Pain Research* 11 (October): 2477–89. https://doi.org/10.2147/JPR.S172828.

Chapter 23

Pain Management in Fracture Reduction

Kaulin J. Ervin*, DO

Touro College of Osteopathic Medicine, New York, NY, USA

Fractures have long been viewed as a debilitating injury with a painful and extensive recovery process, but with an effective pain regimen one can mitigate such unwarranted pain. Here, we will aim to discuss up to date information on how to best navigate the reduction of painand promote proper healing and recovery, while keeping in mind the detrimental effects of the ongoing battle against opioids. In this section, the primary focus will be on long bone fractures being treated with closed reduction, in hopes of guiding pain management from the procedure toa full recovery.

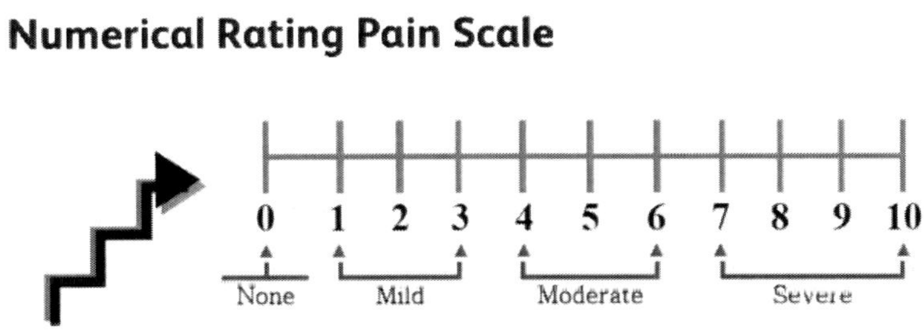

Image 1. (National Institutes of Health Warren Grant Magnuson Clinical Center, 2003).

Pain and its severity are largely subjective; therefore, pain tolerance varies greatly from person to person. An important first step is getting a baseline assessment of pain which can be assimple as utilizing a 0-10 pain scale

* Corresponding Author's Email: kervin2@student.touro.edu.

In: Postoperative Pain
Editors: Indraneil Mukherjee et al.
ISBN: 978-1-68507-971-0

(described to patients as 0 being none and 10 being worst pain you have ever experienced). This type of scale is known as a Numerical Pain Rating Scale (as shown in Image 1), which further breaks down the scale as 0 being none, 1-3 being mild, 4-6 being moderate, and 7-10 being severe. As the scale is divided into graduated subsections, clinicians can easily set pain regimens based on level of severity. In children ages 3 or older, andadults with limited capacity to communicate, a scale known as the Wong-Baker Faces (see Image 2) can be used. This scale utilizes a series of faces and patients are instructed to indicate which face most closely represents the pain they are experiencing. Understanding the patient's level of pain is an important step towards providing relief.

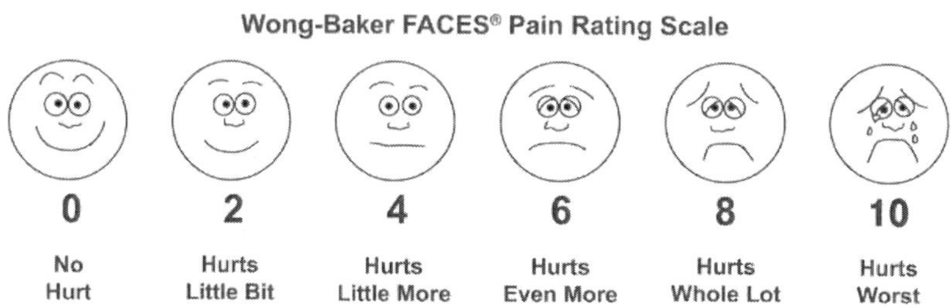

Image 2. (Wong-Baker FACES Foundation, 2020).

Fractures are defined as a complete or partial break in a bone, caused by trauma, overuse,or disease that weakens the bone. Fractures can be classified into many different subtypes including open, closed, transverse, oblique, and pathologic. The general concern about fractures is just how painful these injuries can be. Due to the possible complications associated with delayed treatment, the management of acute fractures is typically initiated in the emergency department. These complications include neurovascular compromise, blood loss, delayed healing, and infection.

Providing adequate analgesia (the lessening or absence of pain) is an important aspect ofacute fracture management. This starts with immobilizing the fracture, utilization of ice, elevation, distraction, and analgesic medications. Initial analgesic medications are given based on the severity of the fracture. For minor fractures, Acetaminophen or Non-Steroidal Anti-Inflammatory Drugs (NSAIDs) are typically enough to provide adequate relief. For major or more severe fractures, Intravenous (IV) morphine has long been the mainstay treatment for providing acute pain relief. However, a more preferred approach involves utilization of a short acting opioid (codeine, hydrocodone, or oxycodone) in combination with acetaminophen or NSAID. This is preferred because it allows a lower dose of the opioid to be used thus reducing the risk of side effects such as respiratory depression, sedation, and addiction.

Much time and research has been spent studying ways to provide pain relief early on in the course of fracture management. This is of great importance because inadequate or lack of treatment in acute pain has been shown to lead to poor patient outcomes and decreased patient satisfaction. An approach that has been proposed is to provide triage nurses with the ability to order pain medication in cases of suspected long-bone fractures (Miller et al., 2018). In triage, the patient reports a pain score and based on the score, medications ranging from Tylenol for mild pain to morphine for severe pain may be administered. Implementing this protocol has shown a significant improvement in the time to which pain management is achieved. Another proposed improvement in suspected fracture cases are periodic meetings with the staff (doctors,nurses, and support staff) in order to allow teamwork and the problem-solving discussions necessary to accomplish timely analgesic administration.

Once initial pain relief is provided, confirming the presence of a fracture is the next orderin management. This starts with a physical exam that assesses for swelling or bruising over a bone, boney deformity, pain worsened by movement or touch, loss of function, loss of sensation,and diminished pulses. Subsequently, imaging studies with plain radiography (x-ray) should be ordered to assess the suspected fracture and surrounding areas. On occasion, fractures can go unnoticed by an x-ray, so if plain radiography continues to be negative but clinical suspicion is high, further imaging tests (bone scintigraphy, magnetic resonance imaging, or computed tomography) may be warranted (Mujoomdar et al., 2012). Once confirmed, the emergency department physician will decide, based on severity, whether to consult orthopedic surgery and thus the next best step in management.

In severe cases where a patient may have an open fracture, diminished pulses, neurovasuclar compromise, or compartment syndrome, urgent surgery is required to preventworsening symptoms. Initial operative management should have the goal of maintaining blood supply and soft tissue health. These cases are best handled by an orthopedic surgeon who will manage the patient in the operating room, often under general anesthesia. This procedure is known as open reduction and internal fixation. In this procedure, a surgeon will make an incisionto re-align the bones and hold them together with hardware like metal pins, plates, rods, or screws (Nunez, 2019). For less severe and hemodynamically stable patients, management can occur outside the operating room with closed reduction and immobilization. Closed reduction procedures can be performed by emergency department physicians, orthopedists, and other physicians trained in the procedure.

Closed reduction is a non-surgical method of treating displaced fractures, usually performed in the emergency department or orthopedic clinic. The procedure is performed using light sedation, analgesia, local anesthetic block, or occasionally general anesthesia. The maneuvers required to gain reduction may vary based on the type of injury, location, and fracture pattern. For example, in a Colles' fracture (distal radius fracture), the steps to reduce the fracture include longitudinal traction followed by palmar flexion and ulnar deviation of the distal fragment (Rajan et al., 2008). This is opposed to reduction of a femoral neck fracture which can be performed with the hip in the flexed position. Traction is then applied, followed by slight adduction of the femoral shaft along the axis of the femur, and finally by circumducting the leg into abduction and bringing it down into extension (Wheeless, 2020). While the exact steps to the different reduction procedures may vary, the goal is focused on gaining realignment of the displaced fragments. After the practitioner is satisfied with the reduction, a repeat x-ray can be performed to confirm proper alignment.

The manipulation and movement required to complete the reduction procedure can further exacerbate the pain of a bone fracture. Thus, management of intra-operative pain is vital before attempting a closed reduction. Some of the possible options for pain relief include opioids, nerve blocks, hematoma blocks, Intravenous Regional Anesthesia (Bier Block), procedural sedation and general anesthesia. The type of sedative or analgesic chosen depends heavily on a multitude of factors including: the physician's familiarity with the agent, type of fracture, suspected length of procedure, patient's anxiety level, pain tolerance, comorbidities, andhospital resources.

Opioids can be administered as solo agents or in combination with other intra-operative anesthetics. In less complicated reduction procedures or procedures of short duration, opioids alone have been able to provide adequate pain control. Opioid medications used intra-operatively are typically administered in the IV form and include morphine, fentanyl,hydromorphone, and tramadol. These medications carry a high risk of both physical dependance and addiction, sedation, loss of consciousness, respiratory depression, and bradycardia.

Nerve blocks are a regional anesthetic technique in which a physician will place a local anesthetic under the skin to create a wheal at the site of needle insertion. With the use of ultrasound, the physician will insert a nerve block needle through the skin wheal (Luftig et al., 2018). The anesthetic agent is then injected within very close proximity to the nerve associated with the fracture. The anesthetic agents used can be shorter acting agents such aslidocaine or longer acting agents like bupivacaine or ropivacaine. Some advantages of the longer acting agents include their ability to provide analgesia throughout the procedure and until it wears off post-procedure. This allows adequate pain control until oral opioid agentscan be started. Side effects include risk of infection, bruising, bleeding, nerve injury, and muscle weakness.

Hematoma Blocks begin with sterilization of the skin with an antiseptic solution, often Chlorhexidine. A syringe filled with lidocaine without epinephrine is inserted into the fracture site. The physician must draw back on the syringe as the needle advances, aspirating until a flash of blood is obtained. This flash of blood indicates that the needle hasreached the hematoma that formed around the fracture. The lidocaine is then injected into the fracture site, making sure to properly disperse the anesthetic throughout. After allowing 5-10 minutes for the anesthetic to take effect, the reduction may be attempted (Emiley et al.,2012). This type of block is great for distal fractures especially of the forearm and wrist. Side effects include neurovascular injury, cellulitis, osteomyelitis, and compartmentsyndrome.

Bier Blocks begin by having an IV catheter placed in the hand, on the side of the fracture. This is followed by a double pneumatic tourniquet with cotton padding which is placed onthe upper arm (when operating on the forearm) or on the forearm (when operating on the hand) (Jeng & Rosenblatt, 2020). The arm is elevated for a few minutes to allow drainage of blood from the area and an Esmarch bandage is wrapped securely from the fingers up to the axilla (Jeng & Rosenblatt, 2020). The distal tourniquet is pumped to between 50 and 100mmHg above systolic blood pressure followed by the proximal tourniquet (Jeng & Rosenblatt, 2020). After palpating for lack of a pulse, the distal tourniquet and Esmarch bandage are removed. Lidociane or Prilocaine are then injected into the previously placed IV catheter (Jeng & Rosenblatt, 2020). Paresthesia starts distally and travels proximal, with complete anesthesia and muscle relaxation in approximately 10-15 minutes. The IV catheteris removed and the reduction procedure is performed with the tourniquet in place. Upon removal of the tourniquet the extremity should regain full sensation within 5 to 10 minutes. This type of block is great for short procedures (between 30 minutes to 1 hour) most commonly of the hand or forearm and less commonly of the foot or ankle. Side effects include tourniquet pain, nerve damage, compartment syndrome, skin discoloration, and thrombophlebitis. Very rare but reported adverse effects include seizures, cardiac arrest, and local anesthetic systemic toxicity (Kraus et al., 2021).

Procedural Sedation and Analgesia (PSA) involves intravenous administration of sedative or dissociative agents, often in combination with short-acting opioids. The preferred agents should have a rapid onset and short duration of action, but every case is different so patients must be evaluated for risk factors and comborbidites prior to administration of any medications. In most cases, one clinician performs the procedure while another administersthe sedative agents and monitors the patient's vital signs and clinical status. Procedural sedation reduces the level of discomfort, apprehension, and potentially unpleasant memories associated with the procedure while facilitating a more ideal environment for theclinician (Hendry, 2017). Side effects of procedural sedation include drowsiness, headache,amnesia, changes in heart rate or blood pressure, aspiration, and respiratory depression.

Some commonly used agents in procedural sedation include propofol, etomidate, midazolam, short-acting opioids, ketamine, methohexital, dexmedetomidine and nitrousoxide.

Propofol: A rapidly acting agent that has both sedating and amnestic effects but no analgesic properties. A therapeutic dose of propofol can take effect in as fast as 40 seconds and has a duration of about 5-10 minutes (Frank, 2020). For procedures longerthan this time, repeat doses of propofol may be required. Patients' most common complaint when using propofol is a burning sensation upon injection. The use of propofol for procedural sedation in children has also been found to be safe and effective.

Etomidate: Another fast-acting sedative agent with similar effects to propofol. Etomidate has an almost immediate onset and a duration of action between 5-15 minutes (Frank, 2020). Due to its lack of analgesic properties, etomidate is often administered with fentanyl. With co-administration of fentanyl and a sedative agentlike etomidate, it is important to watch out for the increased risk of respiratory depression (Frank, 2020). Like propofol, etomidate is also safe and effective in the pediatric population.

Midazolam: A benzodiazepine agent that produces anxiolysis and amnesia but has no analgesic properties (Frank, 2020). Midazolam has an onset between 2-5 minutes, anda duration of action between 30-60 minutes (Frank, 2020). Since midazolam has weaksedative properties, it is often utilized when minimal sedation is required. To achieve a deeper level of sedation and analgesia, one should consider combining it with fentanylor another short acting opioid agent (Frank, 2020). Since other more preferred agents (propofol and etomidate) have become widely available, midazolam has been utilized less often for procedural sedation.

Short-Acting Opioids: Agents such as fentanyl, alfentanil, and remifentanil which havea short onset of action and a short duration of effect. For example, fentanyl has an onset of 2-3 minutes and duration of action between 30-60 minutes (Frank, 2020). These opioid agents produce analgesia but provide no amnestic properties (Frank, 2020). Combining these short-acting opioids with one of the previous agents, such as propofol or etomidate is necessary if sedation is required.

Ketamine: This agent provides the trifecta of sedation, analgesia, and amnesia (Drendel & Helman, 2016). It also has a rapid onset and a short duration of action. Ketamine takes onset within seconds and has a duration of action between 10-20 minutes (Frank, 2020). Due to the many positive effects, this agent is often used in fracture reductions and other brief but painful procedures. Ketamine's sedative, amnestic, and analgesic properties and its relatively low side effect profile makes thisagent the most commonly used agent in pediatric procedural sedation.

Methohexital: This agent has an immediate onset and a duration of action of about 10minutes (Frank, 2020). Like many of the other agents, methohexital provides sedationand amnesia but not analgesia. Of the barbiturate agents, methohexital is the most commonly used agent for procedural sedation (Frank, 2020).

Dexmedetomidine: This is a newer medication that works through agonism of the alpha receptor. It has an onset of about 5-10 minutes and duration of action of 1-2 hours (Malotte et al., 2019). Dexmedetomidine can provide sedation and analgesia without the risk of respiratory depression. This agent has also been found useful for sedation in patients who are being mechanically ventilated in the Intensive Care Unit(ICU) (Frank, 2020).

Nitrous Oxide: An inhaled agent with a very short onset (<30 seconds) and duration ofaction (1-3 minutes) (Stewart & Collins, 2015). Nitrous Oxide can provide sedation, anxiolysis, and analgesia. Nitrous oxide is combined with oxygen and then inhaled, ina concentration of 30-40% N2O which is usually sufficient in most patients (Frank, 2020).

General anesthesia is performed by an anesthesiologist or nurse anesthetist and involves theadministration of medications used to put the patient into a deep sleep so they may avoid feeling pain during the procedure. General anesthesia should be given only after hospitalization, a complete routine history, physical examination, basic lab work, and whileon an empty stomach. In more emergent cases or instances where a quick reduction is preferred, the use of general anesthesia is limited. General anesthesia is also limited by the necessity of an anesthesia team, so it is often necessary to schedule or plan ahead. Side effects and complications include temporary confusion or memory loss, difficulty passing urine, sore throat or laryngeal damage, anaphylaxis, respiratory depression, and cardiovascular collapse (Rull & Tidy, 2019).

Following a properly managed fracture reduction, it is important to inform patients aboutthe possible complications associated with the procedure and adverse events to monitor for post-operatively. When manipulating a fracture, there is a risk of injuring nerves, blood vessels, and soft tissue structures near the injured bone. There is also a risk of new fractures forming due to the forces applied during manipulation. It is possible for blood clots to form and travel to other parts of the body such as the lungs. Another risk is the possibility of an allergic reaction to the pain medications administered during the closed reduction procedure. If the closed reduction procedure is unsuccessful then the patient may need to undergo an open reduction procedure in the operating room. There are some risk factors that increase the likelihood of complications, such as the use of steroids, birth control, insulin; history of smoking, older age, diabetes, and thyroid conditions (Ma & Zieve, 2020).

After the fracture is reduced, it is important to immobilize and protect the injured limb.

This will allow for proper healing and the reduction of pain. Immobilization can be accomplished by either splinting or casting depending on the acute vs chronic nature of the injury. For more acute injuries, splinting, which is a non-circumferential immobilizer, is preferred as it can accommodate the anticipated swelling (Boyd et al., 2009). Casts are circumferential immobilizers which allow for better immobilization but are associated with higher complication rates (Boyd et al., 2009). Casting is typically preferred five to seven days after the injury, once the post-traumatic swelling has subsided. Casts are generally reserved for chronic injuries and more definitive fracture management. Complications associated with the different immobilization techniques consists of loss of reduction, pressure necrosis, compartmentsyndrome, deep vein thrombosis, pulmonary embolism, chronic pain, muscle atrophy, and complex regional pain syndrome (Boyd et al., 2009). Follow up visits after splint or cast placement should be scheduled every 2 weeks to assess proper bone alignment, function, and progression of healing. It is important to inform patients of these complications and instruct them to visit the emergency department if they suspect one of these complications or any other alarming symptoms.

Research suggests that postoperative pain is often under-treated, leaving a significant proportion of patients in moderate to severe pain after their operation (Ossendorp et al., 2013). One goal of postoperative pain management involves providing a smooth transition between intra- and post-operative pain control. Pain immediately after the fracture and the reduction procedure will normally begin to subside slowly, typically within hours to days following the completion of the reduction. While the bone and soft tissue are healing, residual pain can be felt weeks after the injury. This is termed sub-acute pain which can happen for many reasons, such aslack of movement causing muscle weakness, atrophy, and stiffening of the surrounding soft tissue (Osteoporosis Canada, 2019). Additional effects may include inflammation and scarring which can contribute to the stiffness, lack of mobility, and lasting pain. Chronic pain is pain lasting longer than 12 weeks. Typically, this is pain that persists after the fracture and surrounding soft tissue have healed. Contributing factors to chronic pain may be the result of nerve damage, scar tissue development, or aggravation of underlying arthritis, just to name a few(Osteoporosis Canada, 2019).

To limit the risk of opioid abuse, one approach that has been proposed is the utilization ofa multimodal approach. In the acute post-operative setting, a multimodal approach would be the administration of two or more different medications to manage pain (American Society of Anesthesiologists, 2018). The use of a nerve block with a long-acting agent such as bupivacaine or ropivacaine, will provide the benefits of pain relief lasting throughout the procedure and until it wears off post procedure. In addition, the patient may alternate between acetaminophen and ibuprofen in the days following the procedure. One caveat to this multimodal approach is that it must be weighed against the risk of the patient not having adequate pain control after discharge, which has its own set of concerns. A patient whose pain is inadequately treated is at a greater riskfor impaired quality of life, delayed recovery time, higher health-care costs, progression to chronic pain, or illegally obtaining narcotics leading to subsequent abuse (Gan, 2017).

Alternatively, providing opioids in addition to one or more pain management methods, has been associated with fewer opioid prescriptions and less complications than with opioids alone (American Society of Anesthesiologists, 2018). This can be accomplished by providing thepatient with a non-opioid medication (NSAIDS, cyclooxygenase-2 inhibitors, or acetaminophen) upon discharge for mild to moderate pain and a limited quantity of oral opioids (≤3 days; 8-12 pills) which are only to be used for breakthrough pain (Centers for Disease Control and Prevention, 2020). It is also important to counsel the patient on the risk of abuse and addiction and encourage the patient to use opioids only if absolutely necessary. The American College of Surgeons offers a pain management guide, which can be shared with patients, to aid them in selecting the proper pain management option based on their level of pain. The patient will answer the question, "How intense is my pain?" Based on their response, a non-medication therapy (rest, ice, heat, transcutaneous electrical nerve stimulation), a non-opioid medication and/or a short acting opioid is indicated (see Image 3). This will allow the patient adequate pain relief while dealing with the acute pain. After this initial 3 days, acetaminophen and NSAIDS should be sufficient to deal with the subacute pain that may occur in the following weeks as the fracture heals.

Pain Management Guide[7-8]

How Intense Is My Pain?	What Can I Take to Feel Better?
• I hardly notice my pain, and it does not interfere with my activities. • I notice my pain and it distracts me, but I can still do activities (sitting up, walking, standing).	**Non-medication therapies** + **Non-opioid, oral medications** You may take these to control mild to moderate pain when needed
• My pain is hard to ignore and is more noticeable even when I rest. • My pain interferes with my usual activities.	**Non-medication therapies** + **Non-opioid medications** You may be told to take them regularly throughout the day rather than as needed
• I am focused on my pain, and I am not doing my daily activities. • I am groaning in pain, and I cannot sleep. I am unable to do anything. • My pain is as bad as it could be, and nothing else matters.	**Non-medication therapies** + **Around-the-clock non-opioid medications** + **Short-acting opioids** (for a few days) Call your surgeon if your pain continues

Image 3. (American College of Surgeons, 2018).

In cases of chronic pain, it is important to properly assess and manage the pain as it can impair the individual's daily activities and quality of life. Management during the chronic pain period should consist of not only medication but also physical therapy and exercise. While theseapproaches may not completely reverse or cure the pain, they will help in controlling and reducing the pain, thus allowing for a better quality of life (Osteoporosis Canada, 2019). Theimportance of effectively treating a patient's chronic pain can positively affect their overall functioning by improving mobility, decreasing weight gain, and improving sleep quality.

A movement toward sustainable and non-addicting pain therapy is one area of continuingresearch. Also highlighted are a few innovative treatment options that pose potential promise in how fracture related pain is treated. Cannabinoids' (CBD) effects on chronic pain and their ability to limit post-procedural opioid use makes them a topic of discussion in fracture recovery. Cannabinoids such as nabilone or dronabinol as adjunctive therapies have shown a reduction in opioid consumption following traumatic injury (Schneider-Smith et al., 2020). Cannabinoids have had mixed studies, with some showing the agents to have possible anti-inflammatory, analgesic, anxiolytic, and properties proposed to strengthen bones and accelerate the healing of fractures (Moore, 2018). CBD's ability to help with healing and strengthening of bone is thoughtto be attributed to its capability to enhance the maturation of the collagenous matrix (American Friends of Tel Aviv University, 2015). This provides the basis for new mineralization of bone tissue, potentially leaving the healed bone harder to break in the future (American Friends of TelAviv University, 2015). These characteristics show potential promise with the use of cannabinoids as adjunctive therapy in the acute setting and as primary therapy in the chronic stages of fracture pain and healing. Continued research on cannabinoids is necessary as current research has shown promising but overall unclear results.

Lastly, progress has been made in understanding mechanisms that drive skeletal pain andmolecules involved in the regulation of skeletal repair. Such research has found anti-NGF (anti- nerve growth factor), TrkA (tropomyosin receptor kinase A) inhibitors, and anti-sclerostin antibodies as therapies which show potential in the treatment of fractures and other skeletal related pain (Mantyh, 2014). Whether these therapies ever reach approval will depend largely ontheir safety and side-effect profile.

While there are many different post-operative pain treatments available, several of whichhave yielded positive results, it is important to understand the differences among individual fracture cases. Individuals differ in age groups, pain tolerance, risk factors, drug allergies, contraindications, etc. While it is great to have a standard of care in place, it is also important to know that there is no one size fits all plan for dealing with post-operative pain. It is best to look at the patient as a whole and keep in mind the plethora of treatment options when choosing whatis best suited for each individual.

Certain aspects that can further complicate a post-operative pain regimen is the fact that certain commonly prescribed pain medications may delay bone healing in patients. In the short- term, inflammation plays an important role in the body's response to injury and helps the body heal (NYU Langone Health, 2021). This process may be interrupted by the use of certain medications which block the body's natural ability to respond to injury. Anti-inflammatory medications which include corticosteroids and NSAIDs (ibuprofen, naproxen, and aspirin), blockinflammation and slow blood flow, which could lead to delayed or incomplete healing (NYU Langone Health, 2021).

Opioids are another class of medication with potentially negative effects on bone healing,especially when used long-term. The negative effects include nonunion of fractures and reduced bone mass density (Coluzzi et al., 2020). Opioids and anti-inflammatory drugs have their share of complications, for that reason, some physicians prefer acetaminophen during the healing phase of fractures.

The inclusion of the patient's overall health is underestimated as it pertains to the healingof injuries. In the healing phase of acute fractures, improving the body's ability to recover by including alternative therapies can improve long-term healing outcomes (Tabish, 2008). A physically healthy body can better reduce the risk of continuing complications and decrease the time patients require pain medications, thus facilitating a more rapid time to full recovery. A number of adjunctive therapies for fracture healing are available but few rigorous studies have been performed so the appropriate role of such treatments remains undetermined.

One such area of research includes the use of vitamin D and calcium supplementation forpatients with healing fractures. There has been limited research regarding the positive effects of vitamin D and calcium supplementation but evidence has shown that deficiencies in calcium and vitamin D negatively influence fracture healing (Fischer et al., 2018). For this reason, supplementation has been thought to be beneficial for individuals suffering from osteoporosis, deficiencies in vitamin D and calcium, and for the elderly (Fischer et al., 2018).

Other pharmacologic agents are being studied with the hopes of accelerating fracture healing. Examples of these therapies include Growth Hormone (GH), Bone Morphogenetic Proteins (BMP), Parathyroid Hormone (PTH), platelet-derived growth factor, and bisphosphonates (Beutler & Titus, 2019). Similarly, local injections of platelet-rich therapies are also being investigated for their ability to speed up the recovery process (Beutler & Titus, 2019).

Finally, a non-pharmacologic option to improve bone healing is Low Intensity Pulsed Ultrasound (LIPUS), which has been approved by the Food and Drug Administration (FDA) fortreatment of acute fractures and nonunions (Beutler & Titus, 2019). Despite being approved foruse, the efficacy of this therapy is still a debatable topic. Ongoing research in regard to fracturehealing is mounting with optimism that post-procedure therapies can be combined with pain management to accelerate healing and further aid in the reduction of complications and chronic pain.

References

American College of Surgeons. (2018). *Safe and Effective Pain Control After Surgery*. Chicago, IL. https://www.facs.org/-/media/files/education/patient-ed/safe_pain_control_adult.ashx.

American Friends of Tel Aviv University. (2015, July 16). No bones about it: Cannabis may be used to treat fractures: Tel Aviv University researcher finds non-psychotropic compoundin marijuana can help heal bone fissures. *ScienceDaily*. Retrieved May 31, 2021 from www.sciencedaily.com/releases/2015/07/150716124359.htm

American Society of Anesthesiologists. (2018, March). *Multimodal Approach to Pain Management Reduces Opioid Use, Prescriptions After Joint Replacement*. American Society of Anesthesiologists. https://www.asahq.org/about-asa/newsroom/news-releases/2018/03/multimodal-approach-to-pain-management-reduces-opioid-use.`

Argoff, C. (2007). *Tailoring Chronic Pain Treatment to the Patient: Long-Acting, Short-Acting,and Rapid-Onset Opioids: Selecting Opioids: Long-Acting, Short-Acting, and Rapid- Onset Agents*. Medscape. https://www.medscape.org/viewarticle/554015_4.

Bell, D. J., & Hacking, C. (2020). *Closed reduction: Radiology Reference Article*. RadiopaediaBlog RSS. https://radiopaedia.org/articles/closed-reduction?lang=us.

Benyamin, R., Trescot, A. M., Datta, S., Buenaventura, R., Adlaka, R., Sehgal, N., Glaser, S. E.,& Vallejo, R. (2008). Opioid Complications and Side Effects. *Pain Physician, 2s; 11*(3;2s). https://doi.org/10.36076/ppj.2008/11/s105

Bergenstock, Marika & Min, William & Simon, Ann & Sabatino, Christopher & O'Connor, J..(2005). A Comparison Between the Effects of Acetaminophen and Celecoxib on Bone Fracture Healing in Rats. Journal of orthopaedic trauma. 19. 717-23. 10.1097/01.bot. 0000184144.98071.5d.

Beutler, A., & Titus, S. (2019, March 12). *General principles of definitive fracture management*. UpToDate. https://www.uptodate.com/contents/general-principles-of-definitive-fracture- management? search=fracture+management&topicRef=237& source=related_link#H64687126.

Boyd, A. S., Benjamin, H. J., & Asplund, C. (2009). Splints and casts: indications and methods. *American family physician*, *80*(5), 491–499.

Campagne, D. (2021, April). *Overview of Fractures.* Merck Manuals. https://www.merckmanuals.com/home/injuries-and-poisoning/fractures/overview-of-fractures.

Centers for Disease Control and Prevention. (2020, May 6). *Postsurgical Pain.* Centers for Disease Control and Prevention. https://www.cdc.gov/acute-pain/postsurgical-pain/index.html.

Coluzzi, F., Scerpa, M. S., & Centanni, M. (2020). The Effect of Opiates on Bone Formation and Bone Healing. *Current osteoporosis reports*, *18*(3), 325–335. https://doi.org/10.1007/s11914-020-00585-4

Cravero, J. P., & Roback, M. G. (2020, April 14). *Selection of medications for pediatric procedural sedation outside of the operating room.* UpToDate. https://www.uptodate.com/contents/selection-of-medications-for-pediatric-procedural-sedation- outside-of-the-operating-room.

Drendel, A, Helman, A. (2016, February). Pediatric Procedural Sedation. Emergency Medicine Cases. https://emergencymedicinecases.com/pediatric-procedural-sedation/. Accessed 05/31/2021.

Emergency Care Institute. (2020, December 3). *Anaesthesia - Haematoma block.* Emergency Care Institute (ECI). https://www.aci.health.nsw.gov.au/networks/eci/clinical/clinical-resources/procedures/procedures/576176.

Emiley, P., Schreier, S., & Pryor, P. (2012, September 7). *Hematoma Blocks for Reduction of Distal Radius Fractures: Emergency Physicians Monthly.* EPM. https://epmonthly.com/article/hematoma-blocks-for-reduction-of-distal-radius-fractures/.

Farcas A, Bode, J. (2020, April 6). Clinical Question: are we impeding our patients' fracture healing by giving them NSAIDs?Retrieved from http://www.nuemblog.com/blog/fx-nsaids

Fink R. (2000). Pain assessment: the cornerstone to optimal pain management. *Proceedings (Baylor University. Medical Center)*, *13*(3), 236–239. https://doi.org/10.1080/08998280.2000.11927681

Fischer, V., Haffner-Luntzer, M., Amling, M., & Ignatius, A. (2018). Calcium and vitamin D in bone fracture healing and post-traumatic bone turnover. *European cells & materials*, *35*,365–385. https://doi.org/10.22203/eCM.v035a25

Frank, R. L. (2020, July 14). *Procedural sedation in adults outside the operating room.* UpToDate. https://www.uptodate.com/contents/procedural-sedation-in-adults-outside-the-operating-room?search=CLOSED+reduction&source=search_result&selectedTitle=7~150&usage_type= default&display_rank=7#H34.

Gan T. J. (2017). Poorly controlled postoperative pain: prevalence, consequences, and prevention. *Journal of pain research*, *10*, 2287–2298. https://doi.org/10.2147/JPR.S144066

Houghton Mifflin Company. (2012). *Analgesia.* Dictionary.com. https://www.dictionary.com/browse/analgesia.

Howe, A. S. (2018, May 31). *General principles of fracture management: Early and late complications.* UptoDate. https://www.uptodate.com/contents/general-principles-of-fracture-management-early-and-late-complications.

Jeng, C. L., & Rosenblatt, M. A. (2020, October 20). *Upper extremity nerve blocks: Techniques*. UpToDate. https://www.uptodate.com/contents/upper-extremity-nerve-blocks- techniques?sectionName=INTRAVENOUS+REGIONAL+ANESTHESIA +%28BIER+BLOCK%29&search=bier+block&topicRef=399&anchor=H182122941 6&s ource=see_link#H1821229416.

Johns Hopkins Medicine. (2021). *Procedural Sedation*. Johns Hopkins Medicine. https:// www.hopkinsmedicine.org/health/treatment-tests-and-therapies/procedural-sedation.

Joseph, T. N., Turley, R., & Wojcik, S. (2021). *Fractures*. Cedars-Sinai. https://www. cedars-sinai.org/health-library/diseases-and-conditions/f/fractures.html.

Kraus, G. P., Fitzgerald, B. M., & Rondeau, B. (2021, May 4). *Bier Block*. StatPearls [Internet].https://www.ncbi.nlm.nih.gov/books/NBK430760/.

Lewis, S. (2021, April 15). *Nerve Block*. Healthgrades. https://www.healthgrades.com/ right-care/nerve-block.

Luftig, J., Mantuani, D., & Nagdev, A. (2018, October 23). *How to Effectively Block an AcutelyFractured Distal Radius*. ACEP Now. https://www.acepnow.com/article/how-to- effectively-block-an-acutely-fractured-distal-radius/5/?singlepage=1.

Ma, C. B., & Zieve, D. (2020, July). *Closed reduction of a fractured bone*. Mount Sinai Health System. https://www.mountsinai.org/health-library/selfcare-instructions/ closed- reduction-of-a-fractured-bone.

Malotte, K., Walker, K., & Rosielle, D. A. (2019, March 4). *Dexmedetomidine*. Palliative CareNetwork of Wisconsin. https://www.mypcnow.org/fast-fact/dexmedetomidine/.

Mancini, M. C., Zieve, D., & Conaway, B. (2019, January 31). *General anesthesia*. MedlinePlus. https://medlineplus.gov/ency/article/007410.htm#:~:text=General% 20anesthesia%20is%20treatment%20with,what%20is%20 happening%20around%20you.

Mantyh, P. W. (2014). The neurobiology of skeletal pain. *European Journal of Neuroscience*,*39*(3), 508–519. https://doi.org/10.1111/ejn.12462

Mariano, E. R. (2021, May 26). *Management of acute perioperative pain*. UpToDate. https://www.uptodate.com/contents/management-of-acute-perioperative-pain?section Name=STRATEGY+FOR+PERIOPERATIVE+PAIN+CONTROL&search=Anes thesia+in+fracture+reduction&topicRef=100073&anchor=H447933291&source=see _link#H447933291.

Miller, G., Ballejos-Campos, C., Smith, A., Velez, P., Basiliere, C., & Navedo, S. (2018, April 9). *Nurse-Initiated Pain Protocol Improving Treatment for Long Bone Fracture*. Vituity. https://www.vituity.com/blog/implementation-of-nurse-initiated-pain-protocol-in- improving-time-to-pain-treatment-for-long-bone-fracture/.

Moore, M. (2018, November 9). *Cannabidiol Enhances Fracture Healing: Cannabis Sciences*. Labroots. https://www.labroots.com/trending/cannabis-sciences/8584/ cannabidiol-enhances-fracture-healing.

Mujoomdar, M., Russel, E., Dionne, F., et al. (2012). *Diagnosis of Fracture*. Optimizing Health System Use of Medical Isotopes and Other Imaging Modalities [Internet]. https://www.ncbi.nlm.nih.gov/books/NBK174863/#:~:text=Imaging%20of%20 suspected%20fracture%20usually,visible%20immediately% 20on%20x%2Dray.

National Institute for Health and Care Excellence. (2016, February). *Initial pain management*. Fractures (Non-Complex): Assessment and Management. https://www.ncbi.nlm.nih.gov/books/NBK368141/#_ncbi_dlg_citbx_NBK368141.

National Institutes of health warren grant magnuson clinical center. (2003, July). *Pain intensityinstruments*. National Institutes of health warren grant magnuson clinical center. https://acne.gr/wp-content/uploads/2016/06/PainNumericRatingScale.pdf.

Nunez, K. (2019, January 16). *ORIF Surgery: Open Reduction Internal Fixation for Broken Bones*. Healthline. https://www.healthline.com/health/orif- surgery#:~:text=%E2%80%9COpen%20reduction%E2%80%9D%20means%20a%20sur geon,ORIF%20is%20an%20urgent%20surgery.

NYU Langone Health. (2021). *Nonsurgical Treatment for Nonhealing Fractures*. Patient Care at NYU Langone Health. https://nyulangone.org/conditions/nonhealing-fractures-in-adults/ treatments/nonsurgical-treatment-for-nonhealing- fractures#:~:text=Although%20nonsteroidal%20anti%2Dinflammatory%20medications,f low%20and%20delay%20bone%20healing.

Ossendorp, R., Forouzanfar, T., Ashton-James, C. E., & Bloemers, F. (2013). Protocols for treating the postoperative pain of fractures in Dutch hospitals. *Journal of pain research*, *6*, 635–639. https://doi.org/10.2147/JPR.S43729

Osteoporosis Canada. (2019, March 1). *General Information about Pain After A Fracture: Osteoporosis Canada*. Osteoporosis Canada. https://osteoporosis.ca/bone-health-osteoporosis/living-with-the-disease/after-the-fracture/general-information-about-pain- after-a-fracture/.

Pruthi, S. (2020, February 22). *Pain medications after surgery*. Mayo Clinic. https://www.mayoclinic.org/pain-medications/art-20046452.

Rajan, S., Jain, S., Ray, A., & Bhargava, P. (2008). Radiological and functional outcome in extra-articular fractures of lower end radius treated conservatively with respect to its position of immobilization. *Indian journal of orthopaedics*, *42*(2), 201–207. https://doi.org/10.4103/0019-5413.40258

Richard Buckley, M. D. (2021, April 29). General Principles of Fracture Care Treatment & Management: Approach Considerations, Elements of Initial Fracture Management, Nonoperative Therapy. https://emedicine.medscape.com/article/1270717-treatment.

Rull, G., & Tidy, C. (2019, June 28). *Important Complications of Anaesthesia*. Patient. info.https://patient.info/doctor/important-complications-of-anaesthesia#.

Schiller EY, Goyal A, Mechanic OJ. Opioid Overdose. [Updated 2020 Nov 20]. In: StatPearls [Internet]. Treasure Island (FL): StatPearls Publishing; 2021 Jan-. Available from: https://www.ncbi.nlm.nih.gov/books/NBK470415/

Schneider-Smith, E., Salottolo, K., Swartwood, C., Melvin, C., Madayag, R. M., & Bar-Or, D. (2020, February 1). *Matched pilot study examining cannabis-based dronabinol for acutepain following traumatic injury*. Trauma Surgery & Acute Care Open. https://tsaco.bmj.com/content/5/1/e000391.

Stewart, L. S., & Collins, M. (2015, December 16). *Nitrous Oxide as Labor Analgesia: Clinical Implications for Nurses*. Nursing for Women's Health. https://www.sciencedirect.com/science/article/abs/pii/S1751485115306978?via%3Dihub.

Tabish S. A. (2008). Complementary and Alternative Healthcare: Is it Evidence-based?. *International journal of health sciences*, *2*(1), V–IX.

Wheeless, C. R. (2020, July 22). *Femoral Neck Frx: Techniques of Closed Reduction*. Wheeless' Textbook of Orthopaedics. https://www.wheelessonline.com/joints/femoral-neck-frx- techniques-of-closed-reduction/.

Willacy, D. H. (2019, May 13). *Complications from Fractures. Information and treatment*. Patient.info. https://patient.info/doctor/complications-from-fractures#.

Wong-Baker FACES Foundation (2020). Wong-Baker FACES® Pain Rating Scale. Retrieved [05/31/2021] with permission from http://www.WongBakerFACES.org. Originally published in *Whaley & Wong's Nursing Care of Infants and Children*. © Elsevier Inc.

Chapter 24

Psychiatric Comorbidities with Pain

Jennifer Puthota and Joseph Kennedy*, MD
City University of New York School of Medicine, New York, NY, USA

The often overlooked but all too important aspect of pain management is the underlying psychological well-being of the patient. After all, pain can be a manifestation of various psychological pathologies, and underlying psychiatric conditions in a patient puts that patient not only at risk for suffering from chronic pain but also makes their pain more difficult to treat. In the intensive care setting, where pain is a very prevalent complaint amongst patients, psychological morbidity can play a key role in the exacerbation of a patient's pain. Particularly in this setting, patients can be prone to developing post-traumatic stress disorder (PTSD) just from their stay within an intensive care unit (ICU), a diagnosis more formally known as post-intensive care syndrome (PICS). Clinical providers must be aware of the relationship between pain and psychological health, and thus, take adequate steps to not only properly identify the presence of underlying psychological distress in a patient with pain but also to take adequate measures to prevent and treat their patient's psychological pathologies.

In this chapter, we will discuss in further detail the strong interconnected relationship between pain and psychiatric illness as it relates to pain management, both within and outside the perioperative setting. Additionally, we will examine the epidemiology, pathophysiology, diagnosis, treatment, and prevention of PICS and PTSD in the context of patients suffering from chronic pain. Lastly, we will review the gaps in the literature and discuss potential avenues for further research on these topics.

* Corresponding Author's Email: joekennedy96@gmail.com.

In: Postoperative Pain
Editors: Indraneil Mukherjee et al.
ISBN: 978-1-68507-971-0

Pain and Psychiatric Illness

When examining nociceptive physiology and the mechanisms underlying the varying acute and chronic pain states, it is important to remember that pain itself is a complex biopsychosocial concept that can be quite difficult to categorize and understand as it is a highly individualized experience (IASP). Important factors like development, age, gender, geography, socioeconomic status, and culture play a role in the patient's perception and expression of pain. It has been shown that effectively reduced acute pain has been associated with reduced incidence of chronic pain (Yelle). To best treat pain, these said factors must be considered especially considering how poorly controlled psychosocial issues may facilitate acute pain's transition to chronic pain (Turk, Martel, Wolf). With an ever-increasing prevalence of chronic pain, it is important to recognize an underappreciated aspect: underlying psychological aspects of said pain and psychiatric comorbidities. It has been estimated that nearly 50% of patients within a pain management clinic will have a comorbid psychiatric diagnosis (Kaufman). Chronic pain and psychological disorders have been shown to have a bidirectional association: not only are patients suffering with chronic pain more likely to develop said psychological pathologies, but patients with a psychiatric diagnosis are at increased risk of developing chronic pain (Higgins). Thus, these psychiatric and behavioral conditions have been defined as a comorbidity for chronic pain due to their close relationship. These conditions include depression, anxiety, mood disorders, and, when opioids and other controlled substances are introduced in chronic pain management, substance use disorders (paper?). Depression is most common amongst these, with one study finding that individuals with chronic pain were 4 times as likely to have anxiety or depression than those without chronic pain (Kaufman, Gureje et al.). Furthermore, studies have also shown that patients with both depression and pain are less likely to have successfully treated depression (Higgins). Thus, when evaluating a patient with acute or especially chronic pain, it is important to also conduct a psychological evaluation with emphasis on screening for depression to better understand the pain syndrome and enhance management.

The close relationship between pain and behavioral disorders has also revealed itself in the successful treatment of various forms of pain using antidepressant medications. This class of medications has been shown to be effective in decreasing the pain associated with low back discomfort, diabetic neuropathy, postherpetic neuralgia, fibromyalgia, and migraines (Higgins). Of note, the medications that have shown the most success include those that affect norepinephrine and serotonin reuptake, including tricyclic antidepressants and serotonin-norepinephrine reuptake inhibitors. Duoloxetine, for example, which is an SNRI, has been FDA approved for the treatment of diabetic neuropathy. These findings may be due to several mechanisms, including but not limited to treatment of the patient's behavioral disorder, enhancement of descending nociceptive abatement pathways, and from pain perception modulation via cortical mechanisms. Similarly, nonpharmacological psychological therapies including cognitive behavioral therapy and mindfulness-based stress reduction have been shown to be effective through slight persistent reductions of pain as well as improving outlook and acceptance for patients with chronic pain (Turner, Flynn). These different treatment modalities traditionally targeted for behavioral pathologies have shown efficacy in the treatment of chronic pain syndromes, and further support the importance of recognizing the psychological aspect of evaluating and treating pain.

Of note, however, not all psychiatric conditions predispose patients to chronic pain. Patients with schizophrenia have been shown to have a decreased pain sensitivity (Higgins, Engels). While the evidence is limited, some studies have been able to elucidate specific pain response profiles in patients with schizophrenia (Potvin, Levesque). However, these findings are not ubiquitous as patients with a schizophrenia phenotype characterized by more positive symptoms have also been found to exhibit hyperalgesia (Levesque). Thus, due to the lack of high-quality evidence and poorly understood mechanisms, it is difficult to determine whether these findings are secondary to the underlying schizophrenia, to the psychotropic medications, or to a patient's flat affect that prevents pain expression (Engels). Of note, studies have shown that relatives of patients with schizophrenia and individuals with a family history of schizophrenia also have elevated pain thresholds and tolerance, indicating a possible genetic predisposition or mechanism that could explain this phenomenon (Higgins). Elucidating the relationship between pain and schizophrenia is important as currently patients with schizophrenia are less likely to be diagnosed with a chronic pain diagnosis (Owen-Smith). While it is possible that patients with schizophrenia may have higher pain thresholds and thus less likely to develop chronic pain, it is also possible that chronic pain and pain in general is underrecognized in this patient population and subsequently undertreated. Additionally, patients suffering from schizophrenia are also more likely to be diagnosed with substance use disorder, which might even precede the onset of psychotic symptoms, making the treatment of pain even more difficult (Khokhar). Thus, more research is needed to determine the relationship between pain and schizophrenia and its application to clinical practice.

When considering patients with dementia, it is important to recognize that pain is often underrecognized and thus subsequently undertreated (Flo). While patients with dementia might self-report lower levels of pain, patients tend to be elderly and thus susceptible to the development and prevalence of chronic pain. In addition, elderly patients with dementia are at increased risk of requiring ICU stay, which in itself could lead to delirium. Pain can have neuropsychiatric manifestations including agitation, aggression, mood disturbances, sleep difficulties and others, but in this population, it is frequently mistaken for dementia or delirium; thus, it is crucial to be able to differentiate between pain, delirium, and dementia. The underdiagnosing of pain can and has led to further underrecognition and undertreatment of these patients' pain. On the other hand, due to aging's associations with pharmacokinetic changes and polypharmacy, it is also important to critically consider the pharmacological management of pain in this population as these medications carry significant interactions and side effects that can worsen morbidity and mortality.

Due to the complexity of the biopsychosocial context of chronic pain, pain management should include addressing the psychological and social complexities of the patient's pain experience through a multidisciplinary approach. When a behavioral or psychosocial component of pain is recognized, nonpharmacologic and noninvasive treatment modalities such as cognitive behavioral therapy and mindfulness-based stress reduction techniques should be employed in conjunction with other modalities to fully manage a patient's pain (Flynn, Turner).

Post-Intensive Care Syndrome (PICS), PTSD and Pain

While no formal definition of PICS exists at this time, many agree that PICS can be defined as a deterioration of cognitive, mental, or physical well-being either during or after receiving intensive or acute care. PICS-F refers to the physical, cognitive, and mental deterioration of close friends and family members whose relatives had undergone intensive or acute care (Inoue, Needham). As it is not clearly defined and thus not properly recognized, the exact prevalence of PICS or PICS-F is unknown, but some literature has indicated that nearly half of patients leaving ICUs will suffer some form of PICS many months and even years after discharge (Pandharipande, Griffiths).

When focusing on the mental and cognitive aspects of PICS, the main psychiatric impairments seen in critical care survivors are post-traumatic stress disorder (PTSD), anxiety disorder and depression (Desai, Boede). These disorders have significant symptom overlap, can present together, can aggravate each other, and can be associated with chronic pain (Boede, Outcalt, Bair). Importantly, studies have shown that the presence of these psychological disorders in critical care survivors is associated with decreased quality of life and increased mortality months and years after receiving critical care intervention (Hatch). Patients requiring stay within a critical care setting are a high-risk population for the development of behavioral disorders that are associated with the development of and exacerbation of chronic pain. Thus, the critical care setting should serve as a critical intervention point for diagnosis and treatment of both pain and behavioral disorders.

An important development within critical care has been the COVID-19 pandemic. As of this writing, more than a year has passed since the height of the pandemic, which has been characterized by over 170 million cases and more than 3 million lives lost worldwide (Hopkins). The pandemic interrupted care for many individuals, including those suffering from mental illness and chronic pain. Literature has emerged focusing on the potential "second pandemic" of mental illness that would be brought about by the pandemic as evidenced by prior epidemics (Imam Covid19 textbook). As more research comes out about the potential effects, both direct and indirect, of COVID-19 on mental health and cognition, concerns have also been raised about the potential increase in chronic pain after the COVID-19 pandemic (Clauw). This could potentially be through many different pathways: patients with chronic pain who had their usual care interrupted, mental health exacerbations in the population could further exacerbate chronic pain, the dramatic increase in ICU patients and survivors increased the prevalence of PICS which in turn could potentiate pain with a large psychosocial component, and many more (Shanthana, Clauw). As the issues of mental health and quality of life after critical illness become more emphasized, more research will reveal better diagnostic tools to risk-stratify patients who could best be served by both preventive and therapeutic measures for the development of pain and its psychological aspects.

References

Bair, Matthew J., Rebecca L. Robinson, Wayne Katon, and Kurt Kroenke. 2003. "Depression and Pain Comorbidity: A Literature Review." *Archives of Internal Medicine* 163 (20): 2433–45. https://doi.org/10.1001/archinte.163.20.2433.

Boede, Monique, Jochen S. Gensichen, James C. Jackson, Fiene Eißler, Thomas Lehmann, Sven Schulz, Juliana J. Petersen, Florian P. Wolf, Tobias Dreischulte, and Konrad F.R. Schmidt. 2021. "Trajectories of Depression in Sepsis Survivors: An Observational Cohort Study." *Critical Care* 25 (1). https://doi.org/10.1186/s13054-021-03577-7.

Breivik, Harald. 2002. "International Association for the Study of Pain." In *Journal of Pain and Symptom Management*, 24:97–101. https://doi.org/10.1016/s0885-3924(02)00465-7.

Clauw, Daniel J., Winfried Häuser, Steven P. Cohen, and Mary Ann Fitzcharles. 2020. "Considering the Potential for an Increase in Chronic Pain after the COVID-19 Pandemic." *Pain* 161 (8): 1694–97. https://doi.org/10.1097/j.pain.0000000000001950.

Coronavirus Resource Center. 2021. "COVID-19 Dashboard by the Center for Systems Science and Enginee." *Johns Hopkins University & Medicine*. https://gisanddata.maps.arcgis.com/apps/opsdashboard/index.html#/bda7594740fd40299423467b48e9ecf6.

Desai, Sanjay V., Tyler J. Law, and Dale M. Needham. 2011. "Long-Term Complications of Critical Care." *Critical Care Medicine* 39 (2): 371–79. https://doi.org/10.1097/CCM.0b013e3181fd66e5.

Engels, Gwenda, Anneke L. Francke, Berno Van Meijel, Johanna G. Douma, Heidi De Kam, Wubbien Wesselink, Wim Houtjes, and Erik J. A. Scherder. 2014. "Clinical Pain in Schizophrenia: A Systematic Review." *Journal of Pain* 15 (5): 457–67. https://doi.org/10.1016/j.jpain.2013.11.005.

Flo, Elisabeth, Christine Gulla, and Bettina S. Husebo. 2014. "Effective Pain Management in Patients with Dementia: Benefits Beyond Pain?" *Drugs and Aging*. https://doi.org/10.1007/s40266-014-0222-0.

Flynn, D. M. n.d. "Chronic Musculoskeletal Pain: Nonpharmacologic, Noninvasive Treatments. *Am. Fam. Physician*."

Griffiths, John, Robert A. Hatch, Judith Bishop, Kayleigh Morgan, Crispin Jenkinson, Brian H. Cuthbertson, and Stephen J. Brett. 2013. "An Exploration of Social and Economic Outcome and Associated Health-Related Quality of Life after Critical Illness in General Intensive Care Unit Survivors: A 12-Month Follow-up Study." *Critical Care* 17 (3). https://doi.org/10.1186/cc12745.

Hatch, Robert, Duncan Young, Vicki Barber, John Griffiths, David A. Harrison, and Peter Watkinson. 2018. "Anxiety, Depression and Post Traumatic Stress Disorder after Critical Illness: A UK-Wide Prospective Cohort Study." *Critical Care* 22 (1). https://doi.org/10.1186/s13054-018-2223-6.

Imam, S. A., M. Javeed, and J. Kennedy. n.d. "Mental Health Manifestations of COVID-19." Edited by C. Kriz, N. Imam, and S Zaidi. *First Medicine and Global Clinical Partners*. http://www.breakingdowncovid19.org.

Jackson, Peter R. 2016. "The Neuroscience of Clinical Psychiatry: The Pathophysiology of Behavior and Mental Illness." In *Journal of the American Academy of Child & Adolescent Psychiatry*, 3rd ed., 55:632–33. Lippincott Williams & Wilkins. https://doi.org/10.1016/j.jaac.2016.06.001.

Kaufman, David Myland. 2007. "Clinical Neurology for Psychiatrists." In *Clinical Neurology for Psychiatrists*, 8th ed. Elsevier. https://doi.org/10.1016/B978-1-4160-3074-4.X1000-4.

Khokhar, Jibran Y., Lucas L. Dwiel, Angela M. Henricks, Wilder T. Doucette, and Alan I. Green. 2018. "The Link between Schizophrenia and Substance Use Disorder: A Unifying Hypothesis." *Schizophrenia Research* 194: 78–85. https://doi.org/10.1016/j.schres.2017.04.016.

Lévesque, Mylène, Stéphane Potvin, Serge Marchand, Emmanuel Stip, Sylvain Grignon, Lalonde Pierre, Olivier Lipp, and Philippe Goffaux. 2012. "Pain Perception in Schizophrenia: Evidence of a Specific Pain Response Profile." *Pain Medicine (United States)* 13 (12): 1571–79. https://doi.org/10.1111/j.1526-4637.2012.01505.x.

Martel, Marc O., Yoram Shir, and Mark A. Ware. 2018. "Substance-Related Disorders: A Review of Prevalence and Correlates among Patients with Chronic Pain." *Progress in Neuro-Psychopharmacology and Biological Psychiatry* 87 (245): 245–54. https://doi.org/10.1016/j.pnpbp.2017.06.032.

Outcalt, Samantha D., Kurt Kroenke, Erin E. Krebs, Neale R. Chumbler, Jingwei Wu, Zhangsheng Yu, and Matthew J. Bair. 2015. "Chronic Pain and Comorbid Mental Health Conditions: Independent Associations of Posttraumatic Stress Disorder and Depression with Pain, Disability, and Quality of Life." *Journal of Behavioral Medicine* 38 (3): 535–43. https://doi.org/10.1007/s10865-015-9628-3.

Owen-Smith, Ashli, Christine Stewart, Musu M. Sesay, Sheryl M. Strasser, Bobbi Jo Yarborough, Brian Ahmedani, Lisa R. Miller-Matero, et al., 2020. "Chronic Pain Diagnoses and Opioid Dispensings among Insured Individuals with Serious Mental Illness." *BMC Psychiatry* 20 (1). https://doi.org/10.1186/s12888-020-2456-1.

Pandharipande, P. P., T. D. Girard, J. C. Jackson, A. Morandi, J. L. Thompson, B. T. Pun, N. E. Brummel, et al., 2013. "Long-Term Cognitive Impairment after Critical Illness." *New England Journal of Medicine* 369 (14): 1306–16. https://doi.org/10.1056/nejmoa1301372.

Potvin, Stéphane, Emmanuel Stip, Adrien Tempier, Tania Pampoulova, Lahcen Aït Bentaleb, Pierre Lalonde, Olivier Lipp, Philippe Goffaux, and Serge Marchand. 2008. "Pain Perception in Schizophrenia: No Changes in Diffuse Noxious Inhibitory Controls (DNIC) but a Lack of Pain Sensitization." *Journal of Psychiatric Research* 42 (12): 1010–16. https://doi.org/10.1016/j.jpsychires.2007.11.001.

Shanthanna, H., N. H. Strand, D. A. Provenzano, C. A. Lobo, S. Eldabe, A. Bhatia, J. Wegener, K. Curtis, S. P. Cohen, and S. Narouze. 2020. "Caring for Patients with Pain during the COVID-19 Pandemic: Consensus Recommendations from an International Expert Panel." *Anaesthesia* 75 (7): 935–44. https://doi.org/10.1111/anae.15076.

Sims, Lea M. 2006. "Pain Management." In *Journal of the American Association for Medical Transcription*, edited by R. M. Pino and M. A. Albrecht, 9th ed., 25:54. Lippincott Williams & Wilkins.

Turk, Dennis C., and Akiko Okifuji. 2002. "Psychological Factors in Chronic Pain: Evolution and Revolution." *Journal of Consulting and Clinical Psychology* 70 (3): 678–90. https://doi.org/10.1037/0022-006X.70.3.678.

Turner, Judith A., Melissa L. Anderson, Benjamin H. Balderson, Andrea J. Cook, Karen J. Sherman, and Daniel C. Cherkin. 2016. "Mindfulness-Based Stress Reduction and Cognitive Behavioral Therapy for Chronic Low Back Pain: Similar Effects on Mindfulness, Catastrophizing, Self-Efficacy, and Acceptance in a Randomized Controlled Trial." *Pain* 157 (11): 2434–44. https://doi.org/10.1097/j.pain.0000000000000635.

Wolf, Laurie D., Mary C. Davis, Ellen W. Yeung, and Howard A. Tennen. 2015. "The Within-Day Relation between Lonely Episodes and Subsequent Clinical Pain in Individuals with Fibromyalgia: Mediating Role of Pain Cognitions." *Journal of Psychosomatic Research* 79 (3): 202–6. https://doi.org/10.1016/j.jpsychores.2014.12.018.

Chapter 25

VR Glasses for Postoperative Pain

Tanzib Razzaki*
City University of New York School of Medicine, New York, NY, USA

Post-operative pain has been a problem facing patients whenever they are contemplating having a surgical procedure. Studies have shown that the pain after surgery can be debilitating enough to lead to adverse outcomes for the patient and physicians. Pharmacological treatments remain the mainstay for postoperative pain; however, they don't address other stressors patients may face. A patient can feel anxiety toward the outcome of their anesthesia and surgical procedure that carries over after the operation has finished. This psychological stressor has been shown to affect a patient's physical pain, causing complications and prolonging recovery. Virtual reality (VR) is emerging as a means of immersion for patients to help control their pain and anxiety after surgery. With the advent of more affordable, consumer-grade VR equipment like glasses, this kind of intervention has become more feasible for clinicians to provide for their patients. Studies and cases use VR glasses to place patients in a 3D simulation that portrays an environment that can be calming. VR makes it possible for these environments to be interactive and diverts attention away from the pain, acting as a distraction. Studies have yielded both positive and negative results for the use of VR for post-operative pain. Challenges with coming to a consensus include the heterogeneity of the surgical procedures and the use of different pain scores regarding the VR intervention. This review will look to analyze a broad set of cases across different demographics and surgical procedures. Medications still show to be effective for controlling a patient's pain. However, this alternative mainstay

* Corresponding Author's Email: trazzak000@citymail.cuny.edu.

In: Postoperative Pain
Editors: Indraneil Mukherjee et al.
ISBN: 978-1-68507-971-0

which includes opioids carries variable side effects and addictive profiles. Reviewing the efficacy of virtual reality as a means for post-operative pain management can help expand what can be done for pain relief outside of medication.

Post-Operative Pain

For patients who may need surgery, a primary concern is always the risk of complications. Complications can be specific risks associated with the surgery, for instance, bleeding, leaks, or obstruction after abdominal surgery. More general complications can include hypoxia, fever, or sepsis. These risks are made sure to be explained to patients and can be stressful for them from the pre-operative period to the post-operative period. The challenge for providers that are a part of the perioperative treatment is proper management of any stressors that can increase these complications. Managing stressors is imperative since the risks mentioned above can never be ruled out for patients. One of the most common triggers is post-operative pain. Finding creative ways to ease a patient's anxiety and manage their pain is an outlook that can provide benefits for surgical patients moving forward.

A highly prevalent problem that has affected the risk of complications, length of hospital stay, and ultimately patient satisfaction is post-operative pain. Pre-operatively, patients' most common questions are about how much pain they will experience after the surgery. Post-operative pain is defined as an unpleasant physical and psychological experience associated with actual or potential tissue damage caused by the surgery itself. Pain, in general, can be physically and mentally debilitating for any patient. Therefore, after surgery, proper pain management can be the difference between a successful and failed outcome. If a patient's pain is properly managed, then early mobilization after surgery is possible. Early mobilization reduces hospital stays for surgical patients, thus reducing hospital-associated complications. These include falls, pressure ulcers, and hospital-associated infections. Hospital-associated diseases, in particular, can be devastating for patients who are elderly and may be immunocompromised. These patients are encouraged to start walking from their hospital bed as soon as they feel able and using tools like incentive spirometers to prevent any consolidation in their lungs. Studies have shown pain to be one of the three most common medical causes of delayed discharge, with the other two being drowsiness and nausea/vomiting.

All in all, the sequelae of complications from post-operative pain are rooted in physiologic consequences. Inadequately treated pain is associated with natural inflammatory, endocrine, and metabolic responses that help our body compensate for the stressor. These responses are a byproduct of the activation of the autonomic system. The body increases heart rate, peripheral vascular resistance, and myocardial contractility. Untreated pain can cause hypoventilation which leaves our pulmonary system vulnerable to atelectasis and infection. The activation of the autonomic system from increased pain reduces intestinal motility, which explains the prevalence of ileus and obstruction seen after surgery. Our body's hemostatic regulation also reacts to pain leading to increased platelet aggregation. This hypercoagulable state, coupled with lack of mobilization, can precipitate venostasis, explaining the increased risk of deep vein thrombosis and thromboembolism after surgery. A patient's psychological status is affected by pain and the thought of surgery as aforementioned. Post-operative discomfort can worsen anxiety and induce depression if left unmanaged. Despite the overwhelming sentiment behind more effective postoperative pain control, the reality, according to recent studies, suggests we have a ways to go before achieving satisfaction.

Standard of Care and Management of Post-Operative Pain

Pharmacological treatments remain the cornerstone for post-operative pain relief today. Among these treatments, opioids have remained a perennial contender for prompt pain relief, particularly after surgery. The most recent advances in pain pharmacology have been products like extended-release epidural morphine (EREM) and iontophoretic transdermal fentanyl (fentanyl ITS). The advent of EREM is due to studies on current postoperative pain research that state the goal for proper treatment is finding a medication that can work locally to give long-lasting pain relief at the surgical site of focus. Fentanyl ITS is a method of administration that adds to the patient-controlled analgesia (PCA) philosophy that has become a mainstay in recent years. PCA had demonstrated efficacy and patient satisfaction initially as IV administration. However, limitations that presented themselves included the risk of programming errors and the potential to limit patient mobility due to lines and tubing. The patient-controlled fentanyl ITS addresses these concerns by being needle-free, self-contained, and delivering the drug transdermal. Although there have been many advances in pain management's pharmacological side, there are still many disadvantages to this regarding opioid administration. For instance, the side effect profile of opioids has become an issue since patients experience nausea/vomiting, urinary retention, and respiratory depression. Moreover, the recent PCA methods have not been in use for long enough to conclude their efficacy. There aren't ways to currently measure the number of attempts patients try when they control the administration. The PCA technology doesn't let the drug be administered repeatedly after repeated attempts by the patient. However, recording the number of attempts a patient tried would give insight into their level of dependence. Opioid dependence has become a crisis in many parts of the world. This is why this method of pain management can be risky; its side effects coupled with its addictive qualities may not be the best option for post-operative pain moving forward. Due to this risk of dependence, recent studies have also shown instances where providers can be over-cautious not to give opioids to post-surgical patients. As a result, we are at an impasse despite the more nuanced understanding of the mechanisms behind pain and advancements in pharmacology; we are still undertreating post-operative pain. Non-pharmacologic means for post-operative pain may be the future for pain management. Studies have shown success with music therapy and hypnosis. A novel non-pharmacologic treatment that is being studied is virtual reality (VR). This study will look to review recent studies on the efficacy of VR glasses for post-operative pain.

The Advent of Virtual Reality (VR) to Manage Post-Operative Pain

As technology and the application of technology have advanced through the years, virtual reality (VR) has emerged as a non-pharmacologic intervention for pain. This chapter will review how well VR can help patients regarding their pain after surgery and their overall satisfaction throughout their perioperative experience. Virtual Reality (VR) is a computer-generated, simulated experience of a three-dimensional image or environment that a person can interact with. The concept of virtual reality started in the 20th century with an application for entertainment and then for medical, flight, and military training. Current technologies have developed headsets or glasses that a person can wear to immerse themselves in the three-dimensional simulation. These glasses were initially designed for the video gaming industry to give people interactive experiences with their favorite video game titles. Now, VR glasses can provide people with a choice of an environment, real or fictional, to be immersed in gaming purposes and give a realistic trip to that place in time. These recent developments have expanded the use of VR glasses for situations that may help people with their anxiety and pain. The advancements in VR software have made these simulations realistic and drastically different from the humble beginnings that included devices such as the Sensorama. For patients, VR can create a sense of presence and combine interactive scenes to engage the patients in the virtual environment to divert pain. Therefore, VR can work as a distraction to limit a patient's nociceptive stimulation and thus ease their feeling of discomfort. The application of VR glasses on patients is also viable because of the recent advancements in the hardware. Today there is the universality of mobile high-performance computing that has allowed for a reduction in the size of VR hardware as well as cost. With proper research and assessment, there is now an opportunity to use VR as not only a non-pharmacologic method but a cost-effective method for post-operative pain. To date, there is the precedence of VR providing benefits for patients' pain in other medical and procedural settings. Studies have shown VR to help treat anxiety disorders and support physical rehabilitation. VR has shown to be effective during wound care, decreasing pain during bandage changes for severe burns as an alternative to opioids. VR has managed pain for patients during intravenous line placements and dental interventions as well. In all these examples, VR glasses allow patients to enter an environment of their choosing to help blunt the activity of their autonomic system and provide them an experience that takes the focus away from the stress of pain. The options patients have for the type of VR they can participate in varies with the age group and the patient's interests. There have been studies where adult patients prefer to be in a simulation of guided relaxation where they are looking around a scenic mountain or enjoying the beach instead of being given anxiolytics or pain medications. Studies in pediatric populations provide these patients with options for different age-appropriate games. These games include playing sports, feeding animals, or getting past obstacles. Patients in older age demographics were given more complex games that included traversing fantasy worlds and solving problems with fictional characters. Recently, many studies have investigated if these same benefits could be translated to managing post-operative pain. Results from these studies have been varied. Some studies and meta-analyses have reported positive benefits and pain reduction with VR glasses, whereas other studies have reported insignificant or negative correlations with VR glasses. A distinction between the studies that have found success in VR managing different types of pain compared to post-operative pain is that patients undergoing surgical procedures are in a state of severe stress. Most of the time, this level of stress is physiologic and psychologic, a combination that is not prevalent in the setting of wound care or intravenous line placement.

Clinical Application

This chapter will analyze studies investigating virtual reality (VR) across different countries and different surgeries. Limitations of each study will also be kept in mind when comparing the positive correlations with negative or insignificant correlations. VR can be an innovative intervention for postoperative pain, especially in a time with a high prevalence of opioid dependence. However, the theoretical benefit of VR glasses providing a distraction and an escape from pain may also have limitations in actual practice. Therefore, it will be crucial to understand if VR has more potent benefits for certain types of surgeries and specific populations of patients. Moreover, how a patient measures their pain will consist of different scores and metrics across the studies this chapter looks at as well.

Studies spanning the United States, China, India, and Iran all concluded that the use of VR could significantly reduce post-operative pain compared to control groups. Each study looked at procedures in orthopedics, maxillofacial, obstetrics, and cardiac surgery. The orthopedic research out of China investigated the effect VR can have in postoperative and early functional exercise following total knee arthroplasty. The sample size in this study was 66 patients with an average age of 66.45 years. The patients were either going to receive their rehabilitation immersed in the virtual reality environment of their choice or participate in conventional repair at physical therapy sites. Rehabilitation, either conventional or with VR, was done for 30 minutes, three times a day. This study measured its outcome using a postoperative pain score and knee scores that take into account a patient's subjective pain and objective range of motion (ROM). Post-operative pain scores were rated as the higher the score, the more severe the patient's pain. Higher degrees of knee ROM were concluded as positive impacts from the VR interventions. Results showed that postoperative pain scores were significantly lower in the VR group than the control group at 3, 5, and 7 days after the total knee arthroplasty ($p<0.05$). The knee ROMs were significantly higher in the VR group than the control group on days 3, 7, and 14 after total knee arthroplasty ($p<0.05$). Achieving a ROM of 60 and 90 degrees for patients who used VR took 2.45

+/- 0.71 and 13.48 +/- 2.48 days, respectively. In South India, the role of VR was tested in the setting of oral maxillofacial surgery. This study looked at fifty patients and the inclusion criteria were patients who were coming to see the dentist for their first tooth removal. Exclusion criteria were patients with any psychiatric problems, a history of claustrophobia, and a history of epilepsy. The control group, n = 25, were administered local anesthesia without the use of VR. The study group, n = 25, was exposed to VR through the use of a headset display powered by a smartphone. The study group all used the same VR environment to promote relaxation, the patients did not have a choice between different virtual realities. The measures used for this study looked at questionnaires filled out by the patients and vital signs preoperatively, intraoperatively, and postoperatively. Preoperatively, all patients were asked to fill out a Visual Analog Scale, a dental concern questionnaire, and an anxiety assessment form. Preoperative pulse rate and oxygen saturation were measured and these parameters were also measured intraoperatively and post-operatively. Lastly, patients filled out a Visual Analog Scale post-operatively as well. The mean age of the subjects was 39.72 +/- 15.93. The significant findings between the VR group and the control group showed that the VR group had lower intraoperative pulse rates compared to the control group. The results were 77.76 +/- 10.11 in the study group compared to 85.80 +/- 13.30 in the control group with a P-value of 0.020. The study found a significant change when comparing the Visual Analog Scale for pain as well. The postoperative Visual Analog Scale in the control group was 2.60 +/- 1.384 compared to the study group which was 1.28 +/- 0.891 with the P-value in each group being <0.01. Limitations of this study include the fact that the sample size of 50 is relatively small and that a crucial vital sign that is affected by pain, blood pressure, was not measured. The other aspect is that patients were not in control of the VR environment they were being immersed in order to decrease the variability in the efficacy of the VR. However, there may have been instances where the VR of choice was not preferred option by some patients. This study concluded that immersive VR can possibly be an effective distraction tool to alleviate the anxiety of the patient. The benefits of the application of VR include the fact that the technology is now affordable as well as easy to use. The benefit of using fewer pharmacologic analgesics and anxiolytics is noteworthy since many side effect profiles are avoided. In the United States, VR was studied among orthopedic surgeries as not only a means for postoperative pain but also an adjunct to anesthesia intraoperatively. The Department of Anesthesia at Beth Israel Deaconess Medical Center conducted a randomized controlled trial of 40 adult patients who were undergoing surgery on their upper extremity. Patients would be randomly selected to be exposed to an intraoperative VR immersion or usual care. It is important to note that for this study, all these patients received a brachial plexus nerve block prior to their surgery. The study group was designed so that patients would select videos for their immersive VR experience which would be played on their VR headset during surgery. The anesthetist would perform their usual clinical care intraoperatively and would administer anesthetic medications if and when they deemed clinically necessary. The outcomes and measures looked at where the difference in intraoperative propofol dose between the two groups as well as postoperative analgesia requirements and pain scores. The schematic of the study started with each patient taking a baseline survey to assess their preoperative anxiety and pain. The patients would then get randomized into an intraoperative VR group and a control group without any VR. Both groups would get regional anesthetic care dependent upon an anesthetist's clinical assessment intraoperatively. The primary outcome measure would be how much total propofol was needed between the study groups. The secondary outcomes measured had more to do with each patient's post-operative pain, PACU length of stay, and functional status following surgery. Patients were randomized in a 1:1 allocation using block randomization of equal sizes to either the VR group or usual care group. REDCap, the Research Electronic Data Capture randomization module was used to implement the study randomization scheme. The randomization sequence was unknown to research members ahead of time. However, the allocation was informed to research members after the patient was enrolled and assigned. The investigators of this study also deemed that given the nature of the intervention, a protocol for unblinding participants was not applicable. Patients were allowed to voluntarily withdraw from the study and anesthesia providers were allowed to determine a patient's drop-out if they did not meet parameters for a safe surgical procedure, i.e., resistant hypertension above auto-regulation. Analysis of the propofol dosing was normalized to the duration of the procedure. Analysis of PACU stay will include doses of medications across the length of PACU stay. The doses of dexmedetomidine, propofol, remifentanil, hydromorphone, fentanyl, midazolam, morphine, intravenous acetaminophen, ondansetron and ketrolac was all documented. Patient satisfaction and pain scores will be evaluated from a REDCap survey. The results of this study so far have been equivocal but it is known that this study was the first to evaluate the potential for VR technology reduces intraoperative propofol requirements along with reducing post-operative pain. Even though their results have not been conclusive thus far, positive results from a study like this would add to the growing sentiment that VR can be a powerful tool for perioperative care. The limitations of this study included the fact that the anesthesiologists caring for these surgical patients were not blinded. Therefore, they knew which patients were part of the VR group and moreover, the anesthetic care given by the providers was not consistent across cases. Instead, each anesthesia provider was allowed the use of their clinical acumen with regard to different risks that may appear during the surgical case which comes with the nature of an intervention like this. The bias with this is that an anesthesiologist may give a different dose of propofol solely based on whether the patient is wearing a VR headset or not. Virtual reality was also tested in the field of orthopedic surgery in China. The department of Orthopedics in the Central Hospital of Cangzhou City conducted a randomized controlled trial to see if VR could be effective in postoperative rehabilitation after total knee arthroplasty. In their study, investigators had a total of 66 patients with osteoarthritis who were going to be underground a total knee replacement. The patients were then randomly assigned to either a VR rehabilitation group or a control group which would be conventional rehabilitation. The inclusion criteria for all 66 patients were that all patients needed to have a diagnosis of osteoarthritis and had to be undergoing unilateral total knee arthroplasty for the first time. Patients who were excluded included overweight patients, patients with severe osteoporosis, and cases where there was an associated ligament injury or periprosthetic fracture that occurred during the TKA. All patients underwent the same physical therapy exercise plan; however, the study group was given an added VR immersion where they would do physical therapy in the virtual environment. Conventional exercises targeted quadriceps strength and exercises conducting plantar and dorsiflexion. The VR rehabilitation asked patients in the study group to row a boat using knee flexion in an immersive virtual environment for 30-minute periods, three times a day. The measures of outcome used were knee function scores such as WOMAC (Western Ontario and McMaster University osteoarthritis index, HSS (Hospital for Special Surgery knee score, a Visual Analog Scale, and Range of motion by degrees. Each of these assessments was taken from patients at different intervals following surgery. Comparing the 33 patients in the VR group and the 33 patients in the control group, positive significant results appeared with the VR group in terms of the WOMAC and HSS scores measured at 1, 3, and 6 months after surgery. The VR group had significantly lower WOMAC scores than the control group and higher HSS scores than the control group. The WOMAC index evaluates pain, stiffness, and physical functioning of the joints. A lower

WOMAC score indicates better knee function. The HSS knee score deals with knee function and a higher score indicates better knee function. Therefore, this study out of China among anesthesiologists and orthopedic surgeons concluded that a VR intervention in terms of rehabilitation improves functional recovery and pain in OA patients. The last study this review would like to analyze is a study out of Iran and the Department of Midwifery in Mashhad, Iran. The investigator of this study was a team of engineers, anesthetists, midwives, and obstetricians. This group looked at the effect of virtual reality on the pain that women felt during an episiotomy repair. The design of this study was a randomized controlled trial conducted on 30 women in labor. The intervention group received the usual treatment with added VR (video glasses headset and local 5ml of 2% lidocaine) and the control group only received the local anesthetic. The post-operative pain was measured using the Numeric Pain Rating Scale which is 0-100. This was measured before, during, and after the episiotomy repair. Statistically significant results were found when comparing pain scores during episiotomy repair in both groups, with a P-value of P=0.038. To the investigator's knowledge, this was the first study and use of VR in a maternity ward for pain relief. The conclusion made by the group indicates that the clinical use of VR with local anesthesia can reduce pain in terms of an episiotomy repair compared to those receiving standard care. The group also cites two other papers in the Western world that agree with their findings. The Iranian group believes that ultimately the reduction of pain was due to the less perceived pain with the help of the VR headset and this is associated with the fact that patients on the VR headset felt that the perceived repair time was less than 46% of the actual time.

Discussion

Across the handful of studies review by this article, our goal was to look at diverse applications of virtual reality (VR) when it came to dealing with post-operative pain and patient satisfaction. Although this meant not keeping consistent with the type of surgery being review or the homogeneity of a patient population, it did show the easy application of a VR headset across many different fields and surgical procedures. We looked at procedures from orthopedics to obstetrics. Not every study concluded a solely positive correlation with VR and a decrease in post-operative pain and complications. However, most studies did show significant improvement in some parameters that reflected better function or better pain tolerance after the surgery. This was expressed by either better functionality scores when it came to joint range of motion or less need for analgesics after the surgery. Limitations of many of these studies have to do with small sample size and the lack of blinding due to the nature of the surgical or anesthetic interventions. Despite these limitations, we believe there is enough evidence for VR's efficacy as well as its affordability to be a major player in post-operative pain control. The goal we envision for VR is to provide a major supplementary role in perioperative care and not to entirely replace the use of pharmacologic analgesia but instead promote more efficient use of these drugs.

References

Ding, Lingyu, Hongxia Hua, Hanfei Zhu, Shuqin Zhu, Jinling Lu, Kang Zhao, and Qin Xu. 2020. "Effects of Virtual Reality on Relieving Postoperative Pain in Surgical Patients: A Systematic Review and Meta-Analysis." *International Journal of Surgery* 82: 87–94. https://doi.org/10.1016/j.ijsu.2020.08.033.

Faruki, Adeel, Thy Nguyen, Samantha Proeschel, Nadav Levy, Jessica Yu, Victoria Ip, Ariel Mueller, Valerie Banner-Goodspeed, and Brian O'Gara. 2019. "Virtual Reality as an Adjunct to Anesthesia in the Operating Room." *Trials*. https://doi.org/10.1186/s13063-019-3922-2.

Hüppe, M., S. Kükenshöner, F. Bosse, H. R. Casser, T. Kohlmann, G. Lindena, M. Pfingsten, F. Petzke, and B. Nagel. 2017. "Schmerztherapeutische Versorgung in Deutschland – Was Unterscheidet Ambulante Und Stationäre Patienten Zu Behandlungsbeginn? Eine Auswertung Auf Basis Des KEDOQ-Schmerz-Datensatzes." *Schmerz* 31 (6): 559–67. https://doi.org/10.1007/s00482-017-0240-z.

Jahanishoorab, Nahid, Samira Ebrahimzadeh Zagami, Ali Nahvi, Seyed Reza Mazluom, Nahid Golmakani, Mahdi Talebi, and Ferial Pabarja. 2015. "The Effect of Virtual Reality on Pain in Primiparity Women during Episiotomy Repair: A Randomize Clinical Trial." *Iranian Journal of Medical Sciences* 40 (3): 219–24.

Joshi, Girish P., and Babatunde O. Ogunnaike. 2005. "Consequences of Inadequate Postoperative Pain Relief and Chronic Persistent Postoperative Pain." *Anesthesiology Clinics of North America* 23 (1): 21–36. https://doi.org/10.1016/j.atc.2004.11.013.

Li, Xian min, Chun ming Huang, and Cheng fan Zhong. 2016. "Intrathecal Morphine Verse Femoral Nerve Block for Pain Control in Total Knee Arthroplasty: A Meta-Analysis from Randomized Control Trials." *International Journal of Surgery* 32: 89–98. https://doi.org/10.1016/j.ijsu.2016.06.043.

Lundborg, Christopher. 2015. "Why Postoperative Pain Remains a Problem." *Journal of Pain and Palliative Care Pharmacotherapy* 29 (3): 300–302. https://doi.org/10.3109/15360288.2015.1065940.

Mosso-Vázquez, José Luis, Kenneth Gao, Brenda K. Wiederhold, and Mark D. Wiederhold. 2014. "Virtual Reality for Pain Management in Cardiac Surgery."

Cyberpsychology, Behavior, and Social Networking 17 (6): 371–78. https://doi.org/10.1089/cyber.2014.0198.

Spiegel, Brennan, Garth Fuller, Mayra Lopez, Taylor Dupuy, Benjamin Noah, Amber Howard, Michael Albert, et al., 2019. "Virtual Reality for Management of Pain in Hospitalized Patients: A Randomized Comparative Effectiveness Trial." *PLoS ONE* 14 (8). https://doi.org/10.1371/journal.pone.0219115.

Sweta, V. R., R. P. Abhinav, and Asha Ramesh. 2019. "Role of Virtual Reality in Pain Perception of Patients Following the Administration of Local Anesthesia." *Annals of Maxillofacial Surgery* 9 (1): 110–13. https://doi.org/10.4103/ams.ams_263_18.

Vadivelu, Nalini, Sukanya Mitra, and Deepak Narayan. 2010. "Recent Advances in Postoperative Pain Management." *Yale Journal of Biology and Medicine* 83 (1): 11–25.

Won, Andrea Stevenson, Jakki Bailey, Jeremy Bailenson, Christine Tataru, Isabel A. Yoon, and Brenda Golianu. 2017. "Immersive Virtual Reality for Pediatric Pain." *Children*. https://doi.org/10.3390/children4070052.

About the Editors

Editor

Indraneil Mukherjee, MBBS, MD, FACS
Assistant Professor – Zucker School of Medicine/Hofstra/Northwell,
Uniondale, NY, USA
Email: IMukherjee@northwell.edu

Clinical Associate Profession – CUNY School of Medicine, NYC, NY, USA

Clerkship Director
Associate Program Director – General Surgery Residency
Associate Program Director – Fellowship in Advance GI Surgery
Minimal Invasive Surgery, Foregut and Hepato-Pancreato-Biliary
Staten Island University Hospital-Northwell Health, Staten Island, NY, USA

Assistant Editor at *International Journal of Surgery*
256 Mason Ave, 3rd floor Building C,
Staten Island, New York, 10305

Co-Editors

Rayna Walburger, MD
Department of Anesthesia
Icahn School of Medicine at Mount Sinai
1000 10th Ave, New York, New York
Email: rayna3208@gmail.com

Simer Preet Singh, MD, MPH, FAAPMR, FASAM
System Lead Physician for Spine and Pain Medicine
Rochester Regional Health System, Rochester, NY, USA

Clinical Instructor
Physical Medicine and Rehabilitation,
University of Rochester,
Rochester, NY, USA

The Spine Center at Ridgeway
2655 Ridgeway Ave, Ste 440
Rochester, NY, USA 14626
Office Phone: (585) 723-7705

Clinical Assistant Professor
Department of Surgery,
Wright State University, Dayton, OH, USA

Index

N

O

P

Q

R

S

T

U

V

W

X